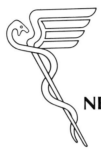

1978
YEAR BOOK OF

NEUROLOGY
AND
NEUROSURGERY

THE 1978 YEAR BOOKS

The YEAR BOOK series provides in condensed form the essence of the best of the recent international medical literature. The material is selected by distinguished editors who critically review more than 500,000 journal articles each year.

Anesthesia
Drs. Eckenhoff, Bruce, Brunner, Holley and Linde.

Cancer
Drs. Clark and Cumley.

Cardiology
Drs. Harvey, Kirkendall, Kirklin, Nadas, Paul and Sonnenblick.

Dentistry
Drs. Hale, Hazen, Moyers, Redig, Robinson and Silverman.

Dermatology
Drs. Malkinson and Pearson.

Diagnostic Radiology
Drs. Whitehouse, Bookstein, Gabrielsen, Holt, Martel, Silver and Thornbury.

Drug Therapy
Drs. Azarnoff, Hollister and Shand.

Endocrinology
Drs. Schwartz and Ryan.

Family Practice
Dr. Rakel.

Medicine
Drs. Rogers, Des Prez, Cline, Braunwald, Greenberger, Bondy and Epstein.

Neurology and Neurosurgery
Drs. De Jong and Sugar.

Nuclear Medicine
Dr. Quinn.

Obstetrics and Gynecology
Drs. Pitkin and Scott.

Ophthalmology
Dr. Hughes.

Orthopedics and Traumatic Surgery
Dr. Coventry.

Otolaryngology
Drs. Strong and Paparella.

Pathology and Clinical Pathology
Drs. Carone and Conn.

Pediatrics
Dr. Gellis.

Plastic and Reconstructive Surgery
Drs. McCoy, Dingman, Hanna, Haynes, Hoehn and Stephenson.

Psychiatry and Applied Mental Health
Drs. Romano, Freedman, Friedhoff, Kolb, Lourie and Nemiah.

Surgery
Drs. Schwartz, Najarian, Peacock, Shires, Silen and Spencer.

Urology
Dr. Grayhack.

The YEAR BOOK of

Neurology and Neurosurgery

1978

NEUROLOGY

Edited by
RUSSELL N. DE JONG, M.D.

Professor and Chairman,
Department of Neurology,
The University of Michigan Medical School

NEUROSURGERY

Edited by
OSCAR SUGAR, M.D.

Professor and Head of the Department of
Neurosurgery, University of Illinois
Abraham Lincoln School of Medicine

YEAR BOOK MEDICAL PUBLISHERS, INC.
CHICAGO • LONDON

Printed in U.S.A.

Library of Congress Catalog Card Number: CD38-24

International Standard Book Number: 0-8151-2418-X

Table of Contents

The material covered in this volume represents literature reviewed up to April, 1977.

6 TABLE OF CONTENTS

Neurosurgery, *edited by* Oscar Sugar, M.D.

Questions for Clinicians

1. Three different types of motor neuron disease have been described. What are the characteristic differences among them? (p. 21)
2. What happens to hyperactive children when they become adolescents and adults? (p. 28)
3. Impairment of size and shape discrimination follows lesions of what area of the brain? (p. 27)
4. Is Sydenham's chorea always a benign, self-limited condition? (p. 43)
5. What is the prognosis for the child who develops seizures in early life? (p. 46)
6. What is the prognosis for the child with absence seizures? (p. 48)
7. How does computerized tomography aid in the diagnosis of dementia? (p. 52)
8. What drug is effective in treating coma due to tricyclic antidepressant overdosage? (p. 243)
9. Compare the results of clinical testing of cutaneous sensation with those of quantitative testing of such sensation in patients with neuromuscular disease. (p. 238)
10. Do death certificates give reliable epidemiologic information? (p. 210)
11. Compare computerized tomography and radionuclide imaging in the diagnosis of stroke. (p. 212)
12. Occlusion of which arteries causes most medullary infarcts? (p. 213 and 215)
13. By what means may one investigate abnormalities of cardiac rhythm and conduction in patients with cerebrovascular insufficiency? (p. 218 and 219)
14. What is the safest and most effective treatment of superior sagittal sinus thrombosis? (p. 224)
15. What are the locations and types of lesions that cause "pure motor hemiplegia"? (p. 225)
16. How effective is glycerol in the treatment of patient with early strokes? (p. 227)

17. What is the prognosis of ischemic strokes in young adults? (p. 228 and 229)
18. What preoperative symptoms influence the prognosis in patients operated on for the treatment of cervical spondylitic myelopathy? (p. 203)
19. What type of nerve injury may follow open heart surgery through a median sternotomy approach? (p. 185)
20. What is the prognostic significance of electrodiagnostic studies in the Guillain-Barré syndrome? (p. 187)
21. What is the prognosis for the patient with diabetic autonomic neuropathy? (p. 196)
22. What are phosphenes and what is their significance? (p. 181)
23. What is Eales' disease and what neurologic involvement may occur with it? (p. 171 and 172)
24. Why is it important to recognize and determine the cause of secondary metabolic encephalopathy? (p. 174)
25. What varieties of central nervous system involvement may occur in patients with diabetes mellitus? (p. 177)
26. How does the childhood type of dermatomyositis differ from that which occurs in adults? (p. 161)
27. How effective is the long-term administration of corticosteroids in myasthenia gravis? (p. 150)
28. What are histocompatibility antigens and how does knowledge about them relate to multiple sclerosis? (p. 132)
29. Are mental changes ever early features of multiple sclerosis? (p. 142)
30. What are the major causes of excessive daytime sleepiness? (p. 122)
31. Is central pontine myelinosis always a fatal disease? (p. 126)
32. What are the neurologic and psychologic consequences of decompression illness? (p. 127)
33. What household pets may be host reservoirs of lymphocytic choriomeningitis virus? (p. 101)
34. What is the long-term effect of levodopa therapy in Parkinson's disease? (pp. 80 and 81)
35. What is the incidence of ulcer after steroid therapy? Is this a serious consideration in deciding on steroid therapy? (p. 266).

36. What measure(s) can be taken to minimize the risks of postoperative brain swelling in patients who have received nitrous-oxide-halothane gas mixtures for craniotomy? (p. 272)

37. Why should nitrous oxide be used as the gas for pneumoencephalography in pediatric patients? (p. 276)

38. How can CT scanning be used to reduce angiography and determine the site of bleeding in a patient with multiple aneurysms? (p. 280)

39. What technique could be used routinely as a noninvasive examination to diagnose potential stroke or transient ischemic attack? (p. 291)

40. Under what circumstance, and with what method, might it be worthwhile to enhance the radioactive pickup by the choroid plexus in radionuclide angiography and scanning? (p. 295)

41. When is lumbar epidural venography of value in diagnosis of lumbar disk disease? (p. 297)

42. How can the sitting position for neurosurgical procedures be modified to make it safer and more comfortable? (p. 312)

43. Is there such an entity as "noncommunicating syringomyelia" or do all cases involve opening into the 4th ventricle? (p. 326)

44. What is the most reliable test for thoracic outlet syndrome? (p. 330)

45. Where can the bone be obtained to fuse the spine in thoracotomy for Pott's disease? What happens to the paraplegia in such patients? (p. 334)

46. What antibiotic regimen and operative protocol can be used to reduce primary infections with ventricular shunts to less than 1%? (p. 335)

47. Should calcified intracranial subdural hematomas be operated on? (p. 341)

48. How can the instability of the lumbar spine after fracture dislocation be handled? (p. 345)

49. Can a dominant-hemisphere intraventricular tumor be removed without adding to the neurologic deficit? (p. 365)

50. What are the relative merits of surgical ablative versus decompressive techniques in the management of

pineal region tumors? (pp. 377 and 378)

51. When spasm appears in cerebral arteries after operation, what can be done for treatment? (p. 389)
52. When should arterial hypertension be encouraged in the course of treatment for aneurysms? (p. 390)
53. What are the relative merits of the subtemporal and pterional approaches to aneurysms of the upper basilar artery? (p. 396)
54. Should the hugely dilated "aneurysm of the vein of Galen" be ligated or removed? (p. 400)
55. What are the indications and contraindications for operation on cerebral hemorrhages? (p. 403)
56. If clinical considerations are not enough to establish the diagnosis of cerebellar hemorrhage, what can be done? (p. 404)
57. Under what circumstances is it proper to reopen an occluded cervical carotid artery? (p. 412)
58. Is successful transcutaneous stimulation for peripheral pain a necessary prerequisite for implanting electrodes for more permanent stimulation? (p. 425)
59. What kinds of myelotomy can be used for controlling painful spasms in paraplegics? (pp. 432 and 433)
60. What is the arrangement of the representation of sensation in the postcentral area of the brain (sensory homunculus)? (p. 437)

NEUROLOGY

RUSSELL N. DE JONG, M.D.

Introduction

Two investigators in the field of the neurologic sciences have recently been recipients of major awards for their extremely significant contributions to neurology. One has broadened the scope of our knowledge of the etiology of neurologic disease, and the other has expanded our techniques for the investigation and diagnosis of diseases of the central nervous system.

Dr. D. Carleton Gajdusek, chief of the laboratory of central nervous system studies at the National Institutes of Neurological and Communicative Disorders and Stroke, National Institutes of Health, Bethesda, Maryland, was awarded the 1976 Nobel Prize in Medicine for his discovery of new transmissible virus-like agents—the atypical slow viruses—and the recognition that so-called degenerative disorders of the human nervous system may be caused by such agents, a totally unanticipated discovery (Tower, D. B.: Arch. Neurol. 34:205, 1977). He became interested in kuru, a fatal degenerative disease of the nervous system that appeared to be endemic among the Fore people who live in the eastern highlands of New Guinea. To investigate this disease he lived among these people for 12 months. Studying the pathology of kuru, he noted its resemblance to scrapie, a disease found in Icelandic sheep and discovered to be transmissible. He and his colleagues inoculated bacteria- and protozoan-free suspensions from samples of kuru-affected brains intracerebrally into chimpanzees. After a long incubation period these animals developed manifestations of the disease and pathologically showed evidence of it. Because these diseases, and transmissible mink encephalopathy as well, also resembled a rare, devastating brain degeneration in human beings, Creutzfeldt-Jakob disease, he investigated this disease also, and he was able to demonstrate that it, too, is caused by a slowly developing virus.

As a result of the discoveries by Doctor Gajdusek and his colleagues, it is now firmly established that chronic degenerative neurologic disorders of man can arise by the slow but relentless multiplication of agents of the slow virus group that may cause the disease to develop many years after the initial infection. Such discoveries are viewed by many as having significant implications for other neurologic "degenerations," including multiple sclerosis, amyotrophic lateral sclerosis, Alzheimer's disease and other presenile and senile dementias. In fact, 2 cases of a familial form of Alzheimer's disease have been transmitted to subhuman primates, and the amyloid plaques typically seen in scrapie and kuru appear to be identical with the immunoglobulin-derived amyloid characteristically present in the brains of patients with presenile dementia (Gajdusek, D. C., and Gibbs, C. J., Jr.: in Tower, D. B., and Chase, T. N. [eds.]: *The Nervous System* [New York: Raven Press, 1975] Vol. 2, *The Clinical Neurosciences,* pp. 113–135). Mims has stated, "It seems probable that we have still not gathered the full harvest of the discoveries made by Gajdusek" (Mims, C.: Nature 283:716, 1976).

Diagnosis and patient monitoring in clinical neurology and neurosurgery have been revolutionized by the recent development of a noninvasive brain scanning technique known as computerized axial tomography. This was originally conceived by Dr. William H. Oldendorf, professor of neurology at the University of California in Los Angeles and career investigator at the Brentwood Veterans Administration Hospital in Los Angeles, and was brought to feasibility by Godfrey Hounsfield, an electrical engineer in England. Doctor Oldendorf has recently received the Lasker Award in Medicine for this contribution. The technique combines a rapid scanning of the head (and now of the body) by a narrow x-ray beam coupled with a computer that translates the differences in tissue density detected along the beam path into numerical or pictorial displays. The technique is approximately 100 times more sensitive than conventional x-ray procedures. It provides far greater resolution of the various brain structures and eliminates the need for some of the traditional radiologic procedures with their attendant risk and discomfort. In fact, it is fast displacing pneumoencephalography, cerebral angiography and even radionuclide scanning (Oldendorf, W. H.: The Wartenberg Lecture, American Academy of Neurology, Atlanta, Ga., Apr. 28, 1977). The fluid spaces in the head, the gray and white matter and certain landmarks like the pineal gland and choroid plexus are distinguished readily by computerized tomography, but seldom by conventional radiologic techniques. Tumors, hemorrhage, brain atrophy and edema are among the pathologic conditions that are quickly, easily and more consistently visualized by this technique.

Computerized tomography is rapidly assuming the role of the major technical adjunct diagnostic procedure in neurology and may revolutionize this area because it can be done on an outpatient basis, saving the patient many days of expensive hospitalization. It has had an extraordinary impact on diagnostic neuroradiology and the clinical management of patients with diseases of the nervous system. The technique has already been extended to problems of the eye, where tumors and other masses in the bony orbit behind the eye have been notoriously difficult to diagnose. Dr. Giovanni Di Chiro of the National Institute of Neurological and Communicative Disorders and Stroke and his co-workers have pioneered the use of the technique to study the spinal cord and its disorders. The whole body scanner has now been developed. This permits scanning of the heart, lungs and abdominal organs where an even more rapid scan helps minimize artifacts from heartbeat and respiration.

Advances in synaptic pharmacology have led to new approaches to understanding and attempts to alleviate the disturbances of neurotransmission that occur in Parkinson's disease. Techniques that initially were developed to elucidate normal synaptic phenomena are being used to screen potential therapeutic agents for efficacy, relative potency and neurotoxicity and to analyze the mechanisms of action of antiparkinsonian drugs (Calne, D. B.: Ann. Neurol. 1:111, 1977).

Progress in the drug treatment of parkinsonism has been one of the major neurologic success stories of the decade. For the better part of a century, patients with this condition were ineffectively treated with extracts from the belladonna plant. In the 1950s, experimentation with the use of tranquilizers as a means of controlling hypertension produced much new information on the action of chemical neurotransmittors, many of which were found to produce parkinson-like symptoms when given in large doses. They also reduced the high concentrations of the neurotransmitter chemical dopamine in parts of the brain responsible for motor control. After the discovery that there was a striking shortage of dopamine in the brain of parkinsonian patients at autopsy, it was felt that replacement therapy might be indicated, and the administration of dopamine was suggested as a treatment. Dopamine, however, does not cross the blood-brain barrier. Further study showed that the metabolic precursor of dopamine, levodopa, the preceding link in the chain of reactions leading to its production, does cross the blood-brain barrier and does alleviate the symptoms of Parkinson's disease. Levodopa has been the major drug used in the treatment of this disease in recent years. Its use leads to marked improvement in the symptoms of the disease. Dosage, however, has to be carefully monitored, and there may be significant side effects associated with its use. Some of these are dose related, but others may be idiosyncratic. It was found that the addition of a decarboxylase inhibitor significantly decreases the dose of levodopa needed to control the parkinsonian symptoms and thus minimizes side effects, but they still occur with prolonged administration.

In the search for newer therapeutic agents for Parkinson's disease, Dr. Donald B. Calne and his associates, working first in England and now at the National Institutes of Health, found that another substance, bromocriptine, works more directly than levodopa. Bromocriptine is known to activate dopaminergic receptors in experimental animals. It is a synthetic ergot alkaloid that was first used to suppress puerperal lactation and has also been used in the treatment of such disorders as galactorrhea, infertility and acromegaly. It has the advantage of acting directly on the dopamine receptor without requiring the presence of an aromatic amino acid decarboxylase for effectiveness. It also has the advantage of more prolonged action than levodopa. It is not yet available for general use in the United States; however, when it becomes available, it certainly will add to our therapeutic armamentarium for this incapacitating disease. Current investigations into the pharmacology and therapeutics of parkinsonism may well bring forth other drugs that will further add to the effectiveness of our therapy.

Recent genetic studies have brought out information about what are known as histocompatibility antigens. These are protein molecules present in all cells. Although everyone has histocompatibility antigens, persons have different types depending on the inherited genes that direct their production. Recent important research indicates that there is a much higher incidence of three particular antigens in patients with multiple sclerosis than in people at large. These antigens are the types HL-A3, HL-A7 and LD-7A (McFarlin, D. E., and McFarland, H. F.: Arch. Neurol. 33: 395, 1977). This finding would suggest that certain persons may inherit a tendency to develop multiple sclerosis, possibly by inheriting genes that produce a defective immune defense system against the disease. In addition, studies have shown that the incidence of persons with the HL-A3 antigens seems to follow the peculiar geographic distribution that multiple sclerosis is known to have. Earlier studies have shown multiple sclerosis to be most prevalent in the temperate and colder climates of Western Europe and North and South America, but exceedingly rare in the tropics. The HL-A3 antigens are more prevalent in these same areas. Studies have also shown that the HL-A3 antigen is uncommon among the Japanese, in whom multiple sclerosis is rare, and the antigen is more prominent among northern Europeans, in whom the incidence of the disease is relatively high. The importance of the increased incidence of these antigens in multiple sclerosis patients is not yet known. Genes that produce them have been found in animal models to be linked closely to what are known as immune response genes, which are thought to be responsible for the body's defense against invaders. Therefore, if there are defects in the immune response genes, these defects may predispose to bacterial or viral disease.

In addition to these genetic studies, investigators have shown that some patients with multiple sclerosis have increased levels of antibodies against the measles virus and other common viruses in their blood and cerebrospinal fluid. Althought no specific virus has yet been found to cause multiple sclerosis, it may be possible that a defective immune system may allow a virus to persist in the body for years before some triggering factor spurs it into action. Investigators in Japan and the United States have also found that patients with multiple sclerosis have higher titers of cerebrospinal fluid antibodies to vaccinia virus than their siblings and patients with other neurologic diseases (Miyamoto, M., et al.: ibid., p. 414). They also found that multiple sclerosis patients usually had smaller vaccination scars than their siblings. They hypothesize: "It may be that their initial infection was a mild one, and, as a result, their immune response to vaccinia virus was weak and allowed systemic spread of the virus, perhaps on revaccination. Thus the virus or its soluble antigens might enter the central nervous system and establish chronic low-grade infection, perhaps involving defective or incomplete virus."

In an editorial in the *Journal of the American Medical Association* (J.A.M.A. 235:2630, 1976), it is stated, "If (multiple sclerosis) is indeed a slow virus disease originating in early infection by measles virus or vaccinia virus, with or without a hereditary predisposition, one may anticipate that an unplanned clinical trial may result from the present policy in the United States, whereby infection by vaccinia virus (vaccination) is no longer introduced routinely to the population, and, at the same time, measles immunization is advocated for all children. The outcome should be a substantial decline of (multiple sclerosis) during the years ahead." It is hoped that this information, along with the results of other extensive investigations of this disease now in progress, ultimately will lead to unraveling the complex interrelationship among the genetic, immunologic and virologic factors that seem to be involved in this baffling disorder.

Recent investigations also have shown that myasthenia gravis is an autoimmune disorder in which the victim's own body sets up an immune reaction against itself. Normally acetylcholine is released from nerve endings and crosses the synapse to attach to protein receptors on the muscle endplate and this triggers muscle contraction. In myasthenia gravis this mechanism is impaired. The lymphocytes in the blood of patients with myasthenia gravis interfere with the receptor molecule on the muscle end-plate (Lindstrom, J. M., et al.: Neurology (Minneap.) 26:1054, 1976). It has been possible to induce myasthenia-like weakness in rabbits by immunizing the animals with acetylcholine receptor protein purified from the electric organ of the eel. The results of these studies have been extended to other animal species and represent a new approach for studying the mechanisms involved in the cause and cure of myasthenia gravis.

In commemoration of the 25th anniversary of the National Institute of Neurological and Communicative Disorders and Stroke, a three-volume work entitled *The Nervous System* has been published (Raven Press). The editor-in-chief of the three volumes is Donald B. Tower. Volume 1, *The Basic Neurosciences,* is edited by Roscoe O. Brady; Volume 2, *The Clinical Neurosciences,* is edited by Thomas N. Chase; and Volume 3, *Human Communication and Its Disorders,* is edited by Eldon L. Eagles. A history of the Institute is included with chapters by the three men who have served as its directors: Pearce Bailey, Richard L. Masland and Edward F. McNichol, Jr., with a chapter by Murray Golstein on manpower recruitment and the training programs in the Institute. Individual chapters covering a wide range of topics are written by specialists in the various fields, and the books provide a compendium of important information. Other significant new books include the second edition of *Diagnostic Radiology* by Juan M. Taveras and Ernest H. Wood (Williams & Wilkins Co.), *Radiologic Anatomy of the Brain* by G. Salamon and Y. P. Huhng (Springer-Verlag New York, Inc.), *Principles of Neurology* by R. D. Adams and M. Victor (McGraw-Hill Book Co.), *Computed Tomography of the Brain* by R. Ramsey (W. B. Saunders Co.), *Scientific Approaches to Clinical Neurology* by E. S. Goldensohn and S. H. Appel (Lea & Febiger), four volumes of the *Handbook of Clinical Neurology* edited by P. J. Vinken and G. W. Bruyn (Volume 25, *Injuries of the Spine and Spinal Cord, Part I;* Volume 26, *Injuries of the Spine and Spinal Cord, Part II;* Volume 27, *Metabolic and Deficiency Diseases of the Nervous System, Part I;* and Volume 28, *Metabolic and Deficiency Diseases of the Nervous System, Part II* [North-Holland Publishing Co.]), *Clinical Neuroendocrinology* by J. D. Martin, S. Reichlin and G. M. Brown (F. A. Davis Co.), *Mechanisms of Neurological Disease* by A. J. Lewis (Little, Brown and Co.), *EEG Interpretation: Problems of Overreading and Underreading* by E. S. Goldensohn and R. Koehle (American Academy of Neurology), *Neurology Notes* by A. F. Haerer and R. D. Currier (Little, Brown and Co.) and *Modern Practical Neurology* by P. Scheinberg (Raven Press).

Significant changes were made in the American neurologic publications during late 1976 and 1977. A new journal, *Annals of Neurology,* with Fred Plum as editor-in-chief, assisted by a well-chosen editorial board, appeared in January, 1977; it is the official journal of the American Neurological Association. Maurice W. Van Allen succeeded Doctor Plum as editor-in-chief of the *Archives of Neurology* in October, 1976, and a new editorial board was appointed. Lewis P. Rowland succeeded Russell N. De Jong as editor-in-chief of *Neurology* in January, 1977, and a major portion of the members of the editorial board completed their terms of appointment at that time, resulting in many new appointments to the editorial board of this journal also.

RUSSELL N. DE JONG, M.D.

Amyotrophic Lateral Sclerosis

Familial Motor Neuron Disease: Evidence for at Least Three Different Types. Familial amyotrophic lateral sclerosis has eluded clear definition but the clinical heterogeneity of the condition suggests that more than 1 distinct entity may be found, as has been true for the muscular dystrophies, spinal muscle atrophies, familial spastic paraplegias and cerebellar ataxias. William A. Horton, Roswell Eldridge and Jacob A. Brody[1] (Natl. Inst. of Health) evaluated 14 families seen during 1974–75 in which at least 2 members had progressive motor neuron disease. The patients had had progressive motor dysfunction with predominantly lower motor neuron signs and were ascertained through several sources. Families whose members mainly had spastic symptoms, lacked pyramidal tract signs after more than 5 years of disease or showed significant dementia or cerebellar or extrapyramidal signs were excluded from study.

No particular geographic area or ethnic group predominated. In 7 families, at least 2 consecutive generations were affected. In 4 of the 7 families with only siblings affected, the parents had died at an age too young to exclude their being affected. No family had a history of known consanguinity. Diagnosis was documented by neurologic examination, electromyography or autopsy in 32 of 400 family members and by history alone in 20 others. Of the 27 male and 25 female family members affected, 40 had died. Six of the 12 survivors were examined and 9 of the 40 who had died had autopsy. Two groups of families were distinguished. One, with shorter survival but an older age at onset, had lesions limited to the anterior horn cells, the anterior horn cells and pyramidal tracts or these areas plus the posterior columns. The other group included 1 autopsy showing the same lesions

---

(1) Neurology (Minneap.) 26:460–465, May, 1976.

and also intracytoplasmic hyaline inclusions in surviving anterior horn cells.

Clinical variations in these cases were more marked among than within families. Cases in most well-documented families have followed the short course. Most families have shown an autosomal dominant inheritance pattern, which was true of the families in this study. The first type of disease is clinically and pathologically identical to sporadic amyotrophic lateral sclerosis; the second type seems to be a distinct entity. A third, still heterogeneous type, is distinctive by the length of survival.

► [The finding that there are at least three different types of familial motor neuron disease must be borne in mind when one is attempting to predict the prognosis in patients with the disorder.—Ed.] ◄

Evidence for Immune-Complex Formation in Patients with Amyotrophic Lateral Sclerosis. The etiology of amyotrophic lateral sclerosis (ALS) is unknown but viruses or virus-like agents have been implicated in several degenerative diseases, and some viral infections leading to chronic disorders in animals are associated with manifestations of immune complexes, presumably representing virus-antiviral antibody. M. B. A. Oldstone, C. B. Wilson, L. H. Perrin and F. H. Norris, Jr.[2] examined the blood and renal glomeruli of ALS patients for immune complexes. The ALS was diagnosed independently by at least 2 neurologists. Study was made of 58 patients with classic ALS, 5 with primary lateral sclerosis, 6 with benign ALS and 15 healthy control subjects. Serum or plasma was obtained from 25 patients with ALS and renal tissues from 33. The radiolabeled C1q test was carried out and plasma C3 was measured. Immunofluorescence studies were also performed.

Positive C1q binding was found in 40% of patients with ALS. Four ALS patients had marked amounts of C1q-binding factor(s) in their serums. No significant reduction in C3 was found in any patient. Granular deposits of IgG, IgM and C3 were found in 9 of 33 ALS patients. Deposits of IgG were localized in mesangial areas and in the renal glomerular basement membranes. No Ig deposits were seen outside the renal glomeruli. Eight of 9 patients with significant deposits of host IgG and C3 had rapidly progressive neurologic cours-

(2)   Lancet 2:169–172, July 24, 1976.

es, leading to death within 1 year. Nine of 12 patients without evidence of immune-complex disease had stable or slowly progressive courses and lived longer than 2 years. The 8 patients with fibrinogen deposits also had slowly progressive courses.

Preliminary evidence of immune-complex formation in patients with ALS was obtained in this study. There was no evidence that the deposited complexes in patients with ALS shared immunologic reactivity with poliomyelitis virus.

▶ [This study is significant and may point out pathways toward determining the etiology of amyotrophic lateral sclerosis and other chronic neurologic diseases.

In a study from the Mayo Clinic (Mulder, D. W., and Howard, F. M., Jr.: Patient resistance and prognosis in amyotrophic lateral sclerosis: Mayo Clin. Proc. 51:537, 1976), it is brought out that those patients with amyotrophic lateral sclerosis whose course is more chronic and who live longer than 5 years may have a disease with an etiology that differs from that in those with a more acute course or they may have been subjected to factors that alter their resistance to the disease. — Ed.] ◄

Histocompatibility Typing in Amyotrophic Lateral Sclerosis. The cause of amyotrophic lateral sclerosis remains unknown. Several chronic and subacutely progressive central nervous system diseases are caused by transmissible agents and epidemiologic evidence hints at a link between poliomyelitis and amyotrophic lateral sclerosis. A viral or autoimmune causation has been implicated in most diseases associated with an increased frequency of particular histocompatibility (HL-A) antigens. Jack P. Antel, Barry G. W. Arnason, Thomas C. Fuller and James R. Lehrich[3] (Harvard Med. School) determined the frequencies of particular HL-A antigens in 44 white patients with amyotrophic lateral sclerosis. Most had confirmatory electromyographic findings. The 27 women and 17 men had a mean age of 55. Disease had been present for 6 months to 15 years. One patient had an affected sibling and had been on Guam but none had a history of paralytic poliomyelitis. The control group included 200 volunteer blood donors. Histocompatibility testing was by a two-stage microlymphocytotoxicity trypan blue exclusion assay, with use of 66 HL-A typing serums and measuring of 18 HL-A specificities.

Only HL-A3 was significantly increased and this increase was noted when two independent groups of patients were

(3) Arch. Neurol. 33:423–425, June, 1976.

analyzed separately. An increase in HL-A7 was noted but was not significant, although 10 of 19 patients with HL-A3 also had HL-A7. Of the other HL-A specificities, only HL-A12 showed a suggestive increase. Five of 6 patients with slowly progressive disease had HL-A12, whereas none had HL-A3 and 1 had HL-A7. With these cases excluded, the incidence of HL-A3 in "classic" amyotrophic lateral sclerosis was 50% and the increase in HL-A12 was no longer observed. A significantly increased incidence of HL-A3 and HL-A7 in a study of 111 patients affected with poliomyelitis has been reported.

Epidemiologic data provide evidence both for and against a correlation of HL-A3 with the incidence of amyotrophic lateral sclerosis. Terasaki and Mickey recently reported several differing haplotype frequencies in amyotrophic lateral sclerosis, including overrepresentations of the 1-22, 3-21 and 2-12 haplotypes. The overall incidence of HL-A3 was increased in their study of 70 patients with amyotrophic lateral sclerosis, but not significantly so.

▶ [This carefully executed study hints at a relationship between poliomyelitis and amyotrophic lateral sclerosis, but does not actually show that there is such a relationship. The one rather definite finding is that the HL-A antigens may link with disease severity in amyotrophic lateral sclerosis. — Ed.] ◀

Behavioral Neurology

Personality Patterns in Insomnia: Theoretical Implications. Insomnia is a frequent symptom in patients with psychiatric disturbances. Anthony Kales, Alex B. Caldwell, Terry Anne Preston, Shevy Healey and Joyce D. Kales[4] analyzed the frequency and types of psychopathology present in 77 men and 51 women aged 17–81 years who presented with a primary complaint of insomnia. All completed the Minnesota Multiphasic Personality Inventory (MMPI) and a general questionnaire on sleep. Four subjects were not evaluable.

One or more MMPI scales were elevated to a pathologic degree in 85% of the subjects. The three scales most elevated were, in order, depression, psychasthenia and conversion hysteria. The preponderance of depression was striking. Four common MMPI code types representing various types of depression were observed. The predominant personality types were characterized by the internalization of psychologic disturbances, rather than by acting out or aggression. The rate of MMPI-identified psychopathology was higher than is found in most defined psychiatric patient samples.

It is hypothesized that the mechanism underlying insomnia is a function of the internalization of psychologic disturbances, which leads to emotional arousal and, in turn, physiologic activation during sleep. Insomnia, then, is the wakefulness of sleeplessness that follows from this chronic emotional arousal and physiologic activation. Several studies have provided data to support this hypothesis. Insomniac patients most typically have personality types characterized by an inability to react outwardly and thus to discharge their feelings. In the absence of current serious emotional disturbance and chronic physiologic activation, the conditioning of a fear of sleeplessness presumably occurred during an earlier period of an acute emotional crisis.

---

(4) Arch. Gen. Psychiatry 33:1128–1134, September, 1976.

Repeated rearousal of this fear of sleeplessness produces emotional arousal and physiologic activation at night, which become self-identified as chronic insomnia in subjects who do not otherwise exhibit significant psychopathology.

► [These authors propose, on the basis of this study, that internalization of psychologic disturbances produces a state of constant emotional arousal and resultant psychologic activation and that this process is a psychophysiologic mechanism underlying insomnia. — Ed.] ◄

Cerebral Dominance for Consciousness. Impaired consciousness after acute unilateral cerebral hemispheric infarction is generally thought to result from bilateral dysfunction due to effects of cerebral edema and transtentorial herniation. Martin L. Albert, Ruth Silverberg, Avinoam Reches and Miriam Berman[5] (Hadassah Univ. Hosp., Jerusalem) observed that patients having infarction of the language-dominant hemisphere were more likely to have impaired consciousness than those with infarction of the nondominant hemisphere. A prospective study was carried out to evaluate this observation in patients admitted in a 6-month period with definite unilateral hemispheric disease of an acute cerebrovascular nature. There were 24 patients with right hemisphere brain damage and 23 with left hemisphere brain damage. The respective mean ages were 69 and 71. No medical complications that might have influenced cerebral perfusion were present on initial evaluation.

Initial reduction of consciousness was found in 25% of patients with right hemisphere brain damage. Three of these 6 patients had hemorrhagic cerebrospinal fluid. Initial impairment was noted in 57% of patients with left hemisphere brain damage; none of the 13 had hemorrhagic cerebrospinal fluid. With exclusion of patients with bloody spinal taps, only 3 patients with right hemisphere brain damage had impaired consciousness, and one of these was left-handed. The difference in severity of impairment of consciousness between the two groups closely approached significance.

These results contradict the common view that focal unilateral cerebral hemispheric lesions do not impair consciousness. Differences in lesion size do not appear to explain the findings. Hemispheric asymmetry may exist for consciousness as well as for other neurobehavioral phenom-

(5) Arch. Neurol. 33:453–454, June, 1976.

ena. Ability to make rapid time judgments may be essential for language comprehension, and this ability may be lateralized to the left hemisphere. Perhaps a selective arousal mechanism exists that preferentially alerts the left hemisphere, providing it with the means of making more rapid time judgments. In the course of acquisition of linguistic skills, this preferential capability may facilitate the development of left cerebral dominance for language.

▶ [This study shows that initial impairment of consciousness occurs more than twice as often with left-sided cerebral lesions as it does with right-sided ones. Unilateral cerebral lesions may cause impaired consciousness, especially if the lesion is in the dominant hemisphere. — Ed.]

Astereognosis: Tactile Discrimination after Localized Hemispheric Lesions in Man. Per E. Roland[6] (Univ. of Copenhagen) investigated how precisely patients with focal cerebral lesions transfer complex spatial somatosensory information and mapped out those hemispheric injuries that evoked an abnormal loss in the information transferred. Study was made of 93 patients who had unilateral, well-defined lesions of the cerebral hemisphere. Lesions were mapped from drawings and photographs of the operative field, from lesion measurements and measurements from the lesion to identified sulci, and from the deposition of clips in the limits of the lesion. The testing with 31 spherical size stimuli and 30 shape-discrimination stimuli was purely somatosensory. Shape discrimination of both parallelepipeda and spherical ellipses was examined. A two-alternative, forced-choice design was utilized.

The findings failed to support earlier views of astereognosis. Only direct damage to, or undercutting of, the anterior part of the middle third of the postcentral gyrus caused impairment of size and shape discrimination contralateral to the lesion. There were no ipsilateral defects in any of the tests, whereas a marked defect occurred when a lesion invaded the contralateral sensory hand area. All patients with abnormal informational loss had lesions that invaded or undercut the middle third of the postcentral gyrus. Many patients with adjacent lesions had no defects. Damage to the anterior and deep part of the implicated area seemed to provoke the most marked defect. This area probably corresponds to the sensory hand area of Penfield and Rasmussen.

(6)   Arch. Neurol. 33:543–550, August, 1976.

When the hand is used for stereognostic discrimination, the integration of somatosensory impulse patterns into spatial information about the objects is believed to take place in the contralateral somatosensory hand area. Impairment of size and shape discrimination by lesions of the hand area could result from destruction or disconnection of feature analyzers in the anterior three fourths of the middle part of the postcentral gyrus.

► [The results of the study failed to support earlier views of astereognosis. Only direct damage to or an undercutting of the anterior part of the middle third of the postcentral gyrus caused impairment of size and shape discrimination. — Ed.] ◄

Hyperactives as Young Adults: Preliminary Report. An estimated 4% of school children in North America are hyperactive. It is important to assess whether hyperactive persons function differently as young adults when compared with matched controls and whether the difficulties observed during adolescence persist through young adulthood. L. Hechtman, G. Weiss, J. Finklestein, A. Werner and R. Benn[7] (Montreal) studied 35 hyperactive subjects, 34 men and 1 woman, and 25 control subjects, 24 men and 1 woman, aged 17–24 years. The respective mean ages were 19½ and 18½ years. Hyperactive subjects had been referred 10 years before with a major problem of sustained, chronic hyperactivity at school and at home when aged 6–12 years. All had normal intelligence, were free from epilepsy and cerebral palsy and were living at home with at least 1 parent. No subject had had any specific treatment for any length of time.

Both groups were comparable in height, weight and EEG findings but hyperactive subjects had higher pulse rates than controls and had more difficulties with cognitive style tests. As many hyperactive subjects as controls were in school but most other biographic findings, such as amount of education completed, higher academic standing and fewer grades failed, indicated trends favoring control subjects. Full-time work and job satisfaction were comparable in both groups. Control subjects had committed more drug-related offenses and hyperactive subjects had committed more thefts. No unusual prevalence of psychosis or personality disorder was noted in either group. Brief Psychiatric Rating

(7) Can. Med. Assoc. J. 115:625–630, Oct. 9, 1976.

Scale scores were similar in the groups, except for more tension in the hyperactive subjects. In the California Personality Inventory, hyperactive subjects scored lower on "socialization" and "sense of well-being." Hyperactive subjects felt much more restless and were observed to be so during interviews. The proportions of subjects that desired psychiatric treatment were comparable.

Hyperactive subjects seem to adjust normally to work situations and living arrangements, although restlessness is a problem and socialization skills are poorer. Hyperactive subjects have not shown significantly more antisocial behavior or serious psychiatric disturbances than controls. It is important to determine if this optimistic picture is real and lasting.

▶ [There have been few retrospective studies done to show what happens to the hyperactive child when he becomes an adult. This study, therefore, is important. It appears that hyperactive children continue to have more scholastic difficulty than controls. Restlessness continued to be a problem for the hyperactive subjects and socialization skills and sense of well-being continued to be poorer than in controls. — Ed.] ◄

Cerebrospinal Fluid

Evaluation of Cerebrospinal Fluid Production in Development of Communicating Hydrocephalus. Experimental studies on cerebrospinal fluid (CSF) production early in the development of hydrocephalus and during compensation have given conflicting results. A. Everette James, Jr., Melvin Epstein, Gary Novak and Barry Burns[8] report findings in normal dogs and in dogs studied during and after the development of communicating hydrocephalus. Hydrocephalus was induced in 11 mongrels by injection of a silicone rubber mixture into the basal subarachnoid space via a suboccipital cisterna magna puncture. Five dogs served as controls. Serial cisternography was carried out. Ventriculocisternal perfusion with artificial CSF containing either ^{3}H-polyethylene glycol or ^{14}C-inulin was carried out for $2-4$ hours. Perfusion was performed 2 weeks to 2 months after the silicone injection, when both ventricular nuclide entry and stasis were present and CSF pressures were normal.

The mean CSF production in normal dogs was 3.6 μl per minute per kg, compared with 2.4 in dogs with acute and subacute hydrocephalus, in which CSF pressures were elevated. In chronic hydrocephalus the ventricles were enlarged, CSF pressures were normal and mean CSF production was 2.9 μl per minute per kg. Differences from normal values were not significant. Regression analysis of measured pressure vs. CSF volume production indicated no relation between these parameters.

Production of CSF was normal in dogs with chronic hydrocephalus and normal CSF pressures in this study. Production of CSF tended to be lower in dogs with increased CSF pressures. When CSF absorption is compromised, decreased CSF production does not appear to be a significant compensatory mechanism. It is expected that further studies quantifying movement into the extracellular space of the peri-

(8) Radiology 122:143–147, January, 1977.

ventricular region will only reduce the measured differences, which presently are just at the threshold level.

▶ [Decreased cerebrospinal fluid production is not an adequate compensatory mechanism to prevent the development of communicating hydrocephalus when cerebrospinal fluid absorption is compromised. — Ed.]

Cerebrospinal Fluid γ-Aminobutyric Acid in Neurologic Disease. γ-Aminobutyric acid (GABA) is considered a putative inhibitory neurotransmitter and is present in large concentrations in the vertebrate central nervous system. Disorder of GABA metabolism has been suggested in certain neurologic diseases. V. S. Achar, K. M. A. Welch, E. Chabi, K. Bartosh and J. S. Meyer[9] (Baylor Univ.) measured GABA levels in the cerebrospinal fluid (CSF) in a series of patients with neurologic disorders having lumbar puncture as part of the clinical examination. An enzymatic assay was used. Of the 151 patients studied, 19 had no organic neurologic disease; GABA was not found in the CSF of any of these patients.

Fig 1. — Cerebrospinal fluid GABA levels in patients with cerebrovascular disease, Parkinson's syndrome, dementia and Huntington's disease and in controls without neurologic disease; *V.B.I.,* vertebrobasilar insufficiency; *M.I.D.,* multi-infarct dementia. (Courtesy of Achar, V. S., et al.: Neurology (Minneap.) 26:777–780, August, 1976.)

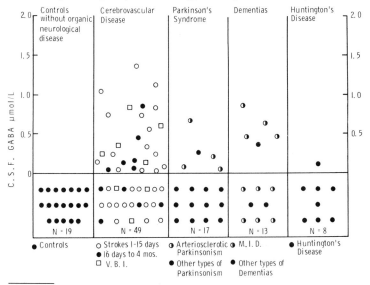

(9) Neurology (Minneap.) 26:777–780, August, 1976.

γ-Aminobutyric acid was found in the CSF of 26 of 49 patients with cerebrovascular disease (Fig 1); the highest levels were found mostly in patients with acute ischemic infarction lasting less than 2 weeks. The severity of neurologic deficit influenced the degree of GABA elevation and its persistence after 2 weeks. Five of 8 patients with vertebrobasilar insufficiency had GABA elevation, as did 5 of 17 with Parkinson's syndrome, 4 of whom had an atherosclerotic origin of disease. Five of 13 patients with various types of dementia had measurable GABA levels; 4 of them had multiinfarct dementia. Three of 6 patients with seizure disorders had detectable GABA (Fig 2). Eight of 29 patients with multiple sclerosis had detectable GABA in CSF; 5 of them had chronic spinal cord lesions. Twenty-two patients without GABA had chronic demyelinating lesions in sites other than the spinal cord; GABA was detected in the CSF of individual patients with various other neurologic disorders. Its detection was unrelated to other CSF abnormalities.

These results suggest the value of continued studies of larger series to evaluate the diagnostic significance of CSF

Fig 2.—Cerebrospinal fluid GABA levels in patients with multiple sclerosis, epilepsy and other neurologic diseases; *T.L.E.,* temporal lobe epilepsy. (Courtesy of Achar, V. S., et al.: Neurology (Minneap.) 26:777–780, August, 1976.)

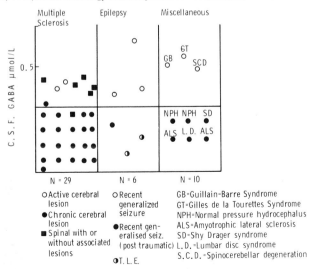

GABA in central nervous system disease and to raise the possibility of a previously unsuspected disorder of GABA metabolism in some neurologic conditions.

► [This study shows that γ-aminobutyric acid is found in patients with various diseases of the nervous system. Further study is necessary, however, to evaluate the significance of this finding. — Ed.] ◄

Evidence for Presence of Vasoactive Substance (Possibly Involved in Etiology of Cerebral Arterial Spasm) in Cerebrospinal Fluid from Patients with Subarachnoid Hemorrhage. D. J. Boullin, J. Mohan and D. G. Grahame-Smith[1] (Oxford, England) obtained cerebrospinal fluid from 34 patients admitted for clipping of cerebral aneurysms after subarachnoid hemorrhage. By means of an isolated human basilar artery test system, the effects of the cerebrospinal fluid on the contractions produced by noradrenaline, 5-hydroxytryptamine (5-HT) and six prostaglandins were examined. The cerebrospinal fluid was obtained 2–10 hours after angiography. Control specimens were taken from 12 patients having myelography for suspected intervertebral disk prolapse.

Twenty-two patients had some degree of arterial spasm, which was largely confined to the internal carotid, middle cerebral and anterior cerebral arteries. Contractile substances were present in the cerebrospinal fluid of 16 of the 22 patients with vasospasm but in only 2 of 12 without spasm. The contractions developed slowly, taking up to 6 hours to reach a maximum. The responses were not blocked by a 5-HT antagonist or by phentolamine. The concentration-dependent contractions induced by K^+ were much smaller than those produced by cerebrospinal fluid, prostaglandins, 5-HT or noradrenaline. Cerebrospinal fluid potentiated the contractile responses to 5-HT and the prostaglandins, especially prostaglandin E_2. Effects on noradrenaline-induced contractions were variable. Atropine failed to modify the cerebrospinal fluid contractile responses.

The unidentified contracting factor in cerebrospinal fluid may play a major role in the production of prolonged spasm in patients with subarachnoid hemorrhage from ruptured aneurysm. Prostaglandins, 5-HT and, possibly, noradrenaline may be involved secondarily, their actions being poten-

(1) J. Neurol. Neurosurg. Psychiatry 39:756–766, August, 1976.

tiated by cerebrospinal fluid containing the contractile substance. Prolonged arterial spasm appears to involve an interaction between these substances and the unidentified agent. The factor is probably derived from blood.

▶ [It is known that patients with subarachnoid hemorrhage may show evidence of cerebral arterial spasm. These authors postulate that there is an unidentified contracting factor in the cerebrospinal fluid of patients who have had a subarachnoid hemorrhage that plays a major role in the production of prolonged spasm of the cerebral arteries. Other substances such as 5-hydroxytryptamine, noradrenaline and certain prostaglandins may be involved in a secondary capacity because their actions are potentiated by contractile substance in the cerebrospinal fluid. The source of the factor is not known but it is probably derived from the blood. – Ed.] ◀

New Ultramicromethod for Concentration of Cerebrospinal Fluid is described by Sidney N. Kahn and E. J. Thompson[2] (Natl. Hosp., London). Routine laboratory electrophoretic methods for analyzing cerebrospinal fluid (CSF) require concentration of the fluid by 20–100 times for 1- to 5-μl applications of protein on support mediums. Current methods of concentration require rather large fluid volumes, which are often unavailable. This method requires no apparatus and permits multiple simultaneous sample processing.

METHOD. – A disk of Diaflo PM 10 ultrafiltration membrane, 62 mm in diameter, is soaked for 2 hours in 50% aqueous glycerol containing 1% Triton X–100 and is allowed to dry thoroughly. The membrane is placed on an absorbent pad of blotting paper on a rigid base and is held firmly in place (Fig 3). The sample is applied to the membrane surface. A 3- to 4-mm area of application is used to concentrate 100 μl, applying 5–10 μl initially. When 10–20% of the initial volume remains, in 2–3 minutes, a second aliquot is applied and the process is repeated until the desired concentration is reached. Microliter syringes and adjustable micropipettes are useful in the procedure.

This method has been used to concentrate single CSF samples to a uniform protein concentration of 10 gm/L before applying 5 μl to an agarose slide for electrophoresis. The method is also applicable to other biologic fluids; it is rapid, easy, economical and makes simultaneous multiple-sample processing possible. The molecular weight cutoff can be varied by selecting different filters. No special apparatus is needed. Reasonable care must be taken to avoid damaging

(2) Lancet 1:1275, June 12, 1976.

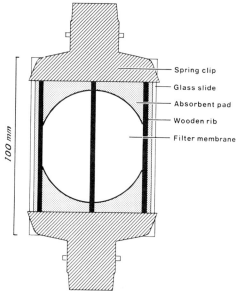

Fig 3.—Complete apparatus showing membrane held in apposition to absorbent pad. (Courtesy of Kahn, S. N., and Thompson, E. J.: Lancet 1:1275, June 12, 1976.)

the membrane; complete drying of the sample must be avoided.

▶ [Concentration of the cerebrospinal fluid is necessary before many important tests can be carried out. The authors describe a method that requires no special apparatus and permits multiple simultaneous sample testing. – Ed.] ◀

Cerebrospinal Fluid Cytology: Diagnostic Accuracy and Comparison of Different Techniques. Bernard Gondos and Eileen B. King[3] (Univ. of California, San Francisco) reviewed 1,021 cases seen in 1967–70 and 1973–74 from which a total of 1,117 cerebrospinal fluid specimens was received. The nucleopore technique was used as the primary method of examining specimens in the earlier period, with Papanicolaou staining of the centrifuged sediment and Wright-stained smears. Subsequently the millipore technique was also used. Recently the cytocentrifuge method has also been used in selected cases. Earlier samples were

(3) Acta Cytol. (Baltimore) 20:542–547, Nov.–Dec., 1976.

generally less than 1 cc in volume; recent ones average over 4 cc. In recent years Wright staining has not been done routinely.

Results were positive in 32.3% of cases of primary central nervous system neoplasm, 24% of cases of tumor originating outside the central nervous system and 42.4% of cases of lymphoma or leukemia. Among cases with autopsy or biopsy verification, 53.5% of those of metastatic tumor and 65.8% of those of lymphomatous or leukemic involvement of the central nervous system yielded positive cytologic findings. Among primary neoplasms, the detection rate was highest for medulloblastoma (61.9%). Leukemia was detected in 61% of cases and lymphoma in 70%. In 16 cases abnormal cells were found in the presence of nonneoplastic conditions. Cases of viral encephalitis, chronic meningitis, demyelinating diseases and recent cerebrovascular accident were most troublesome in this regard. Detection rates were slightly higher in the later review period. Cellularity was greater in the millipore preparations and the quality of cell preservation was more consistent with the millipore filter (Fig 4). The cytocentrifuged specimens showed much greater cell distortion and more variability in cell preservation than those obtained with either type of filter preparation. Specimens of low volume were difficult to evaluate because

Fig 4. – Medulloblastoma. Note dense aggregation and nuclear molding; reduced from ×1600. (Courtesy of Gondos, B., and King, E. B.: Acta Cytol. (Baltimore) 20: 542 – 547, Nov. – Dec., 1976.)

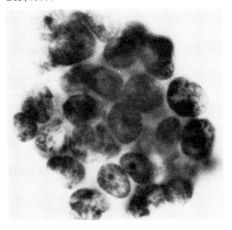

of inadequate cell material, regardless of the technique used.

About half of all metastatic tumors involving the central nervous system can be diagnosed by cerebrospinal fluid cytologic examination. The method is useful in determining the need for local therapy in patients with known systemic lymphoma or leukemia. Accuracy has been slightly better with the millipore filter than with the nucleopore. Experience with the cytocentrifuge method has been disappointing. The usefulness of cerebrospinal fluid cytologic examination depends on collection of adequate material, and preparatory methods have an important influence on the results.

► [These findings indicate that the diagnostic usefulness of examination of cerebrospinal fluid cytology depends on the methods of collection and preparation as well as the anatomical distribution and biologic behavior of the underlying disease. — Ed.] ◄

Pediatric Neurology

Brain Stem and Adrenal Abnormalities in Sudden Infant Death Syndrome. Some victims of sudden infant death syndrome (SIDS) appear to be chronically hypoxemic before death, due to chronic underventilation of the lungs. Some future victims also have abnormalities in respiration, feeding, temperature control and neurologic tests in the neonatal period. Richard L. Naeye[4] (Pennsylvania State Univ., Hershey) undertook a quantitative histologic analysis of astroglial fibers in the medullary reticular formation, where brain stem areas controlling respiration are found, in 28 infants aged 1–12 months who were SIDS victims. Eighteen control infants who died from trauma, carbon monoxide poisoning, suffocation or drowning were also examined. The mean gestational age at birth was 39 weeks in both groups.

In SIDS victims, increases in astroglial density were associated with increases in smooth muscle in small pulmonary arteries, in the number of medial cells in the pulmonary arteries, in brown fat cell retention and in thickness of the chromaffin cell layer of the adrenal medulla (Fig 5). The 5 SIDS victims who had erythropoiesis in the liver were among those with the most astroglial fibers; no controls had hepatic erythropoiesis. Astroglial fibers were generally increased throughout the brain stem in the 14 study patients who had increased densities of such fibers in the reticular formation.

This study showed that SIDS victims with markers of antecedent chronic hypoxemia have increased volumes of adrenal chromaffin cells. Infants with a variety of hypoxemic disorders have increased volumes of these cells in their adrenals, and the greater volume of cells in SIDS victims is apt to be a consequence of chronic hypoxemia. The brain stem and adrenal abnormalities in SIDS are probably both secondary to chronic hypoxemia.

► [The etiology of the sudden infant death syndrome is not definitely

(4)   Am. J. Clin. Pathol. 66:526–530, September, 1976.

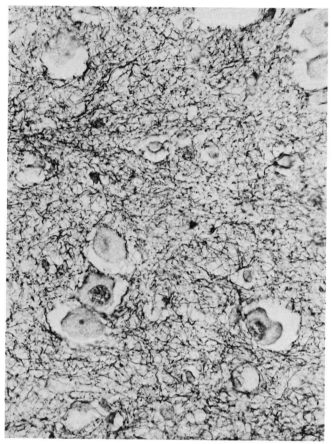

Fig 5. — Marked astroglial proliferation is visible in medulla of SIDS victim aged 3 months. Holzer stain; original magnification, ×600. (Courtesy of Naeye, R. L.: Am. J. Clin. Pathol. 66:526–530, September, 1976.)

known. This study gives important information about possible mechanisms underlying this strange enigma. — Ed.] ◄

Anoxic-Ischemic Encephalopathy in the Human Neonatal Period: Significance of Brain Stem Involvement. Richard W. Leech (Univ. of North Dakota) and Ellsworth C. Alvord, Jr.[5] (Univ. of Washington) found why

(5)   Arch. Neurol. 34:109–113, February, 1977.

human infants sometimes recapitulate the topographic pattern of anoxic-ischemic injury found in experimental animals and other times recapitulate the patterns usually seen in human adults, with a rostrocaudal pattern of selective neuronal vulnerability rather than brain stem and thalamic damage. Study was made of the brains of 16 children with well-defined single asphyxial episodes. All but 5 of the children had had episodes in the immediate perinatal period.

The cerebral cortex was involved variably in most cases, usually by minor patchy or focal neuronal loss. One patient showed frank cystic encephalomalacia and another, sclerotic border zone or watershed-type lesions. The white matter usually reflected the degree of cortical neuronal loss but in 2 infants, white matter damage clearly exceeded that seen in the cortex. The striatum and pallidum were involved variably, but the lateral geniculate bodies and other thalamic nuclei were involved almost always. The ventrolateral and dorsomedial thalamic nuclei were involved more often than other areas. The inferior colliculi showed either loss of neurons with gliosis or ischemic cell changes in 85% of infants. Only 2 of the infants who lived for 1 month or longer showed obvious neuronal loss in brain stem nuclei. The dentate nucleus, cerebellar cortex and substantia nigra were involved variably.

A smaller number of infants appear to have an acute asphyxial episode without significant supervening hypotension or other complications such as acidosis. A larger group of perinatally damaged infants have episodes of prolonged partial asphyxia complicated by hypotension, which produces the cortical injury pattern and leads to mental retardation with cortical nodular sclerosis, ulegyria, status marmoratus and their variations. A third pattern may exist, with extensive white matter damage.

▶ [Many investigators express the belief that the human brain stem is relatively invulnerable to anoxia. This study of 16 instances of a single acute asphyxial episode occurring at or just after birth shows that there are at least two patterns of acute encephalopathy in such patients. In one there is a rostrocaudal pattern of decreasing vulnerability to damage, with the cerebral cortex being the most sensitive and the brain stem the least sensitive. In the other pattern, the damage affects predominantly the brain stem and thalamus. Of the two, the latter pattern appears to follow most of the acute asphyxial episodes in the human neonate and infant. — Ed.] ◀

Neonatal Encephalopathy Following Fetal Distress: Clinical and Electroencephalographic Study. Ischemic-anoxic encephalopathy is the most common neurologic disease of the perinatal period. Harvey B. Sarnat and Margaret S. Sarnat[6] (St. Louis Univ.) attempted a systematic clinical approach to identification of the transitory neurologic signs that appear sequentially after asphyxia near or at birth in relation to prognosis.

Twenty-one infants over 36 weeks' gestational age at birth were studied. None had evidence of congenital heart disease, traumatic cerebral injury, hydrocephalus or infection. Each had a well-defined episode of fetal distress or an Apgar score of 5 or less 1 or 5 minutes after delivery; in no case could this be attributed to drug treatment of the mother. Neurologic examinations were done often for the 1st week and then on alternate days until discharge. Follow-up neurologic and EEG studies were done at 3-month intervals or more often in a few cases.

Three clinical stages of postanoxic encephalopathy were distinguished. Stage 1, lasting less than 24 hours, consisted of hyperalertness, uninhibited Moro's and stretch reflexes, sympathetic effects and a normal EEG. Stage 2 was marked by obtundation, hypotonia, strong distal flexion and multifocal seizures; the EEG showed a periodic pattern, sometimes preceded by continuous delta activity. Infants in stage 3 were stuporous and flaccid and had suppressed brain stem and autonomic functions; the EEG was isopotential or showed infrequent periodic discharges. Only 7 of the 21 infants had features of stage 1, all had stage 2 features and 6 passed through stage 3. Stage 2 lasted a mean of 4.7 days, excluding 2 infants affected for 3 and 9 weeks. Changes in autonomic function were some of the most dramatic contrasts between stages. Seizures occurred in about half the patients.

Four severely affected infants died. Both autopsies showed extensive softening of the cerebrum and cerebellum, with microcystic degeneration of cortical gray and subcortical white matter, extensive neuronal loss and gross atrophy. Infants in whom signs of stage 2 and the EEG reverted to normal within 5 days had a good outcome. Total EEG isopo-

(6) Arch. Neurol. 33:696–705, October, 1976.

tentiality at any time had a poor prognosis, as did a periodic pattern with an isopotential phase between bursts of activity occurring less often than every 6 seconds and a periodic pattern in wakefulness with continuous cortical activity between bursts occurring every 3–6 seconds, lasting a week or longer.

None of these clinical or EEG features are specific for post-anoxic encephalopathy. Quantitation of the clinical and EEG data defines the severity of the brain insult and makes accurate prognosis easier. At least 2 EEGs should be obtained in the 1st week in asphyxiated infants, 2 and 6 days after birth; both wakefulness and sleep should be sampled.

▶ [The prognosis of neonates who have suffered perinatal asphyxia may be determined by careful neurologic observation and electroencephalography.—Ed.] ◄

Follow-up Study of Sydenham's Chorea. In contrast to a lack of physical sequelae, emotional disturbances have been stressed after Sydenham's chorea. Psychosocial difficulties have been described before, during and after acute chorea. Morris T. Bird, Helen Palkes and Arthur L. Prensky[7] (Washington Univ.) compared 25 patients convalescing from Sydenham's chorea with 15 siblings and 20 matched rheumatic fever controls by clinical, EEG, psychometric and psychologic evaluations. Four study patients had two episodes of chorea within 2 years. The siblings were selected by age and sex, and the rheumatic fever controls were selected for age, sex and socioeconomic background. All patients with Sydenham's chorea and rheumatic fever were on penicillin prophylaxis. No patient had evidence of active carditis.

One study patient had persistently reduced myotatic reflexes and 1 control subject had congenital nystagmus. Neurologic signs were more prevalent in both patient groups than in siblings. Ten study patients had two or more neurologic signs on follow-up examination. No significant EEG differences were found between the three groups. Five of the 9 abnormal EEGs in the chorea group were in the 10 most affected patients. Mild diffuse slowing was the usual major abnormality. No significant psychometric test differences were found except for a difference in Bender gestalt visuo-

(7) Neurology (Minneap.) 26:601–606, July, 1976.

motor function results between choreic patients and sibling controls. Psychologic symptoms were comparable in the choreic and rheumatic fever patients but behavioral problems were much more prominent in the choreic group. Behavioral disturbances were not disproportionately localized to the group of choreic patients with the most neurologic signs. Significant differences were not found in those chorea patients who could be matched with their siblings.

Uncomplicated Sydenham's chorea is not necessarily a benign self-limited condition of the central nervous system. Some patients are left with definite, though minimal, neurologic residuals. The many residual motor signs found in patients with Sydenham's chorea and rheumatic fever raises the question of a common effect on the central nervous system in both disorders, possibly to a greater degree in choreic patients.

▶ [Whereas Sydenham's chorea has been a rare disease in the United States during recent years, it generally has been assumed that organic neurologic manifestations rarely follow the disorder, although there may be psychosocial difficulties. This study suggests that uncomplicated Sydenham's chorea is not necessarily a benign, self-limited affliction of the central nervous system, as some patients are left with definite, albeit minimal, neurologic residuals. – Ed.] ◀

Central Monoamines and Hyperkinesis of Childhood. Hyperkinesis is a poorly understood but relatively common disorder of childhood, characterized by excessive motor activity, a shortened attention span and hyperexcitability. It often results in poor motor performance and learning difficulties, even when intelligence test scores remain normal. Analeptic agents have alleviated most of the abnormalities and indirect biochemical observations suggest that monoaminergic mechanisms may relate to the pathogenesis of hyperkinesis of childhood.

Taranath Shetty (Brown Univ.) and Thomas N. Chase[8] (Natl. Inst. of Health) attempted to determine whether hyperkinetic children have abnormalities in resting levels or amphetamine-induced changes in dopamine and serotonin metabolites in the lumbar cerebrospinal fluid. Studies were done on 19 boys and 4 girls aged 2–13 years with typical motor and behavioral features of hyperkinetic syndrome and on 6 control children. The study patients had mild to

(8) Neurology (Minneap.) 26:1000–1002, October, 1976.

moderately severe clinical signs. None had subnormal intelligence or evidence of structural brain disease, and none had received analeptic therapy. Ten patients received 0.5 mg dextroamphetamine per kg daily for 2–14 days and 5 others received placebo tablets.

Steady-state cerebrospinal fluid levels of homovanillic acid and 5-hydroxyindoleacetic acid (5-HIAA) were normal in the hyperactive children. Dextroamphetamine was significantly effective in improving the clinical state of the hyperactive patients. Dextroamphetamine but not placebo led to a substantial (34%) reduction in cerebrospinal fluid homovanillic acid. No consistent change in 5-HIAA levels was noted. The degree of clinical improvement correlated closely with the degree of homovanillic acid reduction in the children given dextroamphetamine (Fig 6).

These findings support the hypothesis that dopaminergic mechanisms contribute to the pathogenesis of childhood hyperkinesis. Increased function in dopamine-containing neural systems is implicated by preclinical studies but this would be compatible with pharmacologic observations only if it is assumed that the therapeutic effect of dextroamphetamine derives mainly from its effect on presynaptic dopa-

Fig 6.—Relationship between dextroamphetamine-induced change in cerebrospinal fluid content of homovanillic acid and improvement score for male *(solid circles)* and female *(open circles)* patients. (Courtesy of Shetty, T., and Chase, T. N.: Neurology (Minneap.) 26:1000–1002, October, 1976.)

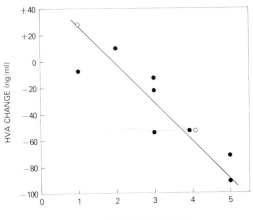

IMPROVEMENT RATING

mine-containing neurons, rather than at postsynaptic dopamine receptor sites, where amphetamine presumably exerts a stimulatory effect. Possibly the pharmacologic actions of amphetamine in part reflect disease-related alterations in central neurohumoral mechanisms.

▶ [These results support the view that an alteration in central dopamine-mediated synaptic function may occur in children manifesting the hyperactive syndrome. — Ed.] ◀

Childhood Seizures: A 25-Year Follow-up — Social and Medical Prognosis is reported by R. M. Harrison and D. C. Taylor[9] (Park Hosp. for Children, Oxford, England) for a group of children originally identified as having had at least 1 seizure in early childhood. Records on 628 children first seen during 1948–53 were available. The age of ascertainment ranged from 1 day to 14 years. A 20% random reduction left 498 subjects, 207 of whom were selected for a stratified sample; of these, information was obtained on 179 subjects. The ratio of boys to girls was about 6:4 in the achieved sample.

Twenty-seven subjects had died (10.1%); 30% of deaths were from seizures. The mortality for seizures in the 1st month of life was 57.1%. Fifteen patients were in institutions and had been there for a mean time of 12 years; 9 other subjects were invalids at home. The rate of continuing epilepsy was 21.8% of the sample and 24.2% of survivors. Only about half the subjects with epilepsy were self-supporting in the community. The overall educational achievement of the sample was good but there were many educational problems. Continuing epilepsy was associated with greatly reduced educational and occupational achievements compared with the group in remission.

This study shows the considerable cost of epilepsy to the community in both human and material terms and why epilepsy is regarded as a frightening illness. Seizures in childhood can be the start of serious social and medical problems. One in 10 children in this series has died and among survivors, slightly more than 1 in 10 are permanently confined in an institution. Two thirds of the group suffered minimal or no ill effects but the consequences for the other third are so serious as to explain why epilepsy is so frightening.

(9) Lancet 1:948–951, May 1, 1976.

▶ [This study shows that the outlook for children in whom seizures have developed in early life must be considered seriously. It also reveals the considerable cost of epilepsy to the community in both human and material terms. It is easy to understand why parents are upset when told that their child has epilepsy. – Ed.] ◀

Predictors of Epilepsy in Children Who Have Experienced Febrile Seizures. Febrile seizures occur in 2–5% of children, and all relevant studies agree that these children are more likely than others to become epileptic. Karin B. Nelson and Jonas H. Ellenberg[1] (Natl. Inst. of Health) examined the frequency of afebrile seizures, recurrent or isolated, and the risk factors for their development by age 7 years in children who had had febrile seizures.

Of about 54,000 children born at 12 hospitals during 1959–66, 1,821 had febrile convulsions; information was available on the status at age 7 years for 1,706 of them (94%). Of the children followed to age 7 years, 65% had no subsequent seizure of any type by this age, whereas 32% had one or more other febrile seizures but no afebrile seizures. Fifty-two children had at least one asymptomatic afebrile seizure by age 7 years; 34 of these 52 children, or 2% of those followed to age 7 years, had recurrent, active, asymptomatic afebrile seizures.

The development of epilepsy was unrelated to a low Apgar score or to low birth weight. None of the study patients had obvious malformations. Epilepsy developed in significantly more children whose first febrile seizure was complex. Children with febrile seizures whose status was abnormal before any seizure were 3 times more likely than the others to be epileptic by age 7 years. Children whose prior status was abnormal had an increasing epileptic rate when three or more seizures occurred, compared to those having two or less. Epilepsy was more frequent in children whose febrile seizures began in the 1st year and especially in the first 6 months of life. Afebrile seizures most often supervened in the year after the first febrile seizure. Seven study children had cerebral palsy and mental retardation and 7 others were mentally retarded.

Prior neurologic and developmental status and characteristics of the first febrile seizure are important predictors of epilepsy after febrile seizures. If subgroups of children at

(1) N. Engl. J. Med. 295:1029–1033, Nov. 4, 1976.

high risk can be identified, it may be reasonable to consider long-term therapy for a minority of children with febrile convulsions who are in special jeopardy. Whether or not chronic anticonvulsant therapy can prevent the emergence of afebrile seizure disorders after febrile seizures is unknown.

▶ [Prior neurologic and developmental status and characteristics of the first febrile seizure are important predictors of the possibility of epilepsy developing in children who have had febrile seizures. – Ed.] ◄

Prognostic Factors in Absence Seizures. Susumu Sato, Fritz E. Dreifuss and J. Kiffin Penry[2] reviewed data on 52 patients hospitalized during 1966–68 with absence seizures. The 25 male and 27 female patients had a mean age of 10.5 years and a mean duration of illness of 3.6 years. Forty-eight patients were followed in 1974; 2 patients were lost to follow-up and 2 had died, 1 by drowning and 1 of lung abscess. The average interval since initial study was 6.9 years. The 22 male and 26 female patients followed had a mean age of 17.3 years and a mean duration of illness of 7.9 years.

Twenty-seven patients were seizure-free at follow-up, 6 had absence seizures only, 9 had both absence and generalized tonic-clonic seizures, 5 had generalized seizures only and 1 had persistent simple partial tonic seizures and generalized tonic-clonic seizures. No patient had partial seizures with complex symptomatology. The persisting absence seizures were similar to those noted initially. There was no age difference between subjects with and those without persistent absence seizures. Only 7 of 22 patients who initially had absence and generalized seizures had stopped having seizures at follow-up, compared to 18 of 23 who initially had absence seizures only. Differences in duration of illness were slight. Multivariate analysis showed the significant prognostic factors for absence seizures to be normal or above-normal intelligence and normal EEG background activity. For any seizure type, significant prognostic factors included a negative history of generalized tonic-clonic seizures, normal or above-normal intelligence and a negative family history of seizure disorders. Nearly 90% of patients with all significant prognostic factors for both absence seizures and seizures of all types ceased having seizures.

Multiple factors influence the prognosis of absence seizures. The most important factor for good prognosis of either absence seizures or seizures in general in this study was a normal or above-normal intelligence quotient.

▶ [For any seizure type, significant factors for a good prognosis were a negative history of generalized tonic-clonic seizures, normal or above normal intelligence and a negative family history of seizure disorders; for absence seizures, they were normal or above normal intelligence and normal EEG background. Nearly 90% of patients with all these significant prognostic factors for both absence seizures and seizures of all types ceased having seizures. – Ed.] ◀

Benign Myoclonus of Early Infancy. C. T. Lombroso and Natalio Fejerman[3] (Harvard Med. School) report data on a small series of infants who might have been diagnosed as having infantile spasms but who exhibited clinical and laboratory features of a distinct subgroup with benign myoclonus of early infancy.

The 16 infants were seen during the past 10 years. All had tonic-myoclonic seizures involving either axial or limb musculature, generally briefly, but often occurring in series or "flurries." Often the neck musculature was predominantly affected. Eight infants had mainly cephalic involvement and 8 had both cephalic and limb involvement. Only rarely were the legs involved. The age of onset was 3 – 8½ months. Generally more attacks occurred early in the morning during feeding or play; none was noted during sleep. Four infants had equivocally abnormal neurologic signs when first seen; only 2 had residua on follow-up. One patient had an unsustained elevation of cerebrospinal fluid protein. The EEGs gave negative results. The spells usually became more frequent over a few weeks or months after their onset but they abated rapidly and no child had episodes after age 2. One child had breath-holding spells. Even infants given no treatment did well.

These infants had little to suggest the presence of the serious specific disorders causing myoclonus. The presenting features were entirely consistent with the so-called cryptogenic or idiopathic form of infantile spasms. Cephalic involvement was frequent. No regression or arrest of developmental milestones was observed, as is usually the case in infantile spasms. Other seizure patterns did not develop

(3)   Ann. Neurol. 1:138–143, February, 1977.

once the spasms had ceased. The term benign myoclonus of early infancy is suggested for this disorder. Etiologic and pathophysiologic mechanisms are not known at present but recognition of the disorder is worthwhile for therapeutic and prognostic guidance.

▶ [The development of myoclonus in infancy usually forebodes an ominous future, with progressive neurologic and intellectual deterioration and uncontrollable seizures. These authors tell us that myoclonus in infancy may not always have such a grave prognosis and that the condition may be self-limited. — Ed.] ◀

Dementia

Prevalence and Malignancy of Alzheimer's Disease: A Major Killer. Robert Katzman[4] (New York) states that the argument that Alzheimer's disease is a major killer rests on the assumption that the disease and senile dementia are one process. Both are progressive dementias with similar clinical features and the pathologic findings are identical.

Ultrastructural studies have established the identity of the neurofibrillary tangle and the senile plaque. Most studies indicate that the neurofibrillary tangle in both disorders is characterized by the twisted tubule that represents two neurofilaments joined in a helical fashion with a periodicity of 800 Å. Quantitative correlation has been established between the number of tangles and senile plaques in the cerebral cortex and the degree of dementia. Genetic analysis has, however, shown many relatives with senile dementia but none with a diagnosis of Alzheimer's disease in the same kindred. The incidence of the Alzheimer-senile dementia complex is strongly age related, even among the elderly. Only age has distinguished the two disorders and the author believes that it is time to drop the arbitrary age distinction and adopt the single designation, Alzheimer's disease.

Studies of patients with Alzheimer's disease show a marked decrease in life expectancy, depending on the age at onset of symptoms. Based on the prevalence of severe forms of dementia and life expectancy, from 60,000 to 90,000 persons with senile dementia die each year, not counting persons under age 65 or those in whom moderate forms of dementia may shorten life expectancy. Mild memory deficit may be relatively common in older persons but these minor changes do not result in the functional disability or increased mortality that can be attributed to Alzheimer's disease. Senile and presenile forms of Alzheimer's disease are

(4) Arch. Neurol. 33:217–218, April, 1976.

one entity, a disease whose cause must be determined and whose course must be aborted and, ultimately, a disease to be prevented.

▶ [There are both senile and presenile forms of Alzheimer's disease — there is no clinical or pathologic difference between the two. Most instances of so-called senile dementia are probably instances of Alzheimer's disease. The etiology of Alzheimer's disease has not been determined. It is important to determine the cause of the disease in the hope that its course may be aborted and its development prevented. — Ed.] ◀

Correlation between Computerized Transaxial Tomography and Radionuclide Cisternography in Dementia. Earlier reports have recognized the value of noninvasive computerized transaxial tomography (CTT) in visualizing the ventricular system and the sulci over the convexities. M. H. Gado, R. E. Coleman, K. S. Lee, M. A. Mikhael, P. O. Alderson and C. R. Archer[5] (Washington Univ.) compared CTT patterns with cisternographic patterns of cerebrospinal fluid (CSF) pathways in 44 patients with dementia. The CTT scans were done with an EMI scanner and cisternograms were done by the lumbar intrathecal administration of $250-500$ μCi ^{111}In-diethylenetriamine pentaacetic acid (DTPA); imaging was done with a gamma camera. Images were recorded 4, 24, 48 and often 72 hours after nuclide injection.

Cisternograms showed cerebral atrophy in 21 cases, communicating hydrocephalus in 12, an intermediate pattern in 9 and normal findings in 2. The CTT scans showed lateral ventricular dilatation in all 12 patients with a cisternographic pattern of communicating hydrocephalus. Moderate ventricular dilatation was seen in 11 patients with a pattern of cerebral atrophy; severe dilatation was seen in 1. Third ventricular dilatation was more frequent in the group with a cisternographic pattern of communicating hydrocephalus. When visualized, the 4th ventricle differed more between the two groups. The cerebral sulci were dilated in half the patients with a cisternographic pattern of cerebral atrophy and were prominent in 10% of those with communicating hydrocephalus.

Visualization of the sulci on CTT does not depend on filling the sulci with contrast medium (air). Cisternography and CTT are complementary to each other. Despite their agreement in a high percentage of cases, CTT does not provide the physiologic dynamic information offered by the cisternogram. Both studies are essential in evaluating dementia. The role of cisternography should not be diminished by the availability of CTT.

► [This article reveals that computerized transaxial tomography can replace pneumoencephalography for evaluating patients with dementia. Cisternography often contributes complementary information. – Ed.] ◄

Dementia in Parkinson's Disease. Reijo J. Marttila and Urpo K. Rinne[6] (Univ. of Turku) studied the occurrence of dementia in a parkinsonian population consisting of all traceable patients living in a defined area of southwest Finland, with a population of about 400,000, in 1972 and 1973. Of 484 patients alive on the prevalence day, 444 were examined. The diagnosis of Parkinson's disease was based on the presence of at least two cardinal signs. The overall occurrence of dementia was 28.8%. No significant differences were found between the idiopathic and the postencephalitic groups regarding the frequency of dementia, but the postencephalitic sample was small.

About half the demented patients were considered to be in the first stage, whereas about 20% were severely demented. Similar medical treatment had been given the demented and nondemented patients, although the former had received levodopa less often. Females were demented slightly more often than males. Dementia was more frequent in older patients and in patients with clinical arteriosclerosis. Nondemented patients exhibited severe disability less frequently in all age groups. Demented patients had slightly more severe tremor than the others, but differences in rigidity and hypokinesia scores were more marked. The severity of disease tended to decrease in the demented patients after age 70 years. Severity scores were generally lower in the demented patients with arteriosclerosis than in patients without arteriosclerosis.

The findings corroborate the concept of dementia as part of the clinical picture of Parkinson's disease. Cerebral atrophy has often been considered to be responsible for dementia in Parkinson's disease, but subcortical structures may be partly responsible. That levodopa does not alter the progress

(6) Acta Neurol. Scand. 54:431–441, 1976.

of dementia and often accentuates dementia might suggest that other neurotransmitter systems are involved in the pathophysiology of dementia in Parkinson's disease.

▶ [The association between dementia and the degree of motor involvement is considered to suggest the role of subcortical structures in the pathophysiology of dementia in Parkinson's disease. — Ed.] ◀

Epilepsy and the Convulsive Disorders

Depth and Direct Cortical Recording in Seizure Disorders of Extratemporal Origin. Monitoring of extratemporal structures may be necessary sometimes in patients with seizures refractory to all medical management whose lives are significantly and adversely affected by the disorder. The mesial aspect of the hemisphere and the orbitofrontal cortex occasionally are the source of focal attacks but cannot be monitored adequately by scalp EEG. B. I. Ludwig, C. Ajmone Marsan and J. Van Buren[7] (Natl. Inst. of Health) implanted extratemporal or a combination of temporal and extratemporal electrodes in 28 patients with intractable seizures to localize the epileptogenic process.

Eighteen patients had only extratemporal electrodes implanted. Electrodes were placed in the most probable areas of ictal onset, based on localizing data from clinical, electrographic and radiologic parameters. Depth electrodes with nine platinum-iridium contacts have been inserted stereotactically during the past 10 years. Implants are left in place for 7–10 days and recordings are made for at least 2–3 hours daily.

The mean age at onset of seizures was 10 years and at depth EEG study, 23 years. The etiopathology was unknown in 64% of cases. Neurologic examination results were normal in 61% of patients; the roentgenologic findings were normal in 54%. In most cases, the exact location and extent of the epileptiform disorder varied considerably. Several patients had prominent independent spike activity over different regions and were thought to have true multifocal lesions. Four subjects had no convincing interictal paroxysmal activity on electrography. Interictal epileptiform activity was far more evident on intracranial than on scalp EEG recording. Brief electrographic seizures were commonly

---

(7)   Neurology (Minneap.) 26:1085–1099, November, 1976.

seen and often corresponded to auras or minor motor phenomena. The epileptogenic process was localized from ictal phenomena in 17 cases and from interictal activity or the results of electric stimulation studies, or both, in the others. Partial cortical resections were done on 13 patients and a hemicorticectomy on 1; 1 of the former patients also subsequently had a hemicorticectomy. Fourteen patients were inoperable.

Electrode implantation in patients with seizure disorders of probable extratemporal origin can be of diagnostic value in certain situations, but in most cases the technique demonstrates the complexity of an apparently simple case or might tend to oversimplify very complex cases. Focal epilepsy in the absence of gross pathology is an ingenuous concept, the simplicity of which tends to deemphasize the true complexity of the disorder and the incomplete knowledge of its pathophysiology.

► [The authors conclude that the use of implanted electrodes in seizure disorders of probable extratemporal origin can be of real diagnostic benefit in certain specific situations. In most cases, however, this technique simply serves to demonstrate the complexity of an apparently simple case or, of greater clinical consequence, might tend to simplify cases that are actually extremely complex. In many respects this study raises some doubts about the validity of the classic concept of "focal" epilepsy. — Ed.] ◄

Regional Cerebral Blood Flow in Focal Cortical Epilepsy. Epileptic seizures are associated with increased metabolism and blood flow in the nervous tissue involved in the paroxysmal discharge. Kjeld Hougaard, Tadato Oikawa, Edda Sveinsdottir, Erki Skinhøj, D. H. Ingvar and Niels A. Lassen[8] (Copenhagen) measured regional cerebral blood flow (rCBF) by intra-arterial radioxenon injection in 10 patients with focal cortical epilepsy. A multidetector gamma camera was used in the studies. Regional ^{133}Xe clearance curves were processed on-line on a digital computer. The seizures in all cases showed no or only minimal generalization and were not related to alcohol or drug withdrawal. All patients had a normal social life. Four patients (group 1) were studied during clinical seizure activity and 6 (group 2), only in the interictal phase. Three group 1 patients were also studied during the interictal phase.

(8) Arch. Neurol. 33:527–535, August, 1976.

The 4 patients studied during clinical seizures showed marked focal hyperemia, with rCBF values 2–10 times above those of nonfocal regions in the same hemisphere. Autoregulation was abolished in the most hyperemic part of the focus in 1 of the 2 patients so tested. The localization of the hyperemic focus corresponded well to the clinically involved brain region. Interictal studies in 9 patients showed intermittent light-induced activation associated with a marked focal flow increase in regions that became hyperemic during seizures. Focal hyperemia occurred in all 9 patients, either spontaneously or during light stimulation. Resting flow patterns were essentially normal. Autoregulation of rCBF was normal in 3 of 5 cases, lost focally in 1 case and lost diffusely in 1.

Localization of cortical epileptic foci by the rCBF method is more precise than crude localization by EEG. It remains to be seen how often subictal hyperemic foci will be found by this technique in a larger series of patients with epilepsy caused by focal cortical epileptogenic lesions. Both the relatively gross spatial depth resolution with this technique and the trauma of carotid puncture could be eliminated by using a three-dimensional, section-scanning method for clearance of a diffusible nuclide, but such a method is not yet available.

▶ [It appears that cerebral blood flow studies can be valuable diagnostic tools in the investigation of patients with cortical epileptogenic lesions. There were changes in cerebral blood flow during seizures even in patients who had no distinct epileptic EEG foci during such seizures.—Ed.] ◀

Immunoglobulin A Deficiency, Epilepsy and Hydantoin Medication. Preliminary observations have suggested that hydantoin medication often is associated with selective IgA deficiency. A. Fontana, P. J. Grob, R. Sauter and Helen Joller[9] (Zurich) confirmed this association and found that a predisposition to hydantoin-induced low IgA levels occurs only in epileptic patients in whom constitutional factors are present.

Blood was sampled from 364 consecutive epileptic patients over a 2-month period in 1976. Eighty-four patients had not received hydantoin for at least 5 years before study. Phenytoin or its salts was used most often. Local cerebral

(9) Lancet 2:228–231, July 31, 1976.

factors predominated in 114 patients, while in 250 cases, clinical and EEG study gave generally accepted evidence of constitutional factors. A positive family history was present in 81 of these cases.

Blood IgA levels were significantly reduced in hydantoin-treated patients with constitutional factors present, whether or not a positive family history was obtained. Levels were also reduced in non-hydantoin-treated patients with a positive family history. Levels of IgG and IgM were increased in all epileptic groups compared to a blood donor group but were similar to values of a hospital group. The IgA levels were below 0.6 mg/ml in 12% of the epileptics and were below 0.05 mg/ml in 14 patients. All IgA-deficient patients had constitutional factors and all but 3 had received hydantoin. No other obvious correlations between IgA deficiency and drug therapy were seen. Complement levels and IgE levels were normal in all epileptic groups. The prevalence of recurrent infections, atopic disorders, gastrointestinal diseases and malignant nonbrain tumors was increased in IgA-deficient patients.

Epilepsy with constitutional characteristics may predispose to low IgA but IgA deficiency occurs only when hydantoins are given. Whether or not this postulated predisposition is relevant to the cause or pathogenesis of epilepsy is unknown. It is possible that IgA plays an important role not only at the body surfaces but also in the defense system of the brain at the serum-fluid barrier.

► [The data suggest that epilepsy with constitutional characteristics might predispose to low IgA, but that IgA deficiency only exists when hydantoins are given. The authors use the term "constitutional characteristics" in describing epileptics whose disease is known to be secondary to traumatic or infectious events or metabolic disturbances. – Ed.] ◄

Relationships between Intelligence and Electroencephalographic Epileptiform Activity in Adult Epileptics. Electroencephalographic epileptiform activity may be associated with deficits in performance on cognitive-motor tasks but few researchers have evaluated the relationship of epileptiform activity to intellectual abilities. Carl B. Dodrill and Robert J. Wilkus[1] (Univ. of Washington) assessed this relationship in 90 adult epileptics, 57 men and 33 women,

(1) Neurology (Minneap.) 26:525–531, June, 1976.

with an average age of 28.4 years. The mean age at onset of seizures in 88 cases was 12.5 years; the average duration of seizure disorder was 15.9 years. Fifty-five patients had complex partial (psychomotor) seizures; 47 had had generalized tonic-clonic seizures on one or more occasions. Intelligence

Fig 7. – Analysis of WAIS subtest scores in patients grouped according to average rate (low = < 1, high => 1 per minute) and topographic distribution of EEG epileptiform discharges. Differential subtest scores were derived by subtracting individual subtest values from average mean performance of each subject; the results were averaged for each group. (Courtesy of Dodrill, C. B., and Wilkus, R. J.: Neurology (Minneap.) 26:525–531, June, 1976.)

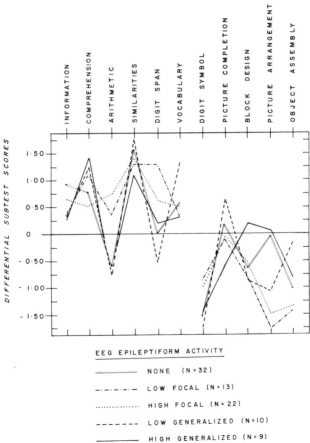

was assessed using the Wechsler Adult Intelligence Scale (WAIS).

Patients without discharges did best on all subtests and summary scores. Intelligence scores were lower in patients with generalized discharges than in those with focal discharges. Poorer scores for picture arrangement were obtained in association with discharges over the nondominant hemisphere. Summary scores for verbal, performance and full-scale IQ were progressively poorer in the low focal, high focal, low generalized and high generalized groups of patients. Results of an intra-individual subtest study are shown in Figure 7. The only subtest showing a significant difference was picture arrangement, on which both focal groups did poorest.

The greatest differences in intelligence in this study were found between patients without epileptiform activity and those with such activity. The results do not indicate that epileptiform discharges are causally related to poorer intellectual capabilities. It may simply be that the EEG abnormalities indicate the relative severity and distribution of cerebral pathologic or physiologic changes among different groups.

▶ [The results suggest that EEG epileptiform activity is significantly related to intellectual functioning in epileptics. − Ed.] ◀

Gelastic, Quiritarian and Cursive Epilepsy: Clinicopathologic Appraisal. Laughter and episodic running are extremely uncommon epileptic phenomena, and the combination of "gelastic" (laughter) and "cursive" (running) forms in the same person is rare. Only 3 such cases have been reported, all resulting from diffuse cerebral disorder. P. K. Sethi and T. Surya Rao[2] (Lucknow, India) describe an individual with episodes of epileptic laughter, running and crying, occurring alone or in combination, in association with a discrete neoplastic lesion in the left temporal lobe.

Man, 33, a soldier, had had episodic seizures for 1½ years. Four to six seizures occurred each day, lasting 30−60 seconds. Crying, laughter and the combination were observed, as were episodes of running. No convulsive movements were noted, and the patient never fell unconscious to the ground. The episodes could sometimes be induced by hyperventilation. There was no history of trauma or any febrile episode, and no family history of epilepsy. A right cen-

(2)   J. Neurol. Neurosurg. Psychiatry 39:823−828, September, 1976.

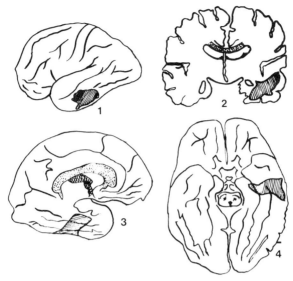

Fig 8. – Diagrammatic representation of extent of tumor (*hatched areas*). (Courtesy of Sethi, P. K., and Rao, T. S.: J. Neurol. Neurosurg. Psychiatry 39:823 – 828, September, 1976.)

tral type of facial asymmetry was the only abnormality. The EEG showed generalized spike discharges during seizures induced by hyperventilation, with an epileptogenic focus in the left temporal lobe. Carotid angiography showed a mass lesion in the anterior and middle temporal area. A tumor was found in the middle and inferior temporal gyri, extending subcortically inferomedially toward the uncus. It was excised and found to extend up to the pole just short of 2 cm and up to the vein of Labbe (Fig 8). The patient has been asymptomatic on anticonvulsant therapy for 6 months since surgery.

Involuntary laughter or crying may occur as a release phenomenon due to a destructive lesion or as an epileptic event. The inferior and medial portion of the temporal lobe has come to be considered a seat of emotions. In the present case, the tumor also extended inferiorly and medially, and the role of the temporal lobe in producing the epileptic discharges was clearly demonstrated. The precise location of laughter, crying and running in the temporal lobe, however, remains uncertain.

▶ [This is an interesting case report. In the same journal issue, M. I. Offen et al. report paroxysmal attacks of weeping and lacrimation associated with head turning and followed by confusion and amnesia (J. Neurol. Neurosurg. Psychiatry 39:829, 1976). They use the term "dacrystic epilepsy." In their case this was associated with atrophy of the right temporal region. — Ed.] ◄

Study of Epilepsy by Computerized Axial Tomography of the Encephalon. H. Gastaut, J.-L. Gastaut, H. Régis, Ch. Raybaud, Ph. Farnarier, P. Michotey and B. Michel[3] (Marseilles, France) used an EMI scanner reserved for use in epileptic patients to examine 500 patients. Among these, 401 (80.2%) could be classified, according to the international classification of epilepsy proposed by Gastaut (1969), as having generalized (147) or partial (198) epilepsy or epilepsy of another type (56). Results of the study could be divided into two large groups from the tacoencephalographic data according to the electroclinical type or the etiology of the epilepsy.

Among the electroclinical varieties, the tacoencephalogram (Taco EG) was normal in 73 (90%) of the patients with primary generalized epilepsy and showed a cerebral lesion in 74 (61%) of those with secondary generalized epilepsy. In partial epilepsy, the Taco EG showed a cerebral lesion in 63% of the subjects (97 focalized and 28 diffuse lesions). Also, the Taco EG was normal in all 15 children with benign epilepsy and in 10 of 25 with late grand mal epilepsy studied.

Among the etiologic groups, tumoral epilepsy involved 53 patients. Ten cases had already been established by neuroradiology, 20 were suspected clinically and/or by EEG, 17 were unsuspected and 6 were diagnosed as normal by neuroradiologic examination. Tacoencephalography was by far the best method for diagnosis because it showed the tumors in their entirety.

Man, 41, for 10 years had had right-sided hand-mouth seizures with anarthria. Initial EEG, angiographic, pneumoencephalographic and scintigraphic examinations were normal. Repeat angiography at age 32 years indicated the possibility of a left temporal expansive process. Surgery did not reveal the tumor but was followed by paretic sequellae and aggravated epilepsy. In the next 8 years, a new angiogram and 6 scintiscans were normal, but the EEG showed a temporal focus, apparently resulting from the oper-

(3) Nouv. Presse Med. 5:481–486, Feb. 21, 1976.

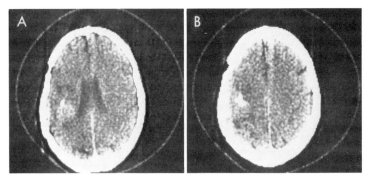

Fig 9. – **A,** in contact with the posterior part of the roof of the left lateral ventricle, which is neither deformed nor displaced, there is an expansive process which appears as a rounded dense zone about 2.5 cm in diameter. The zone is surrounded by an area of hypodensity corresponding to peritumoral edema. **B,** the supraventricular section shows that the tumor, which appears to involve only the oval center, comes in contact with cerebral cortex and has a focus of calcification. Bony sequelae of the operative flap can be seen in both sections. (Courtesy of Gastaut, H., et al.: Nouv. Presse Med. 5:481 – 486, Feb. 21, 1976.)

ation. Tacoencephalography indicated a left centroparietal tumor (Fig 9) situated closely behind the surgical approach.

Among the other etiologic groups, there were 27 cases of verified posttraumatic epilepsy, in which the Taco EG showed lesions 33 times (85%) – 4 diffused and 19 focal cases. There were 20 cases of postischemic epilepsy, i.e., 5% of the population, 7 cases of postinfectious epilepsy and some cases due to various other causes (Bourneville and Sturge-Weber syndromes, and others).

▶ [This study shows the value of transverse axial tomography in patients with seizures. It makes possible an increase in the percentage of cases of epilepsy in which the etiology is determined. – Ed.] ◀

Clonazepam in Treatment of Epilepsy: Controlled Clinical Trial in Simple Absences, Bilateral Massive Epileptic Myoclonus and Atonic Seizures. Bent Mikkelsen, Erik Birket-Smith, Sven Brandt, Per Holm, Mogens Lund, Ingrid Thorn, Svein Vestermark and Poul Zander Olsen[4] conducted a controlled study of clonazepam in outpatients with different forms of epilepsy, using a single-blind crossover design with sequential analysis.

Consecutive patients coming for routine ambulatory con-

(4) Arch. Neurol. 33:322 – 325, May, 1976.

trol, who had had 6 or more seizures monthly despite adequate conventional antiepileptic therapy, were included in the trial. Placebo was given for 4 weeks, followed by 4 weeks of clonazepam therapy. Tablets of 2 mg were used for patients over age 6 years and a 0.25% solution of clonazepam in propylene glycol was used for younger patients. Patients over age 6 years received 1 mg clonazepam daily initially and 6 mg daily for maintenance; the maintenance dose was reached in 2 weeks. Patients aged 3–6 years received 0.4 mg clonazepam daily initially and then 3 mg daily; those under age 3 years received 0.4 mg daily initially and then 1.5 mg daily.

Clonazepam was superior to placebo as adjunctive therapy in 10 patients with simple absences or pychoepilepsy; 6 of these patients received ethosuximide during the trial. Eight patients became free from simple absences during the trial; none had grand mal seizures. Nine patients had side effects, mostly in the form of sedation. Ten patients were treated for bilateral massive epileptic myoclonus and atonic seizures; 1 also had grand mal epilepsy and most had many daily attacks. Clonazepam was superior to placebo as an adjunct to established therapy in this group also. Seven patients became free or nearly free from seizures during the trial. Three patients had long-lasting side effects and 2 had transient side effects, mostly varying degrees of sedation. In 1 case, clonazepam was withdrawn because of somnolence, behavior disturbances and drug inefficacy.

Patients with myoclonic atonic seizures and those with simple absences refractory to conventional anticonvulsant agents should receive additional treatment with clonazepam.

► [According to this study, the use of clonazepam as an adjunct to the medications taken by patients with poorly controlled absence and myoclonic seizures gave "remarkably good" results. Side effects usually subsided spontaneously or could be controlled by reduction or slow increase in dosage. Similar results were obtained by another investigator (Browne, T. R: Arch. Neurol. 33:326, 1976).—Ed.] ◄

Anticonvulsant Drug Mechanisms: Phenytoin, Phenobarbital and Ethosuximide, and Calcium Flux in Isolated Presynaptic Endings. Inhibition of Ca^{2+} uptake at nerve terminals, with resulting impairment of neurotransmitter release, might explain the ability of a drug to suppress seizures. Phenytoin inhibits Ca^{2+} uptake by presynaptic endings from rat brain, and barbiturates inhibit Ca^{2+} uptake by stimulated autonomic ganglia. Richard S. Sohn and James A. Ferrendelli[5] (Washington Univ., St. Louis) studied the effects of four anticonvulsants and a central nervous system stimulant on the uptake of ionized calcium chloride by synaptosomes isolated from rabbit neocortex.

Calcium influx produced by depolarizing concentrations of K^+ (69 mM) was inhibited 7–63% by phenytoin, phenobarbital and procaine hydrochloride, whereas ethosuximide was ineffective. Decreased Ca^{2+} influx was noted with as little as 0.08 mM phenytoin and 0.04 mM phenobarbital. In contrast, 4 mM procaine was required to produce an effect. The central nervous system stimulant pentylenetetrazol had no effect on ^{45}Ca uptake by synaptosomes at concentrations up to 4 mM.

Phenobarbital, phenytoin and procaine inhibit Ca^{2+} uptake by synaptosomes, but ethosuximide does not. An ability to produce membrane stabilization is not a property of all anticonvulsant drugs, because ethosuximide does not inhibit Ca^{2+} uptake, but this property may be essential for the action of drugs that are effective in the treatment of major seizures. Other pharmacologic properties must be responsible for the anticonvulsant action of certain drugs such as ethosuximide, which prevents petit mal seizures.

► [These results lead to the conclusion that the ability to produce membrane stabilization may be essential to the action of drugs effective in the control of major seizures. – Ed.] ◄

Therapeutic and Pharmacokinetic Effect of Increasing Phenytoin in Chronic Epileptics on Multiple-Drug Therapy. Two prospective studies of phenytoin in epilepsy have suggested that maximum seizure control is obtained only when the serum level of phenytoin exceeds 40 μM/L. Wide variations in serum levels are found in different patients on the same dose, however, and serum levels are usually outside the assumed therapeutic range of 40–80 μM/L unless adequate monitoring is carried out.

D. G. Lambie, R. H. Johnson, R. N. Nanda and R. A. Shakir[6] (Glasgow) studied 20 chronic epileptics who were receiving phenytoin and either phenobarbitone or primidone. All had frequent seizures and serum phenytoin levels

(5) Arch. Neurol. 33:626–629, September, 1976.
(6) Lancet 2:386–389, Aug. 21, 1976.

below 40 μM/L. The patients were receiving 200–350 mg phenytoin daily and either 90–180 mg phenobarbitone or 75–100 mg primidone daily. After 4 months of control observations, phenytoin doses were increased using the Richens-Dunlop nomogram, and the study was continued for 4 months more. Fifteen patients obtained therapeutic serum phenytoin levels after one dose increase of 50–100 mg, whereas 5 required further dose increases. Other treatment was continued unchanged during the study.

After increased levels of phenytoin were administered, the number of minor seizures was unchanged but major seizures were reduced. Seven patients had no further major seizures when the serum phenytoin level was increased above 40 μM/L. Major seizures were reduced in frequency in 3 other patients and increased in 3, whereas 3 patients showed no change. Doses of 250–450 mg phenytoin daily were required to reach serum levels above 40 μM/L. In a number of cases the dose required was considerably less than that predicted from the nomogram. Serum phenobarbitone levels increased significantly as the serum phenytoin level was increased.

Adjustment of serum phenytoin levels may be valuable in the treatment of major seizures in patients on multiple-drug therapy. The dose must be adjusted in small increments, with constant measurement of serum concentrations, because methods of predicting dose increases may be unreliable.

► [It is of interest that in these cases the serum concentration of phenobarbital rose with the increasing dose of phenytoin. This may cause deviations from the expected relationship between dose and serum concentrations of phenytoin and would explain instances in which it is difficult to predict the therapeutic dose of phenytoin. – Ed.] ◄

Risks to Offspring of Women Treated with Hydantoin Anticonvulsants, with Emphasis on Fetal Hydantoin Syndrome. A syndrome of unusual facies, distal phalangeal hypoplasia and other defects was recently described in infants exposed in utero to hydantoin anticonvulsants. James W. Hanson, Ntinos C. Myrianthopoulos, Mary Ann Sedgwick Harvey and David W. Smith[7] (Seattle, Wash.) determined the frequency of altered development and growth in a group of 35 children born to 23 women who had

(7) J. Pediatr. 89:662–668, October, 1976.

received hydantoin anticonvulsants during pregnancy. In 15 pregnancies only a hydantoin drug was given, whereas in the rest other drugs, mostly barbiturates, were also given. None of the children was referred because of recognized abnormalities. A matched control evaluation was made of data on 104 children in a national prospective study, whose mothers were given hydantoins continuously throughout pregnancy for convulsive disorders. Control subjects were available for 100 hydantoin cases.

Four of the 35 study infants had abnormalities consistent with the fetal hydantoin syndrome, and 11 other children displayed some abnormalities. Many dysmorphic features of the type seen in the hydantoin syndrome were noted in the cases in the Collaborative Perinatal Project. At least three of four major features (prenatal growth deficiency, postnatal growth deficiency, microcephaly, mental deficiency) were present in 11 children in the hydantoin group and in none in the control group. Six of the 11 children in the hydantoin group exhibited low mental performance. No evidence of a dose-response relationship was obtained. No children born to 17 women who were given barbiturates alone for convulsive disorders had a pattern of features similar to the fetal hydantoin syndrome.

Women with convulsive disorders who are considering pregnancy must be told of the risks to the developing fetus from hydantoin therapy. More recently, Shapiro et al. (1976) reported that it may be the epileptic parent, rather than exposure to hydantoin drugs in utero, who is responsible for the increased risk of malformation in the offspring. Only 5 of 23 patients seen with the fetal hydantoin syndrome would have been detected in a search for major birth defects.

► [Women being treated with hydantoin anticonvulsants should be told of the nature and magnitude of risk to the developing fetus before they consider a pregnancy. There should not be undue alarm, however, because statistically only a small percentage of infants born to mothers receiving hydantoinates have congenital defects. — Ed.] ◄

Eterobarb Therapy in Epilepsy. Eterobarb, a phenobarbital derivative, has been shown to possess anticonvulsant activity in a wide range of animal models of epilepsy and to produce less hypnotic effect than phenobarbital. Richard H. Mattson (VA Hosp., West Haven, Conn.), Peter D. Williamson and Elene Hanahan[8] (Yale Univ.) conducted a double-

(8) Neurology (Minneap.) 26:1014–1017, November, 1976.

blind crossover trial comparing eterobarb and phenobarbital in 27 patients with uncontrolled epileptic seizures.

Before the trial, patients received phenytoin and phenobarbital or eterobarb. Dosages were estimated from past experience to be as close to therapeutic quantities as possible. The dose of eterobarb was 3 times that of phenobarbital and the dosage was increased gradually until toxicity appeared. Medication was crossed over at 12 weeks. The 18 male and 9 female patients were aged 14–59 years. Eighteen had partial complex or psychomotor seizures and 6 had partial elementary or focal seizures. Most patients with partial seizures had a history of secondary generalization.

Seizure frequency was reduced in the 21 patients who completed the trial but there was no significant difference between drugs. Status epilepticus developed in 3 patients when they were changed from eterobarb to phenobarbital. Eterobarb therapy had no serious side effects. The mean drug doses in patients completing the study were 150 mg phenobarbital and 420 mg eterobarb daily. Mean serum barbiturate levels were higher with eterobarb but mean phenytoin levels were about the same.

Eterobarb is a potent anticonvulsant drug with effects on seizure frequency equivalent to those of phenobarbital. The finding that barbiturate levels were higher on eterobarb therapy, despite comparable subjective effects, raises the possibility that metabolites of eterobarb may compete with phenobarbital for brain receptor sites that cause less sedation than phenobarbital.

► [This study showed that eterobarb is a safe and potent anticonvulsant comparable in efficacy to phenobarbital. The superior results obtained in some patients with eterobarb therapy indicate that it may be used as an effective alternative anticonvulsant. – Ed.] ◄

Acetazolamide-Induced Interference with Primidone Absorption: Case Reports and Metabolic Studies. Gaby B. Syversen, John P. Morgan, Michael Weintraub and Gary J. Myers[9] (Univ. of Rochester) studied a hospitalized patient receiving primidone orally who had none of this antiepileptic drug in her blood when concurrently taking acetazolamide orally. Two other patients receiving identical treatment but with some plasma primidone detectable also were

(9) Arch. Neurol. 34:80–84, February, 1977.

studied. Each patient participated in two studies at intervals of 2–17 days. After fasting overnight and during the study day, patients received 500 mg primidone alone in the morning or 250 mg acetazolamide twice, 12 hours before and again with the test dose of primidone.

Apparent interaction between primidone and acetazolamide occurred in 2 patients. Primidone was not detected in the plasma when given orally with acetazolamide in 1 patient; in another, the peak serum concentration was delayed, as was the urinary excretion of primidone and metabolites. Phenylethylmalonamide was undetectable in the plasma or urine of 1 of these patients and in the other, the urinary excretion of phenylethylmalonamide seemed delayed. Phenobarbital was never detected in the plasma or urine of 1 patient. One patient had no acetazolamide-dependent changes in primidone metabolism.

This undesirable interaction between primidone and acetazolamide seems limited to susceptible persons; its incidence is unknown. If clinical seizure control is impaired when acetazolamide is given with primidone, the blood and urine concentrations of primidone should be monitored and appropriate changes should be made.

► [It is always important to bear in mind the possibility of drug interactions when multiple drugs are used in treatment. This article reports an interaction of anticonvulsant medications that apparently has not been noted previously. – Ed.] ◄

Further Observations on Carbamazepine Plasma Levels in Epileptic Patients: Relationships with Therapeutic and Side Effects. Many reports have documented the clinical efficacy of carbamazepine in the treatment of trigeminal neuralgia and convulsive disorders. F. Monaco, A. Riccio, P. Benna, A. Covacich, L. Durelli, M. Fantini, P. M. Furlan, M. Gilli, R. Mutani, W. Troni, M. Gerna and P. L. Morselli[1] studied relationships between the clinical effects of carbamazepine and plasma levels of the drug and of its metabolite, carbamazepine-10, 11-epoxide.

Studies were done over 9 weeks in epileptic patients who had received little benefit from anticonvulsant therapy before plasma drug levels were monitored. Sixteen adult male epileptics and 4 children aged 6–11 years were monitored.

(1) Neurology 26:936–943, October, 1976.

Fifteen patients had secondary generalized epilepsy, 4 had primary generalized epilepsy and 1 had the Lennox-Gastaut syndrome. Ten patients were hospitalized during the entire observation period. Eleven patients had received carbamazepine previously. Carbamazepine was given as tablets or syrup in daily doses of 5 – 24 mg/kg, phenobarbital in doses of 0.9 – 2.5 mg/kg and phenytoin in doses of 0.7 – 5.0 mg/kg.

Fourteen of 20 patients initially had plasma anticonvulsant levels below the therapeutic threshold. A clear effect on seizure frequency was evident after a week of monitoring, and the trend continued to 4 weeks, when the overall seizure frequency tended to stabilize at 10 per week. Carbamazepine alone induced a consistent fall in seizure frequency with plasma levels of about 8 – 10 μg/ml, and metabolite levels of 0.5 – 1.8 μg/ml. Concurrent treatment with phenytoin or phenobarbital had no significant influence on plasma carbamazepine levels. Drug clearance appeared to be increased in children. Neurologic and gastric side effects were infrequent during monitoring. Four patients had a relatively transient leukopenia.

Carbamazepine may have a definite positive effect on seizure frequency in poorly controlled epileptics when plasma drug levels are carefully monitored. The effect is most marked in patients with secondary generalized epilepsy, with grand mal and/or psychomotor seizures. Therapeutic plasma levels range from 4 to 12 μg/ml. The EEG pattern cannot be relied on to correlate with clinical control of seizures.

▶ [The data reported confirm that with the careful monitoring of drug plasma levels, carbamazepine may exert a definite effect on seizure frequency in epileptic patients poorly responsive to prior therapy. – Ed.] ◀

Drug-Induced IgA Deficiency in Epileptic Patients. A preliminary study showed that 25% of adult epileptic patients had low serum IgA and IgM levels. Johan A. Aarli[2] (Univ. of Bergen) correlated serum IgA levels with clinical data in 124 adults and 60 children, aged 10 – 16 years, who were under treatment for epilepsy. Four adults and 10 children were studied before and after receiving anticonvulsant drugs. Phenytoin was being used by 153 patients, by 97 as a single drug; phenytoin had been withdrawn in 11 other

(2) Arch. Neurol. 33:296 – 299, April, 1976.

cases. Serum samples also were taken from 70 healthy adults and 25 healthy children.

Serum IgA levels were subnormal in 42% of 50 children on antiepileptic drugs, while untreated children had normal IgA levels. Twenty-five adult patients had serum IgA levels below 0.60 mg/ml. Salivary IgA was not detected in 5 patients with serum levels below 0.02 mg/ml and the levels in saliva were low in patients with low serum IgA levels. The median IgM level was lower than the normal median in adult patients. Serum IgG levels were lower than normal in treated children. Serum IgA levels fell by 50% or more in several patients given phenytoin. Low IgA levels were found more often in men than in women and in all types of epilepsy. Two of 10 patients with low IgA levels became intoxicated, even on small doses of phenytoin. Serum phenytoin levels remained low despite an increased dosage in 4 of the 10 patients.

Antiepileptic treatment may induce deficiencies of both serum and secretory IgA levels in some patients with epilepsy but it is unknown whether this phenomenon is associated with clinical disturbances. Possibly the IgA anomaly is a contributory mechanism in the pathogenesis of some of the side effects of certain antiepileptic drugs.

▶ [It appears that in certain patients phenytoin administration causes a decrease in the IgA level. This happens most frequently in men and children. The IgA anomaly was not specific for any one type of epilepsy. – Ed.] ◀

Chronic Cerebellar Stimulation in Epilepsy: Clinical and Anatomical Studies.

Irving S. Cooper, Ismail Amin, Manuel Riklan, Joseph M. Waltz and Tung Pui Poon[3] (New York) reviewed the effects of chronic stimulation of cerebellar cortex in 15 patients with intractable epilepsy, who had been under medical treatment for 1–49 years. Six had mainly psychomotor seizures, 6 had grand mal and 3 had myoclonic epilepsy. All patients had definitive EEG abnormalities, an IQ of at least 80 and no demonstrable mass lesion. An electrode plate was applied to the cortex of the anterior or posterior cerebellar lobe via a suboccipital craniectomy and stimulation was provoked by transcutaneous inductive coupling. More recently bilateral anterior lobe electrode placement has been used. Most often, a stimula-

(3)   Arch. Neurol. 33:559–570, August, 1976.

tion frequency of 10 cps has been used, but the stimulation variables have varied from case to case and have been altered in individual cases.

Of the 6 patients with psychomotor epilepsy, 4 have improved markedly on chronic cerebellar stimulation. Of the 6 with focal epilepsy or grand mal, or both, 3 have improved noticeably, whereas 2 showed no response to cerebellar stimulation. Medication has been reduced in 2 of these patients and unchanged in 4. Of the 3 patients with myoclonic seizures, 2 improved markedly and 1 improved moderately. Cerebellar biopsy specimens taken from 5 patients at the time of surgery showed abnormal findings in the molecular layer, which was markedly thinner, with a decreased number of cells in the granular layer and decrease or absence of Purkinje's cells. A specimen from 1 patient who died showed cell loss in areas of electrode placement but no evidence of electrolytic damage to the pia or subjacent cortical tissue. No significant psychologic sequelae of chronic stimulation were noted in the 14 patients given standardized psychologic tests. Patients often reported reduced tension, increased alertness, improved thinking and speech fluency and reduced depression in postoperative interviews. Anger and aggression were reduced when initially present in association with the seizure disorder.

Clinical seizures were modified in 10 of these patients with intractable epilepsy during chronic cerebellar stimulation. Studies are needed to determine which areas of cerebellar cortex are most suitable for seizure inhibition and whether the cerebellum contributes directly to behavior regulation.

► [There is no evidence of any adverse effect of chronic cerebellar stimulation in persons who have undergone stimulation for periods of up to 3 years. There appeared to be definite improvement in seizure control in these patients with intractable epilepsy, but questions continue to be asked about the justification of this procedure from a humanitarian point of view. — Ed.] ◄

Facial Asymmetry in Patients with Temporal Lobe Epilepsy: Clinical Sign Useful in Lateralization of Temporal Epileptogenic Foci. Temporal lobe epilepsy can

Fig 10.—Left to right: at rest, voluntary movement, emotional involvement. **A,** right temporal focus, marked left facial weakness on emotional movement. **B,** left

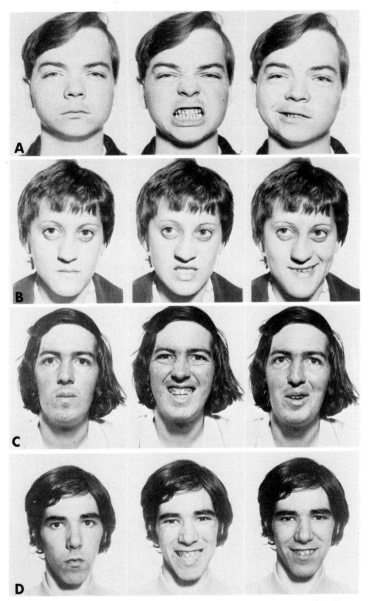

temporal focus, marked right facial weakness on emotional movement. **C,** left temporal focus, moderate right facial weakness on emotional movement. **D,** left temporal focus, mild right weakness on emotional movement. (Courtesy of Remillard, G. M., et al.: Neurology (Minneap.) 27:109–114, February, 1977.)

Extrapyramidal Diseases

Primary Sensory Symptoms in Parkinsonism. Aching, burning and other subjective sensory phenomena are often mentioned in descriptions of parkinsonism. Stuart R. Snider, Stanley Fahn, William P. Isgreen and Lucien J. Cote[5] (Columbia Univ.) prospectively interviewed and examined 105 ambulatory outpatients with parkinsonism to determine the extent to which sensory symptoms are related to various factors in this condition.

No patient was seriously ill or had other significant illness. Analysis of idiopathic sensory complaints was carried out in 64 other persons, including spouses of patients, residents of a home for the elderly and medical staff. Forty-three of the patients with parkinsonism had sensory symptoms without an apparent somatic etiology, as did 5 (8%) controls.

Pain occurred in 67% of the symptomatic study patients, usually as an intermittent, poorly localized, cramplike or aching sensation, not affected by motion or pressure. It was often proximal and in the limb with the greatest motor deficit. Burning paresthesia was sometimes related to antiparkinson therapy. Sensations of tingling or numbness occurred more often in the distal extremities. Nine patients had a sensory complaint that antedated the diagnosis of parkinsonism; 5 of these had pain preceding tremor or rigidity in the limb that was the site of the first motor disorder.

Motor deficit scores and medications are compared in the patients with and without sensory symptoms in Figure 11. Except for motor signs of parkinsonism, few abnormalities were found in the patients with sensory symptoms. Treatment was complicated in these patients because antiparkinson medications sometimes caused the sensory symptoms to become worse. Decreasing the medication produced varying, often incomplete relief, although in some patients amelioration of pain was attributed to levodopa or anticholinergic

(5) Neurology (Minneap.) 26:423–429, May, 1976.

	WITHOUT SENSORY SYMPTOMS	WITH SENSORY SYMPTOMS
NUMBER OF PATIENTS	58	17♀ 41♂	24♂ 19♀ 43
AGE (YEARS)	64.3 ± 1.0	65.1 ± 1.4
DURATION OF ILLNESS (YEARS)	9.3 ± 0.9	11.2 ± 1.8
RIGIDITY	1.31 ± .14	1.37 ± .15
BRADYKINESIA	1.40 ± .15	1.51 ± .15
TREMOR	1.47 ± .16	1.26 ± .13
POSTURE	1.47 ± .11	1.42 ± .17
TOTAL DISABILITY SCORE	5.64 ± .40	5.56 ± .38
% TAKING LEVODOPA	81%	81%
% TAKING ANTICHOLINERGICS	47%	58%
% TAKING AMANTADINE	21%	30%

Fig 11. — Motor deficit scores and medications in parkinsonism patients without and with sensory symptoms; mean ± SE. No significant differences (t test after analysis of variance). Motor deficit is rated on 0 (no deficit) to 4 (maximum deficit) scale. Total disability score of each patient was obtained and mean for all total scores in group was calculated. Percentage figure for medication refers to percent of patients taking medication at time of interview. Average dose of levodopa was 4.1 ± 0.4 gm in patients without symptoms and 4.0 ± 0.4 gm in patients with symptoms (not significant). Anticholinergic medication doses between groups were not significantly different. (Courtesy of Snider, S. R., et al.: Neurology (Minneap.) 26:423–429, May, 1976.)

medication. Stellate ganglion block in 2 patients was ineffective but symptomatic therapy benefited about 20% of the patients.

At least some sensory symptoms originate within the nervous system as a manifestation of parkinsonism and are not secondary effects of the motor disorder.

▶ [Whereas the manifestations of Parkinson's disease usually are considered to be limited to the motor system, this study shows that at least some sensory symptoms do occur and that they originate within the nervous system as specific manifestations of the disease process and are not secondary to the motor disorder. — Ed.] ◀

Dysautonomia in Parkinsonism: Clinicopathologic Study. Autonomic dysfunction has been described in Parkinson's disease, and parkinsonian features may occur in multiple-system atrophy, of which progressive autonomic failure may be a predominant feature. A. H. Rajput and B. Rozdilsky[6] (Univ. of Saskatchewan) evaluated autonomic

(6) J. Neurol. Neurosurg. Psychiatry 39:1092–1100, November, 1976.

function in 6 patients with idiopathic paralysis agitans and 1 patient with multiple-system atrophy. One patient with brain tumor was used as a control.

Woman, 72, had become dizzy on standing at age 58 years and at age 62 had had moderate rigidity and bradykinesia but little tremor. Anticholinergic drugs were administered. Memory deficit and intermittent confusion were noticed at age 69, and orthostatic hypotension was more marked on levodopa therapy. After 4 weeks off all drugs the patient had moderate seborrhea but no sweating on the face or feet and had considerable fluctuations in the supine blood pressure. Intermittent diplopia developed 3 months before death and myoclonic jerks in the upper limbs a month before death. Occasional urinary incontinence was also present. Death was due to acute bronchopneumonia.

Autopsy showed slight cerebral atheromatosis and severe cell loss in the substantia nigra. Less severe changes were seen in the locus ceruleus and dorsal vagal nucleus. Slight nerve cell loss was seen in the intermediolateral column of the cord. The sympathetic ganglia showed striking loss and degenerative changes of nerve cells, collections of round cells (nodules of Nageotte), diffuse fibrosis, axon swellings and numerous Lewy bodies (Fig 12). Areas of recent demyelination were present in the middle of the pons.

Orthostatic hypotension in multiple-system atrophy is believed to be due to cell loss in the intermediolateral column of the spinal cord. In 5 of these cases of Parkinson's dis-

Fig 12. — Lewy bodies in nerve cell processes within stellate ganglion. Nissl; reduced from ×280. (Courtesy of Rajput, A. H., and Rozdilsky, B.: J. Neurol. Neurosurg. Psychiatry 39:1092 – 1100, November, 1976.)

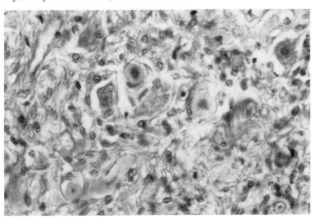

ease, Lewy bodies, with or without cell loss, were found in the sympathetic ganglia. Three of these patients had orthostatic hypotension, and its degree correlated approximately with the severity of the lesion. Lesions of the sympathetic ganglia may play a major role in the production of orthostatic hypotension in idiopathic Parkinson's disease.

▶ [Lesions of the sympathetic ganglia appear to play a major role in the production of orthostatic hypotension in Parkinson's disease. – Ed.] ◀

Coincidence of Schizophrenia and Parkinsonism: Some Neurochemical Implications are discussed by T. J. Crow, Eve C. Johnstone and H. A. McClelland[7] (Newcastle upon Tyne). The view that the extrapyramidal effects of phenothiazine drugs are a necessary concomitant of their use in the treatment of schizophrenia has been widely debated. If the ability to block dopamine receptors confers both extrapyramidal and antipsychotic actions on these drugs, schizophrenic symptoms should not arise in the setting of established parkinsonism. The authors, however, report 4 cases in which patients developed an illness with schizophrenic features in the setting of long-standing Parkinson's disease. All 4 patients had typically schizophrenic symptoms, including auditory hallucinations and paranoid delusions. The features could not be explained by mood change or altered consciousness.

Although these cases appear to conflict with the view that increased dopamine release in the striatum is necessary for the expression of schizophrenic psychopathology, they do not rule out the possibility that increased transmission may occur at other dopaminergic sites in the brain. The dopamine receptor blockade hypothesis of the therapeutic effects of neuroleptic drugs cannot be maintained with respect to an action in the striatum, in view of the differences between the actions of thioridazine and chlorpromazine in this structure, but it may be tenable for actions at extrastriatal sites. Further studies of the actions of these two drugs on dopaminergic mechanisms in the corpus striatum, nucleus accumbens and cerebral cortex are needed.

▶ [These findings appear to conflict with the view that increased dopamine release in the striatum is necessary for the expression of schizophrenic psychopathology. However, they do not exclude the possibility that increased transmission may occur at other dopaminergic sites in the

(7)   Psychol. Med. 6:227–233, May, 1976.

brain, for example, the nucleus accumbens, tuberculum olfactorium and cerebral cortex. – Ed.] ◄

Aging and Extrapyramidal Function. Patrick L. McGeer, Edith G. McGeer and Joane S. Suzuki[8] (Univ. of British Columbia) measured some enzymes concerned with neurotransmitter synthesis in human brain samples to relate aging with extrapyramidal function. Human brains were obtained as soon after death as possible, and the substantia nigra was sectioned for histologic evaluation. Enzyme data were obtained on some 55 areas of 28 control brains from patients dying without known neurologic concomitants.

Tyrosine hydroxylase (TH), glutamate decarboxylase (GAD) and choline acetyltransferase (CAT) showed significant decrements with aging in a high proportion of the brain regions evaluated. The most dramatic effect was shown by TH in the caudate, putamen and nucleus accumbens, all areas with high concentrations of dopaminergic nerve endings. Cell bodies in the substantia nigra were significantly reduced in number with age, but the loss from ages 5 to 25 years was not as dramatic as that of TH activity in the striatal nerve endings. The cells tended to be plump in young children and more shriveled in older subjects. All four parkinsonian samples had low values, but the single choreic brain examined had a normal cell count. Both CAT and GAD activities also decreased significantly with age in the caudate, and GAD activity was significantly correlated with age in the putamen.

Cell loss by itself seems unlikely to explain the sharp decline in TH activity occurring in the striatum between ages 5 and 25 years. This is the time at which the human substantia nigra becomes heavily pigmented, and the pigment itself may inhibit proper functioning of these neurons. Ratios of TH to CAT activity in the putamen indicate a parkinsonian-like condition with aging. Recent animal studies suggest that the dopaminergic nigrostriatal tract may have a role in mental function quite apart from those associated with control of movements. Much more work is needed before a role in such behavior can be ascribed to this tract in human beings, but methods of protecting the tract against the deleterious effects of aging may be well worth investi-

(8) Arch. Neurol. 34:33–35, January, 1977.

gating. Studies are under way in guinea pigs to determine whether agents that inhibit melanin formation can inhibit the loss in dopaminergic function with age.

► [It is possible that the loss in striatal tyrosine hydroxylase activity may account for some of the difficulties in movement seen in aging persons. — Ed.] ◄

Parkinsonism and Levodopa: Five-Year Experience. Initially, the response of parkinsonian patients to levodopa therapy is dramatic, but subsequently the patient's condition tends to deteriorate, and treatment is limited by complications including psychiatric disorder and abnormal involuntary movements. Peyton Delaney and Joseph Fermaglich[9] (Georgetown Univ.) reviewed the therapeutic responses of 70 parkinsonian patients to uninterrupted levodopa therapy for 5 years. The patients were treated in 1969–74. The daily dose of levodopa did not change significantly after the induction phase. The maintenance dose was kept as high as possible to the point of tolerable side effects throughout treatment. Many patients were taking anticholinergic agents or amantadine, or both, initially, and these were continued in most cases.

Sixty-three patients (90%) improved during the initial 6–12 months of treatment, whereas 7 failed to respond. Rigidity and bradykinesis improved the most, often by over 75%. Subsequently, 24% of patients continued to improve and maintained good functional ability, 28% stabilized and 48% had a gradual worsening of their parkinsonism. The 12 patients who had had stereotactic brain surgery responded like the other patients. Nausea and emesis decreased during continued treatment. Orthostatic hypotension occurred in only 3 patients. Abnormal involuntary movements increased during treatment, and they restricted therapy in 35% of cases. Only 5 patients had episodic bradykinesis (on-off effect) during treatment. Psychiatric complications tended to occur more frequently in the later course of treatment. Dementia was present initially in 19% of patients and in 36% after 5 years of levodopa therapy. The antiparkinsonian effect of levodopa usually decreased when the dose was reduced to allow mental aberrations to clear.

The reasons for early improvement and later deteriora-

(9)   J. Clin. Pharmacol. 16:652–659, Nov.–Dec., 1976.

tion in parkinsonian symptoms during levodopa therapy remain unclear. Parkinson's disease may not be simply a striatal dopamine-deficiency syndrome, and treatment with levodopa may be more than replacement therapy. An intracellular molecular approach to the study of parkinsonism and its treatment is essential.

► [The data presented herein confirm the clinical impression that levodopa is an extremely helpful drug in Parkinson's disease but that its effectiveness seems to wane and complications seem to develop as treatment progresses. The reason for early improvement and subsequent deterioration of parkinsonian symptoms and signs despite levodopa therapy remains unexplained. This suggests that continued research is needed to develop other drugs for use in treatment of Parkinson's disease. Bromocriptine, which has been used in England and at the National Institutes of Health, is one of these drugs. Unfortunately it is not yet available for general use. — Ed.] ◄

Six Years of High-Level Levodopa Therapy in Severely Akinetic Parkinsonian Patients. André Barbeau[1] (Univ. of Montreal) reviewed data on 80 parkinsonian patients initially described in 1969. The 58 men and 22 women had a mean age of 59.1 years at the start of study; 10 had a history and symptoms of epidemic lethargic encephalitis and 70 had "idiopathic" disease. Eighteen patients had had thalamotomies or pallidotomies.

The average duration of idiopathic disease before study was 4.3 years. The most prominent symptom was bradykinesia in 73% of patients. In 68% of cases, akinesia was the first symptom to appear and remained the dominant feature. Seventeen other parkinsonian patients with equally severe disease did not receive levodopa; akinesia was the dominant symptom in this group also. Levodopa was given in daily doses of 1.5 – 7 gm. Most patients also received either anticholinergic or antihistaminic medications, or both, for part or all of the 6-year study. No patient received a peripheral dopa decarboxylase inhibitor during the primary study.

Nineteen patients died of unrelated illnesses during the study. No death was directly attributable to levodopa therapy. Eighteen patients stopped taking levodopa for various reasons. About 80% of the patients had over 50% improvement in function after 2 months of treatment; this percent-

(1)   Arch. Neurol. 33:333–338, May, 1976.

age has declined steadily since then, only 29% of patients
having good results (greater than 50% improvement) after 6
years. Another 25% had fair results (20–49% improvement).
The rate of good results in patients still taking levodopa
after 6 years is 53%. About 20% of patients were functionally independent at follow-up, compared with only 1 of the 17
control patients. Dyskinesias were apparent in half the patients after 2 months of therapy. A few severely ill patients
have shown diphasic dyskinesias after more than 3 years of
treatment. Oscillations in performance have included end-
of-dose akinesia, "on-off" phenomena and akinesia para-
doxica or "hypotonic freezing."

Levodopa retards some of the early disability of Parkinson's disease due to infections and immobility but does not
reduce mortality or arrest disease progression. Levodopa is
the best available treatment of Parkinson's disease because
it allows worthwhile improvement in the patient's quality of
life.

► [The results of this review by an early and long-term investigator of the
efficacy of levodopa in parkinsonism lead him to conclude that even with
its drawbacks, levodopa is still the best available treatment of akinetic
parkinsonism; this is despite the fact that it does not arrest disease progression or reduce the mortality and despite the difficulties encountered
in levodopa administration. It would be interesting to compare the results
of this study with those of a similar one in which a peripheral dopa decarboxylase inhibitor also was used. C. D. Marsden and J. D. Parkes also have
reported recently on the success and problems of long-term levodopa
therapy in Parkinson's disease. Their results and conclusions are similar
to those of Barbeau. The major problems, according to them, are the insidious and progressive loss of benefit from levodopa and the appearance
of progressively more severe fluctuations in disability. They express the
belief that progression of the underlying pathology of the disease is probably responsible for both of these (Lancet 1:345, 1977). – Ed.] ◄

**Thrombocytopenia Associated with Long-Term Le-
vodopa Therapy.** William M. Wanamaker, Sonja J. Wanamaker, Gastone G. Celesia and Arlan A. Koeller[2] (Univ. of
Wisconsin) describe a man on long-term levodopa therapy in
whom severe thrombocytopenia developed due to an autoimmune process, presumably similar to that induced by the
chemically similar drug methyldopa.

Man, 63, was given 15 mg procyclidine daily for bradykinesia
and rigidity, but symptoms of Parkinson's disease worsened steadily; levodopa was given in a dose of 4.5 gm daily, with an excellent

    (2) J.A.M.A. 235:2217–2219, May 17, 1976.

clinical response. After more than 3 years of such treatment, easy bruising and nosebleeds developed and worsened and a platelet count of 2,600/cu mm was found. Levodopa and procyclidine were discontinued and prednisone was given in a dose of 45 mg daily. The platelet count rose steadily and was 134,000/cu mm after the dosage of prednisone was decreased to 10 mg daily. Parkinsonian symptoms reappeared rapidly when levodopa was discontinued, and trihexiphenidyl was given with little benefit. Prednisone was withdrawn with no adverse effect on platelet count or general status. Challenge with increasing doses of levodopa caused no significant change in platelet count. Prednisone was restarted in a dose of 20 mg every other day and levodopa was begun in a dose of 500 mg daily, increased gradually to 2.5 gm daily. Parkinsonian symptoms regressed dramatically. Prednisone has since been reduced to 10 mg on alternate days and the dose of levodopa increased to 3.5 gm daily. No thrombocytopenia has been seen except for one slightly low count. A Coombs test result was negative. The antinuclear antibody test results remained positive but with a weak or speck-type reaction.

There is evidence that levodopa causes autoimmunity because it is given in unnaturally high concentration. The development of serologic abnormality and hematologic disease is time and dose related. Each patient must be studied carefully before levodopa therapy and followed cautiously during treatment to avoid the definite risk of reinducing an extremely severe thrombocytopenia.

▶ [With prolonged use of any new drug, side effects and complications may become apparent that were not noted earlier. – Ed.] ◀

Comparison of Levodopa with Carbidopa or Benserazide in Parkinsonism. Peripheral decarboxylase inhibitors prevent extracerebral decarboxylation of levodopa. Both carbidopa and benserazide reduce nausea and vomiting associated with levodopa and allow a reduction in dosage to 60–80% of the basal dosage. J. K. Greenacre, A. Coxon, A. Petrie and J. L. Reid[3] (Royal Postgrad. Med. School, London) conducted a blind, randomized, crossover trial of commercially available formulations of levodopa with carbidopa (Sinemet) or benserazide (Madopar) in 14 men and 7 women with idiopathic parkinsonism. Mean patient age was 63.9 years. All had been symptomatic for 2 years or longer. Fourteen were receiving anticholinergic drugs, 4 were on tricyclic antidepressants and 1 was on amantadine;

(3) Lancet 2:381–384, Aug. 21, 1976.

these drugs were continued at the same dose levels during the study.

Patients were allocated to 100 or 250 mg levodopa with 10 or 25 mg carbidopa, and to 100 or 200 mg levodopa with 25 or 50 mg benserazide for a 6-week period before crossover. Two patients were withdrawn because of orofacial and limb dyskinesia on levodopa-benserazide therapy. The average daily dose of levodopa was 605 mg on benserazide and 658 mg on carbidopa therapy. The mean daily dose of benserazide was 151 mg and of carbidopa, 66 mg.

No significant clinical advantages of either regimen were observed. Differences in blood pressures on the two regimens were small. Patient ratings of disability were comparable with the two regimens; the average assessed disability was not great. Comparable numbers of patients preferred the two regimens at the end of the study.

These commercially available combinations of levodopa and a peripheral decarboxylase inhibitor have similar beneficial effects on parkinsonian symptoms and signs, and their ranges and severities of side effects are similar at the same daily intake of levodopa. Central nervous system actions and side effects depend on the daily dose of levodopa, regardless of differing ratios of decarboxylase inhibitors to levodopa.

▶ [Two commercially available decarboxylase inhibitor-containing preparations, carbidopa and benserazide, have been used in combination with levodopa therapy of Parkinson's disease to decrease some of the side effects of this agent and the dose of levodopa needed for relief of symptoms. Carbidopa has been used longer in the United States. In this comparison of the two agents, it is concluded that no significant difference exists in their therapeutic or adverse effects. Central nervous system actions and side effects depend on the daily dose of levodopa regardless of the different ratios of decarboxylase inhibitors to levodopa. − Ed.] ◀

Clinical Picture and Plasma Levodopa Metabolite Profile of Parkinsonian Nonresponders: Treatment with Levodopa and Decarboxylase Inhibitor. About one third of the parkinsonian patients do not improve on levodopa therapy. Leonor Rivera-Calimlim, Deepak Tandon (Univ. of Rochester), Frank Anderson (George Washington Univ.) and Robert Joynt[4] (Univ. of Rochester) determined

(4) Arch. Neurol. 34:228−232, April, 1977.

the plasma metabolic profile of 3 patients who failed to respond to either levodopa therapy or the combination of levodopa and carbidopa.

The 2 men and 1 woman were aged 41–64. They had failed to improve on 4 gm or more of levodopa daily over 6 months before the study. Plasma metabolite levels were determined at intervals up to 5 hours after an oral dose of levodopa and the study was repeated after a month of combined levodopa-carbidopa therapy.

One patient improved slightly on levodopa-carbidopa therapy but not enough to be reasonably functional. Doses could not be increased further because of involuntary movements in 2 patients and muscle cramps in 1. Unusually high baseline 3-0-methyldopa levels were present and the levels increased significantly further during combined therapy. All patients had ratios of 3-0-methyldopa to levodopa exceeding 1, even 2 hours after treatment.

Six parkinsonian patients with dementia who responded to combination therapy and did not exhibit the "on-off" phenomenon had a mean plasma levodopa level of 1.49 and a mean level of 3-0-methyldopa of 0.393 ng/ml. All had plasma 3-0-methyldopa-to-levodopa ratios below 1. Three patients who responded to levodopa alone also had ratios less than 1.

Levodopa-unresponsive patients with parkinsonism have high plasma 3-0-methyldopa-levodopa ratios on levodopa alone and increased ratios during decarboxylase inhibitor-levodopa administration. The ratio of plasma epinephrine to dose of levodopa increased in 2 patients during dopa decarboxylase inhibitor treatment. It appears important to determine whether a 3-0-methyldopa-to-levodopa ratio above 1 is in fact a good index of whether a patient will experience "on-off" phenomena or involuntary movements or will fail to improve clinically on levodopa therapy, with or without a decarboxylase inhibitor.

▶ [The patient with Parkinson's disease who does not respond to levodopa or to a levodopa-decarboxylase inhibitor combination is a therapeutic enigma. This study suggests that high plasma concentrations of 3-0-methyldopa may be responsible for such nonresponse and that the ratio between levodopa and 3-0-methyldopa concentrations should be established in patients who do not respond to the usual therapeutic dose of levodopa. —Ed.] ◀

Effect of Amantadine on Drug-Induced Parkinsonism: Relationship between Plasma Levels and Effect was studied by G. M. Pacifici, M. Nardini, P. Ferrari, R. Latini, C. Fieschi and P. L. Morselli[5] in 15 women aged 31 – 62 years with various psychiatric syndromes and behavioral changes. All were being treated with neuroleptic and anticholinergic drugs. An extrapyramidal syndrome had been poorly controlled by classic anticholinergic drugs Anticholinergic medication was replaced by a placebo, whereas neuroleptics were continued in the usual doses. After 1 week, amantadine was given for 15 days in a dose of 200 mg, followed by placebo for 4 days.

Amantadine led to a rapid, marked improvement in extrapyramidal symptoms in most cases. Rigidity and tremor improved the most, and hypokinesia and vegetative disturbances to a lesser extent. Marked differences were noted within individual patients (Fig 13). The effects were not related to the severity of extrapyramidal symptoms. No side effects were noted. Extrapyramidal symptoms re-emerged within 48-72 hours of the discontinuance of amantadine.

Fig 13. — Effect of amantadine (200 mg/day) on clinical rating score before *(open columns)* and after *(closed columns)* 15 days of treatment. (Courtesy of Pacifici, G. M., et al.: Br. J. Clin. Pharmacol. 3:883 – 889, October, 1976.)

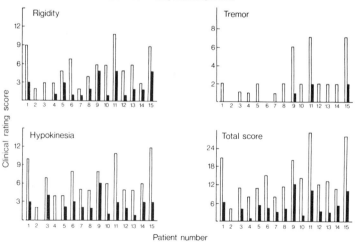

(5)   Br. J. Clin. Pharmacol. 3:883 – 889, October, 1976.

Plasma amantadine levels of 400–900 ng/ml were achieved within 4–7 days, but marked interindividual variability was noted. After the drug was discontinued, plasma levels declined monoexponentially. A trend toward a longer half-life in older patients was observed. An increase in morning plasma amantadine levels mirrored a concomitant decrease in mean clinical rating scores, and the inverse was true after amantadine was discontinued. When amantadine disappeared more rapidly, extrapyramidal symptoms were more severe.

These data suggest a direct effect of amantadine on dopaminergic receptors. The significant relationship found between worsening of the clinical picture and the plasma levels present 48 hours after discontinuance of amantadine suggests a competitive antagonism at the receptor level.

► [A significant relationship was found between the plasma levels of amantadine and the effects on the extrapyramidal symptomatology caused by neuroleptic drugs. The data suggest that there is a direct effect by amantadine on dopaminergic receptors. – Ed.] ◄

Studies with Bromocriptine. *–Part 1. "On-off" phenomena.* –The variable gastrointestinal absorption of levodopa and its short plasma half-life lead to marked fluctuations in blood drug levels that may contribute to "on-off" phenomena. The use of multiple small doses and control of dietary protein intake have only partially reduced the frequency and severity of the fluctuations between akinesia and choreoathetoid movements. Bromocriptine is a dopamine receptor agonist, which is effective in the treatment of idiopathic parkinsonism. Ronald Kartzinel and Donald B. Calne[6] (Natl. Inst. of Health) evaluated bromocriptine in 9 patients with idiopathic parkinsonism, 7 men and 2 women aged 49–64 years, who had had on-off phenomena of moderate to marked severity over 1½–3 years. They had received levodopa for 3–10 years. Six patients were also taking carbidopa at the start of the study. Initially medications were adjusted to give optimal results. In the levodopa phase of the study, bromocriptine placebo was started and the optimum dose of levodopa (with or without carbidopa) was continued. In the transition phase, bromocriptine was increased (by substituting active drug for placebo) and levodopa was re-

(6)   Neurology (Minneap.) 26:508–510, June, 1976.

duced. In the bromocriptine phase, the optimal dose of bromocriptine or a maximum of 25 mg 4 times daily was given, with levodopa added only if necessary. Each phase lasted 10–30 days.

All patients continued to have on-off episodes while they were taking 100 mg bromocriptine daily, but fluctuations in clinical state were significantly reduced, and parkinsonism scores were significantly reduced. Dyskinesia scores, however, were increased significantly. An 82% reduction in the dose of levodopa was necessary during the bromocriptine phase, and 3 patients were able to stop levodopa entirely. All patients were subjectively improved on bromocriptine, compared with levodopa. The clinical half-life of bromocriptine appeared to be 6–8 hours. Adverse reactions included gastric distress and nausea in 2 patients, orthostatic hypotension in 1, and ventricular premature beats in 1. These responded to a reduction in dosage and a later, slower increase in dosage.

Bromocriptine significantly reduced the frequency of on-off responses in parkinsonian patients in this study. The patients were generally less parkinsonian but more dyskinetic during treatment, but they preferred dyskinesia, because this allowed them greater mobility.

Part 2. Double-blind comparison with levodopa in idiopathic parkinsonism. – Bromocriptine may be more effective than levodopa in some patients with parkinsonism. Kartzinel, Ira Shoulson (Univ. of Rochester) and Calne[7] performed a double-blind, crossover study of bromocriptine in 12 hospitalized patients with idiopathic parkinsonism. All had received optimal antiparkinsonism medication for at least 3 months. The initial dosage of bromocriptine was 2.5 mg 4 times daily, which was increased by 5–20 mg daily according to tolerance to a maximum of 100 mg daily. In the 8 patients on levodopa, dosage of this drug was reduced by about 25% for each 20-mg increase in bromocriptine dosage, with a placebo substituted for the levodopa. The placebo and drug phases each lasted 2–4 weeks.

Tremor and rigidity were both significantly improved by bromocriptine. Bradykinesia decreased insignificantly. Several other variables improved and parkinsonism scores de-

(7) Neurology (Minneap.) 26:511–513, June, 1976.

clined significantly during bromocriptine therapy, particularly in patients who had previously been taking levodopa. Three fourths of patients improved on bromocriptine therapy. Two patients who responded had been withdrawn from levodopa because of adverse reactions. Side effects of bromocriptine were dose dependent and resembled those experienced with levodopa. No hematologic or biochemical abnormalities developed during bromocriptine therapy. Three patients had orthostatic hypotension.

Bromocriptine was superior to previous optimal drug treatment, including levodopa, in this trial. It promises to be an effective drug for the treatment of Parkinson's disease, but it must be given cautiously, because long-term therapy has induced hallucinations and delusions, which in some instances lasted 2 or 3 weeks after the drug was discontinued. Ankle edema and tenderness have also been observed in patients given bromocriptine.

Part 3. Concomitant administration of caffeine to patients with idiopathic parkinsonism. — Caffeine, which inhibits the action of the enzyme hydrolyzing cyclic adenosine monophosphate, potentiates the actions of levodopa and dopamine receptor agonists in rats with nigral lesions induced by 6-hydroxydopamine. Similar results have been obtained with the new dopamine receptor agonist bromocriptine, which is effective in the treatment of idiopathic parkinsonism. Kartzinel, Shoulson and Calne[8] used caffeine as a phosphodiesterase inhibitor in an attempt to potentiate the action of bromocriptine in 6 patients with idiopathic parkinsonism. The 3 men and 3 women, aged 45–64 years, had previously responded favorably to bromocriptine. Four had been treated previously with 4–7 gm levodopa daily. After observation for at least 10 days on 100 mg bromocriptine daily, the dosage was reduced to 40 mg daily, and caffeine was begun in a daily dose of 400 mg and then increased to 1 gm in 4 divided doses. The placebo and caffeine phases each lasted 2 weeks.

Disability scores for the cardinal signs of parkinsonism and parkinsonism scores increased when the dose of bromocriptine was reduced, but not significantly. Addition of caffeine did not prevent this deterioration, and a significant

(8)   Neurology (Minneap.) 26:741–743, August, 1976.

increase in tremor and rigidity followed introduction of caffeine. The increase in parkinsonism scores approached significance. Four patients had anxiety and restlessness when given caffeine and 2 had insomnia. These effects disappeared when caffeine was withdrawn. No significant ECG, hematologic or blood chemistry changes were observed during the study.

Caffeine failed to potentiate the antiparkinsonism actions of bromocriptine in this study. The pharmacologic actions of caffeine are complex, and some of them may have induced the adverse effects that limited its dosage. These untoward effects could have accounted for the increased clinical deficits recorded during caffeine therapy, because anxiety commonly exacerbates parkinsonian signs. Further trials with more specific inhibitors of phosphodiesterase might be more successful in manipulation of the nigrostriatal dopaminergic system in patients with idiopathic parkinsonism.

▶ [This series presents the first articles published in the United States on the studies that Doctor Calne and his associates first started in England. Bromocriptine appears to represent a therapeutic advance in the treatment of Parkinson's disease. Other recent articles on the efficacy of this compound are those by Parkes et al. (J. Neurol. Neurosurg. Psychiatry 39: 1101, 1976) and by Lieberman et al. (N. Engl. J. Med. 295:1400, 1976). — Ed.

Drug Therapy of Tardive Dyskinesia is discussed by Ronald M. Kobayashi[9] (VA Hosp., San Diego, Calif.). Drug-induced tardive dyskinesia is a major side effect that limits the long-term use of antipsychotic drugs and responds poorly to treatment. The phenothiazines and haloperidol are most often associated with development of the syndrome. Up to 40% of elderly, chronically institutionalized patients may be affected.

Typically, there are involuntary and repetitive movements, especially affecting orofacial structures but possibly involving the limbs and trunk also. Dyskinesia is particularly frequent after antipsychotic medication is stopped and tends to persist after discontinuance of drug therapy. Chronic receptor blockade may result in a state of denervation hypersensitivity. Worsening of tardive dyskinesia by L-dopa is further evidence that dyskinesia reflects dopaminergic hyperactivity.

The most effective way to reduce the frequency of tardive

dyskinesia may be by avoiding the long-term, high-dose use of antipsychotic drugs, especially in elderly patients, unless they are clearly needed. The antipsychotic drug should be stopped when dyskinesia first appears and, if necessary, another drug should be considered, such as thioridazine or clozapine. Anticholinergic drugs should be stopped at the first sign of dyskinesia. Most treatments have been directed toward reducing brain dopamine levels or blocking dopamine action on receptors. Haloperidol is one of the most potent dopamine-receptor antagonists. Lithium also has been effective in dyskinetic patients. Anticholinergic drugs have been beneficial in some cases but further clinical trials of such agents as deanol are necessary. Clonazepam has been reported to improve dyskinesia.

Attempts to treat tardive dyskinesia with specific agents have not been encouraging; no drug has emerged as the agent of choice. Several different types of drugs that act relatively rapidly might be tried in dyskinetic patients, such as cholinomimetic drugs and dopamine-blocking agents. The responses may then suggest a longer, more extensive treatment course with agents of a particular type.

► [Attempts to treat tardive dyskinesias with specific agents have not been encouraging, and no single drug has emerged as an agent of choice. The author suggests that an appropriate approach might be to challenge dyskinetic patients with several categories of drugs with rather rapid action, including cholinomimetic drugs and dopamine-blocking agents. Evaluation of the response to such a series of drugs may then suggest a longer, more extensive therapeutic course with agents of a particular group. – Ed.] ◄

Prevalence of Huntington's Chorea in Area of East Anglia. A general study of Huntington's chorea in East Anglia, begun in 1972, showed a much higher prevalence than was suggested by previous work. Adrian J. Caro[1] (Norfolk, England) attempted to assess as completely as possible the prevalence of Huntington's chorea in the northern part of East Anglia, in an area with an arc of radius about 40 miles centered on Cromer, Norfolk. Cases were found by searching death and discharge records at mental hospitals, indices of general hospitals, records of general practitioners in the area, parish registers and family visits. Other methods of detection such as interviewing retired psychiatrists and hearsay also were used.

(1)   J. R. Coll. Gen. Pract. 27:41 – 45, January, 1977.

Using progressively more stringent methods of ascertaining prevalence, the figure rose to 9.24/100,000. The disease was unevenly distributed in the area, with a considerable pocket in Lowestoft. The prevalence is greater than anywhere else in the world except Tasmania.

A small number of affected persons in known families could be the forefathers of a large number of present-day patients with Huntington's chorea. In some areas of East Anglia the rates are much higher than in other local areas of England. Information of this type may be of value if positive action is contemplated for limiting the propagation of such disease.

▶ [Historical studies tell us that the first cases of Huntington's chorea in the United States came to colonial New England from East Anglia. It is interesting that this study indicates that this area of England has the highest known prevalence for the disease. — Ed.] ◀

Huntington's Chorea: Changes in Neurotransmitter Receptors in the Brain. In contrast to the dopamine deficiency in Parkinson's disease, dopamine levels are normal in the corpus striatum of patients with Huntington's chorea, and L-dopa exacerbates and dopamine antagonists alleviate the choreic movements. Salvatore J. Enna, Edward D. Bird, James P. Bennett, Jr., David B. Bylund, Henry I. Yamamura, Leslie L. Iversen and Solomon H. Snyder[2] (Johns Hopkins Univ.) measured choline acetyltransferase and glutamic acid decarboxylase activities, muscarinic cholinergic, β-adrenergic, serotonin and γ-aminobutyric acid (GABA) receptor binding in the caudate nucleus and cerebral cortex of 16 patients with Huntington's chorea and 16 control brains. Muscarinic receptors were assayed by measuring the membrane binding of ^{3}H-quinuclidinyl benzilate.

An 85% reduction in glutamic acid decarboxylase activity was found in the caudate nucleus in Huntington's chorea, with a 50% fall in acetylcholine activity (Fig 14). Muscarinic cholinergic receptor binding was significantly reduced by about 50% in the caudate of choreic patients. Lysergide and serotonin binding were also reduced by about 50% in caudate tissue from choreic patients. Dissociation constants were similar in patients and controls. Binding was not altered in cerebral cortical membranes of choreic patients,

(2) N. Engl. J. Med. 294:1305–1309, June 10, 1976.

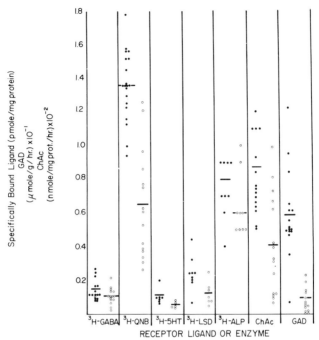

Fig 14. – Neurotransmitter receptor binding and choline acetyltransferase *(ChAc)* and glutamic acid decarboxylase *(GAD)* activity in caudate nucleus of control *(closed circles)* and choreic *(open circles)* brains. Values of ³H-dihydroalprenolol *(³H-ALP)* are ×10⁻¹. Differences between means *(bars)* of enzyme activities and receptor binding for control versus choreic samples are significant as follows: ³H-quinuclidinyl benzilate *(³H-QNB)*, P<0.01; ³H-5-hydroxytryptamine *(³H-5HT)*, P<0.01; ³H-lysergide *(³H-LSD)*, P<0.05; ChAc, P<0.001; and GAD, P<0.001. Ligand concentrations in incubation mediums were ³H-GABA, 25 nM; ³H-5HT, 8 nM; ³H-LSD, 3 nM; ³H-ALP, 1 nM; and ³H-QNB, 1 nM. (Courtesy of Enna, S. J., et al.: N. Engl. J. Med. 294:1305–1309, June 10, 1976.)

further indicating that the decline in muscarinic and serotonin receptor binding in the caudate nucleus of patients is a selective effect and not due to nonspecific postmortem changes.

This study showed a 50% reduction in binding at serotonin and muscarinic cholinergic receptors in the caudate nucleus in patients with Huntington's chorea. Apparently the remaining serotonin receptors, along with a normal supply of endogenous neurotransmitter, can maintain an adequate "serotoninergic" balance in these patients. Treatment with cholinomimetic drugs might be beneficial in Huntington's chorea but the results of trials with physostigmine have been equivocal. The observed variability in the decline of muscarinic cholinergic receptors in the brains of these patients may be related to the variable therapeutic responses to physostigmine.

▶ [These results suggest that despite the loss of γ-aminobutyric acid synthesizing ability in the corpus striatum in patients with Huntington's chorea, γ-aminobutyric acid mimetic drugs may alleviate the hyperkinetic manifestations of the disease. — Ed.] ◀

Bromocriptine in Huntington's Chorea. Huntington's chorea (HC) is an autosomal dominant disease characterized by involuntary movements and dementia. Disordered dopamine-mediated neuronal function has been suggested as the biochemical basis of HC. Levodopa exacerbates the involuntary movements and dopamine receptor antagonists and inhibitors of dopamine synthesis have limited beneficial effects on HC. Tolosa and Sparber (1974), however, reported that apomorphine, a dopamine receptor agonist, reduces the involuntary movements of HC and chorea caused by other factors. Ronald Kartzinel, Robert D. Hunt and Donald B. Calne[3] (Natl. Inst. of Health) studied the effects of another dopamine agonist, bromocriptine, on 6 hospitalized patients with HC, 4 men and 2 women aged 41 – 54 years. All patients had moderately severe involuntary movements. A double-blind crossover study was done over 6 – 8 weeks. Bromocriptine was given in an initial dose of 2.5 mg 4 times daily and increased according to tolerance to a maximum dose of 100 mg daily.

Doses of 45 mg bromocriptine or more daily significantly increased involuntary movements compared to placebo. No significant change in the Zung depression scale or in other neurologic deficits was noted. Insomnia was significantly improved. No significant changes occurred with 40 mg bromocriptine or less daily. The average maximum daily dose of bromocriptine was 75.8 mg. All patients improved when returned to placebo. Adverse reactions included nausea and vomiting in 3 patients, agitation in 2, confusion in 2, and irritability and somnolence in 1 case each. All these

(3)   Arch. Neurol. 33:517 – 518, July, 1976.

effects resolved when bromocriptine was replaced with placebo. No hematologic or biochemical changes were seen.

Bromocriptine, a postsynaptic dopamine receptor agonist in animal models of parkinsonism, aggravates the involuntary movements of patients with HC. The findings support the view that dopaminergic agonists ameliorate parkinsonism and exacerbate chorea and that choreic movements correlate with overactivity in dopaminergic systems.

► [Bromocriptine, a dopamine receptor agonist, produced an exacerbation of symptoms in 6 patients with Huntington's chorea. This finding supports the view that choreic movements correlate with overactivity in dopaminergic systems. — Ed.] ◄

Headache

Clonidine (Catapresan): Double-Blind Study after Long-Term Treatment with the Drug in Migraine. There is no consensus concerning the efficacy of clonidine in migraine prophylaxis. Most researchers have found beneficial initial effects but the long-term effect of clonidine is less certain. Per Stensrud and Ottar Sjaastad[4] (Univ. of Oslo) evaluated clonidine in comparison with placebo in a double-blind study after clonidine had been given for at least 4 months. Twenty-four women and 5 men, aged 25–61 years, with common and classic migraine were studied. The mean period of previous clonidine therapy was 10 months; the patients seemed to have responded well. Patients received the same dose of clonidine, 75–150 µg, and placebo, each for 7 weeks; the last 5 weeks of each period were used for analysis.

Two patients withdrew from the study, 1 because she increased the dosage of clonidine. Headache indices showed that clonidine had a significantly better effect than placebo. In 9 patients, however, various other factors may have influenced the frequency and severity of attacks. Excluding these patients, no significant difference between clonidine and placebo was found.

These results may suggest that the improvement obtained with clonidine persists for a time after discontinuation of treatment or that there was no real clonidine effect at the time of the double-blind study. The long-term results of clonidine therapy seem less favorable than the short-term results; there may be a decreasing effect of clonidine in many instances. Many patients feel a sedative effect in the first 2–3 weeks of clonidine therapy; the initial beneficial effect partly may be due to this sedative effect, which subsides with time.

(4) Acta Neurol. Scand. 53:233–236, 1976.

Short-Term Clinical Trial of Propranolol in Racemic Form (Inderal), D-Propranolol and Placebo in Migraine. The varying results obtained with different β-blockers in migraine prophylaxis may suggest that factors other than the β-blocking properties may be important. Per Stensrud and Ottar Sjaastad[5] (Univ. of Oslo) evaluated propranolol in racemic form (Inderal) and D-propranolol in 20 patients with migraine.

D-Propranolol has only a slight β-blocking effect but both substances penetrate the blood-brain barrier. Of the 14 female and 6 male patients, aged 15–60 years, 17 had common and 3 had classic migraine. Pills containing 40 mg Inderal, 40 mg D-propranolol or placebo were given in randomized sequence for 4-week periods, with a one-week washout period between test periods. The patients were managed as outpatients and were allowed analgesics or, if necessary, ergotamine preparations for migraine attacks.

One patient withdrew from study while on Inderal because of dyspnea and more frequent headache attacks; other side effects were negligible. Both Inderal and D-propranolol were significantly superior to placebo, especially Inderal. Inderal was more effective than D-propranolol in reducing headache indices, but not significantly so. Three patients did better on placebo than on Inderal; extraneous factors might have been responsible in 1 instance. Varying degrees of bradycardia and slight blood pressure reduction were noted during Inderal therapy in almost all cases. The mean pulse rate was 63 with Inderal, 75 with D-propranolol and 77 with placebo.

Inderal is beneficial in migraine prophylaxis. The precise mechanism of β-blocker action in migraine is unknown. A slight positive effect of D-propranolol also was seen. The β-blocking properties of these drugs seem of major significance in this context but further studies are warranted. A substance with properties like Inderal but without the ability to penetrate the blood-brain barrier would be useful for comparison in migraine prophylaxis.

► [This article and the preceding one, the results of studies in the same clinic, show that both propranolol and clonidine are statistically effective in the prophylaxis of migraine. Propranolol appears to act not only through its β-receptor blocking property, but possibly through other

(5) Acta Neurol. Scand. 53:229–232, 1976.

mechanisms as well. Clonidine seems to have a sedative effect, and long-term results seem to be less favorable than short-term results. — Ed.] ◄

Immunologic and Histologic Studies of Temporal Arteries from Patients with Temporal Arteritis and/or Polymyalgia Rheumatica. Erik Waaler, Olav Tönder and Einar-Johan Milde[6] (Bergen, Norway) examined biopsy specimens from the temporal arteries of 45 patients presenting with the clinical picture of temporal arteritis and 35 with polymyalgia rheumatica. The 104 control patients had no indication of active or healed arteritis. Only 2 control patients had weak anti-IgG activity in arterial sections. Only half the patients with polymyalgia rheumatica had active arteritis or older lesions. Anti-IgG activity was not found in these arteries but it was noted in 40 of the 45 patients with temporal arteritis.

Cases were classified as granulomatous inflammation, nongranulomatous mononuclear arteritis, regenerative lesions and scars or minimal noncharacteristic lesions (Fig 15). Strong anti-IgG activity was often present in association with granulomatous arteritis but it was also found with noncharacteristic lesions and old regenerative lesions and scars. There was 1 false positive mixed agglutination reac-

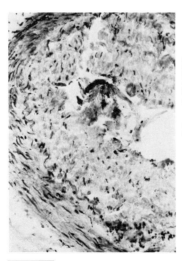

Fig 15. — Frozen section of temporal artery 9 weeks after onset of symptoms, illustrating minimal noncharacteristic lesion. Note thickened intima and small focus in media with lymphocytic infiltration. Hematoxylin-eosin; reduced from ×175. (Courtesy of Waaler, E., et al.: Acta Pathol. Microbiol. Scand. [A] 84:55–63, January, 1976.)

(6) Acta Pathol. Microbiol. Scand. [A] 84:55–63, January, 1976.

tion in an artery without signs of inflammation. Biopsy specimens of 21 arteries exhibited anti-IgG activity of Ig type and complement, mainly C1q; IgA was the dominant component, either alone or together with IgG or IgM, or both. In 6 biopsy specimens, other reactors appeared to be responsible for positive mixed agglutination reactions. All 21 specimens with tissue-bound Ig and complement exhibited granulomatous arteritis. Most biopsy specimens with other reactors exhibited proliferative changes and lymphocytes.

These findings support earlier reports of anti-IgG activities in arteries of patients with temporal arteritis or polymyalgia rheumatica. Immunoglobulin A predominates in granulomatous arteritis. The clinical-histologic picture is definitely related to the presence of anti-IgG activity in the lesions. The mixed agglutination test is an efficient diagnostic tool for temporal arteritis.

▶ [Because the lesions of temporal arteritis easily are overlooked, the mixed agglutination test proved to be a good diagnostic tool in this disease. Arteries without anti-IgG activity showed no signs of temporal arteritis. — Ed.] ◀

Infectious Diseases

The Hamster as a Secondary Reservoir Host of Lymphocytic Choriomeningitis Virus. Interest in lymphocytic choriomeningitis (LCM) has increased with recent reports of infection resulting from contact with the Syrian hamster, kept as a pet. H. H. Skinner, E. H. Knight and L. S. Buckley[7] (Woking, England) documented the ease with which transfer of the infection can occur and confirmed that infected hamsters can be a source of LCM virus, especially hazardous in the home, school or pet shop where they are handled. Hamsters were bred under barrier conditions and kept in cages of 2–4 animals up to age 4 months, after which they were caged singly. Forceps were used for handling infected animals. Experimental bites were made with the use of infective urine and blood from freshly killed Pirbright P(PTI)-strain mice.

Exposure of weaned hamsters to an environment contaminated with LCM virus shed by tolerantly infected mice led to short subclinical infections. If infection occurred in early pregnancy, the young seemed normal at birth but their tissues were highly infective; their bites and urine were also highly infective for 2–3 months. Viremia did not last long enough for successive vertical transmissions of infection to be likely, but viruria persisted for at least 8 months in most prenatally infected hamsters and, under simulated field conditions, was a potent virus source for contact infections, leading to further generations of prenatally infected young.

In the absence of the natural reservoir host, such long-term carriers could have been a major factor in causing the buildup of infection in hamster colonies which, when bought as pets, led to a recent outbreak of human clinical infections in Germany and the United States. The risk of human infection through mucosa or skin contaminated by infected urine or saliva may be high and should be prevented by a high

---

(7) J. Hyg. (Camb.) 76:299–306, April, 1976.

standard of hygiene. The bites and urine of young prenatally infected hamsters are as hazardous as those of tolerantly infected wild or pet mice. When future cases of LCM infection are diagnosed, the possibility of contact with infected hamsters should be considered.

▶ [It has recently been shown that rats and mice are not the only reservoir hosts of the lymphocytic choriomeningitis virus, but that a common household pet, the gerbil, may transmit the disease. This study shows that another common household pet, the hamster, also may transmit the infection. – Ed.] ◀

Ribonuclease Treatment of Tick-Borne Encephalitis. Ribonuclease (RNAse) inhibits RNA synthesis and the reproduction of RNA-containing viruses, including tick-borne encephalitis viruses. Boris N. Glukhov, Alexey P. Jerusalimsky, Valentina M. Canter and Rudolf I. Salganik[8] (Novosibirsk, USSR) conducted clinical trials of pancreatic RNAse in 507 patients with tick-borne encephalitis, corroborated serologically, in 4 endemic areas of the USSR in 1965 – 71. Ribonuclease was given to 246 patients and antiencephalitic γ-globulin to 261. Commercial sterile beef pancreatic RNAse was used. Gamma-globulin was prepared from horse serum from animals hyperimmunized by a mixture of strains of tick-borne encephalitis viruses. The average dose of RNAse was 180 mg daily and 800 – 1,000 mg in a course of treatment, γ-globulin was given for 3 days in a dose of 6 ml daily.

The average serum and cerebrospinal fluid RNAse levels increased more than twofold after intramuscular administration of RNAse. With RNAse treatment the febrile period was shorter, the temperature became normal twice as rapidly and the patient's general condition improved rapidly. Prolonged asthenia was much less frequent in RNAse-treated patients than in those given γ-globulin. Mortality in patients with focal brain lesions was much higher after γ-globulin than after RNAse treatment. Immunogenesis was inhibited by γ-globulin treatment but not by RNAse therapy. Hemagglutinin titers increased from the first days of disease in RNAse-treated patients.

The therapeutic effect of RNAse in tick-borne encephalitis is considerably higher than that of γ-globulin. Immunologic defenses are able to support the beneficial effects of RNAse,

(8) Arch. Neurol. 33:598 – 603, September, 1976.

whereas in contrast, passive immunization with antiencephalitic γ-globulin inhibits immunogenesis. Ribonuclease was recently introduced officially in the USSR as a new antiviral drug for the efficient treatment of tick-borne encephalitis.

► [This study was carried out at the Novosibirsk State Medical Institute and Institute of Cytology and Genetics, Siberian Branch, U.S.S.R. Academy of Sciences. The efficacy of pancreatic ribonuclease was compared with that of antiencephalitic γ-globulin in the treatment of patients with tick-borne encephalitis. The study demonstrated a considerable advantage of the former. With its use, the temperature became normal twice as quickly, and the meningeal symptoms and cerebrospinal fluid pleocytosis regressed rapidly. No adverse reaction or aftereffects were noted. Ribonuclease was accepted as a new, highly effective treatment of tick-borne encephalitis. − Ed.] ◄

Recovery from Rabies in Man. All three reports of recovery from rabies have come from the United States, where rabies exposure is infrequent and relatively few persons receive postexposure vaccination. The exposure risk is greater in most Latin American countries and about 300,000 persons are vaccinated each year. Casimiro Porras, Juan José Barboza, Eduardo Fuenzalida, Héctor López Adaros, Ana María Oviedo de Díaz and Jorge Furst[9] (Mendoza, Argentina) report the only known case of human rabies recovery in Latin America.

Woman, 45, was severely bitten on the arm by a dog that was nervous and had occasional seizures and died 4 days later. Rabies treatment was begun 6 days after the dog died; 14 daily doses of suckling mouse brain vaccine were followed by 2 booster doses. The patient's daughter also was bitten and vaccinated and remained well. The patient had a cerebellar striatal syndrome 21 days after being bitten. Paresthesia in the left arm was the first symptom. The syndrome lasted several months and severe encephalitic symptoms lasted 75 days. The patient had almost completely recovered after 13 months. Her serum and cerebrospinal fluid contained rabies-neutralizing antibodies that reached peak titers of 1 : 640,000 and 1 : 160,000, respectively. Treatment also included diphenhydramine, diazepam, biperiden, phenytoin, betamethasone and ACTH gel.

Titers of the magnitude found in this patient have not been recorded previously after suckling mouse brain vaccine treatment. This, along with the epidemiologic, clinical and

(9)   Ann. Intern. Med. 85:44−48, July, 1976.

laboratory observations, supports the conclusion of a nonfatal case of rabies in man. The patient recovered from the significant central nervous system damaged caused by rabies.

Intensive Care in Rabies Therapy: Clinical Observations are reported by G. R. Gode, A. V. Raju, T. S. Jayalakshmi, H. L. Kaul and N. K. Bhide[1] (New Delhi, India). Rabies is almost always fatal. Every year about 15,000 deaths from rabies are reported in India and over 3 million persons are exposed to the risk. Intensive treatment of rabies has been tried since 1969.

Two early patients were treated intensively with discouraging results because facilities were inadequate; later, 5 patients with clinical rabies were treated in a special intensive care room by volunteers protected by preexposure immunization against rabies. Hypoxia from muscle spasms was prevented by intermittent positive-pressure ventilation, facilitated by muscle relaxants and sedatives. Other measures included nutritional maintenance, correction of fluid-electrolyte and acid-base balances, antiviral agents, immunologic stimulation and intensive nursing care. Cytosine arabinoside and Freund's emulsion also were tried.

All 7 patients were male and had been bitten by stray dogs. Maximum survival was 17 days. Unconsciousness was not deep except terminally or when respiratory or cardiac complications supervened. Temperature monitoring in 3 cases showed a distinct tendency toward poikilothermy. Several ECG changes were noted in the 3 patients monitored. Complications of tracheostomy and long-term ventilation were significant. There were considerable variations in urine output during the course of illness in the long-survival cases. Blood cell counts fell progressively during the illness. Two of the 3 autopsies showed a large number of Negri bodies in the temporal, parietal and hippocampal regions. Inclusion bodies were found in cerebellar Purkinje cells. Degenerative changes were seen in pyramidal cells and basal ganglion in 1 case.

The helplessness felt in attempts to treat earlier cases of rabies has been replaced by the hope of eventually saving some patients.

(1) Lancet 2:6–8, July 3, 1976.

► [It has been generally accepted that human rabies patients usually die within 3–10 days after the first appearance of symptoms. The preceding article reports the recovery of a patient with clinical rabies, even though some central nervous system manifestations persisted for a long period.

In this article from India, an intensive-care regimen for patients with rabies is outlined. All 7 of the patients so treated died, but 2 lived for 16 days and 1 for 17 days. The authors express hope that the use of this technique may eventually make it possible for some patients with rabies to survive. — Ed.] ◄

Successful Protection of Humans Exposed to Rabies Infection: Postexposure Treatment with the New Human Diploid Cell Rabies Vaccine and Antirabies Serum was evaluated by Mahmoud Bahmanyar, Ahmad Fayaz, Shokrollah Nour-Salehi, Manouchehr Mohammadi (Pasteur Inst. of Iran, Tehran) and Hilary Koprowski[2] (Wistar Inst.). After brain tissue vaccine was proved to be almost totally useless in protecting persons severely exposed to rabies in Iran, the use of a combination of serum and vaccine was again recommended by the WHO Expert Committee on Rabies. Adverse reactions to both the serum and the vaccine were observed, but Koprowski et al. then showed that WI-38 cells were the substrate of choice, and human diploid cell vaccine (HDCV) was produced for clinical trials in Iran. Antirabies serum was produced in mules. One dose of the heterologous serum was given intramuscularly to 44 of 45 persons bitten by dogs or wolves in rural areas of Iran in 1975 and 1976. Vaccine was given simultaneously or within 1 hour, and a total of 5 doses of HDCV were given subcutaneously within 30 days, with a booster dose on day 90. Two batches of HDCV were used. Reactions to the inoculations of vaccine were mild.

Except for a man aged 90, who died of a heart attack 5 months after exposure to rabies, all the treated patients are well 6–12 months after exposure. The predicted mortality in this group without treatment was at least 35%. The occasionally unpleasant side effects of the heterologous antirabies serum would have been avoided had rabies immune globulin of human origin been available.

A major breakthrough has been achieved in the postexposure treatment of human beings exposed to rabies infection. The number of injections has been reduced from 14–21 to 6

(2) J.A.M.A. 236:2751–2754, Dec. 13, 1976.

or less, and the HDCV used causes virtually no side effects and is highly immunogenic. All patients in this series were protected against rabies. Almost a century after postexposure treatment of human beings was begun, an effective means of protecting man against rabies has been developed.

▶ [This contribution describes a major breakthrough in the postexposure treatment of human beings exposed to rabies infection. The procedure, however, is dependent on the availability of an adequate number of donors. — Ed.] ◀

Airborne Rabies Encephalitis: Demonstration of Rabies Virus in the Human Central Nervous System. The observance of Koch's postulates is not always approximated in instances of known alleged viral disease of the nervous system. John P. Conomy (Cleveland Clinic), Albert Leibovitz, William McCombs and James Stinson[3] (Scott and White Clinic, Temple, Texas) describe a patient who died of rabies encephalitis in whom the means of disease contact was unusual, perhaps unique, and in whom Koch's postulates were fulfilled.

Man, 56, a veterinarian, had vomiting, diarrhea, weakness and headache and became confused. He was febrile when seen, with a white blood cell count of 13,600/cu mm with a shift to the left. Stupor and delirium ensued. The lumbar cerebrospinal fluid had an opening pressure of 300 mm and contained 131 white blood cells/cu mm, 53% of them polymorphonuclear cells. The patient was comatose the next day, with decerebrate posturing and left-sided hyperreflexia; he remained comatose with intractable seizures and central ventilatory dyscontrol until death on day 9 of the illness.

The patient was employed by a firm preparing commercial veterinary vaccines and had homogenized rabid goat brain 2 weeks before the onset of symptoms. He had probably removed his mask when pipetting aliquots of the homogenate from a blender. He had last been immunized against rabies 13 years previously and no antibody was detected in the serum on testing 1 year later. The serum rabies antibody titer rose from less than 1 : 5 to 1 : 45 over the acute phase of illness.

Autopsy showed spongy cerebral cortical changes, cuffing of capillaries and venules by inflammatory cells and acute anoxic neuronal damage with moderate astrocytosis. Virions were abundant and tended to be located in synaptic zones. The virions were consistent with rabies virus morphologically.

Airborne rabies is rare; only 2 other possible cases have

(3) Neurology (Minneap.) 27:67–69, January, 1977.

been reported, both in persons who had explored bat caves. This patient had used a blender of the type known to produce a lingering aerosol or viral cloud after tissue mixing. Formed rabies virions were identified in the synaptic zones of the olfactory glomeruli in this patient. Experimental disease production and tissue cytopathic effects of virus recovered from the brain fulfilled Koch's postulates.

An affinity of rabies virions for synaptic structures and the resultant transmission interference may be related to some of the symptoms of rabies seen before multitudes of individual neurons are destroyed.

► [As far as is known, this is the first confirmed report of airborne rabies encephalitis. The investigative studies done fulfill Koch's postulates in this unusual incidence of virus disease of the nervous system. — Ed.] ◄

Mollaret's Meningitis: Report of Three Cases. Benign, recurrent aseptic Mollaret's meningitis has been recognized most often in Europe; only 1 case has been reported from North America, although cases reported as forms of "periodic disease" may not differ from Mollaret's meningitis. Barton F. Haynes (Natl. Inst. of Health), Richard Wright and Joseph P. McCracken[4] (Durham, N.C.) report 3 cases with unusual manifestations of this disease. Postpartum pituitary necrosis was an antecedent event in 1 case. One case occurred in an otherwise healthy woman aged 82 years, and 1 patient was thought to have *Histoplasma* meningitis. An association with seizures at the onset of the syndrome, as in 1 of the present cases, is not unusual. Fever was not present in 1 case. In 1 case the initial cerebrospinal fluid culture was reported as positive for *Histoplasma capsulatum*.

Recurrent aseptic Mollaret's meningitis is an uncommon disease, with a benign but often prolonged course. The episodes last 2–3 days, with symptom-free intervals of variable duration. Symptom intensity may vary, and the episodes may occur periodically or may be related to the menstrual cycle. No viral agent has been found in many well-studied cases. No definite immunologic abnormality has been detected in Mollaret's meningitis, but detailed immunologic studies have not been performed. The cerebrospinal fluid protein level usually does not rise above 100 mg/100 ml.

Attempts to treat Mollaret's meningitis with steroids,

(4) J.A.M.A. 236:1967–1969, Oct. 25, 1976.

diphenhydramine, procaine and meprobamate have not succeeded. Colchicine has been reported to be of use in 1 case. The rarity of cases and the variable intervals between attacks make evaluation of therapy difficult. The pathophysiology of Mollaret's meningitis remains unclear, and treatment at present consists of supportive care.

▶ [Is Mollaret's meningitis a real clinical entity? Many feel that the term is used for those cases in which the clinician is unable to find the etiologic organism by culture and present-day laboratory techniques. Perhaps in some of these cases antibiotics have been given early and as a result no growth appears on the cultures. It is up to those who choose to make the diagnosis of Mollaret's meningitis to prove that there is such an entity. — Ed.] ◀

Evolution of Cerebral Abscess: Correlation of Clinical Features with Computed Tomography: Case Report. Brain abscess is often not diagnosed until it has become encapsulated or until rupture or herniation has occurred. Computed tomography (CT) is a sensitive means of detecting minimal changes in brain density. Robert A. Zimmerman, Larissa T. Bilaniuk, Paul M. Shipkin, Donald H. Gilden and Fredrick Murtagh[5] (Univ. of Pennsylvania) used CT to follow the evolution of a brain abscess from the stage of cerebritis to that of a well-developed abscess. This is the first documentation of the evolution of a brain abscess from a nonspecific focal inflammation to precisely defined, encapsulated purulent material.

Woman, 26, was admitted with headache and behavioral changes 2 weeks after a "cold" and stiff neck. Left arm paresthesias and dizziness had developed 2 days before admission. She had become less responsive and had begun giggling inappropriately. She was not attentive and answered questions slowly. The left visual field was neglected and optokinetic nystagmus was impaired. Bizarre posturing of the left arm was noted, as was an extensive sensory deficit on the left side. An EEG indicated diffuse hemispheric dysfunction, maximal in the right central to posterior temporal regions. A ^{99m}Tc brain scan showed a spherical 4-cm area of activity in the right parietal region, and carotid angiography showed a large avascular mass in this area. The CT scanning showed a mass effect and a large zone of reduced density in the right parietal region. Multiple marginal areas of increased vascularity were noted after contrast injection. Dexamethasone and mannitol were given, as was ampicillin, but she became comatose and decorticate and

(5) Neurology (Minneap.) 27:14–19, January, 1977.

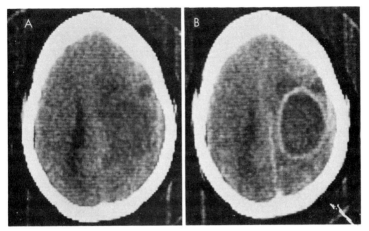

Fig 16.–**A,** CT scan after 2-week interval. Note more homogeneous zone of decreased density still associated with marked mass effect. **B,** after injection of contrast agent, there is oval rim of increased density consistent with abscess capsule. (Courtesy of Zimmerman, R. A., et al.: Neurology (Minneap.) 27:14–19, January, 1977.)

acquired a fixed, dilated right pupil. Emergency hyperventilation and intravenous mannitol reversed the signs completely.

A CT scan done on day 4 showed continuing inflammation. Chloramphenicol was added but left-sided signs persisted and a third CT scan showed a decrease in mass effect but a possible early abscess capsule. A subsequent CT scan showed a well-formed oval abscess capsule (Fig 16). Emergency drainage became necessary; *Staphylococcus epidermidis* was cultured. A CT scan made 3 weeks after drainage showed barium within the collapsed cavity, with no capsule recognizable. Remnants of the abscess were removed at elective craniotomy. A small zone of reduced density was present 14 weeks after removal of the abscess cavity. The patient continued to improve and on prophylactic anticonvulsants has remained asymptomatic and without neurologic signs.

The CT scanning allowed visualization of the active abscess in this patient. Contrast injection was essential for demonstration of the abscess wall. In conjunction with the clinical findings, CT scanning can be helpful in determining the transition from cerebritis to encapsulated brain abscess.

▶ [Computed tomography is more specific than either radionuclide scanning or angiography in the diagnosis of brain abscess and is the only diagnostic tool that is capable of differentiating between acute focal encephalomalacia (cerebritis) and brain abscess. – Ed.] ◀

Subacute Sclerosing Panencephalitis in the Middle East: Report of 99 Cases. Fuad Sami Haddad, Winthrop S. Risk and J. T. Jabbour[6] (American Univ., Beirut) reviewed data on all patients given a differential diagnosis of subacute sclerosing panencephalitis (SSPE) at two major Lebanese medical centers since 1956. A total of 99 cases was available. There were 4 cases in 1956–57 and 95 cases in 1964–75. The prevalence was 1.7 cases per year per million total population in Lebanon.

More than 90% of the patients acquired SSPE between ages 4 and 16. The incidence was 50% higher at ages 4–9 than at ages 10–16. The duration of illness has ranged from 6 weeks to 8 years in the 94 patients followed. Twenty-one patients are still alive. Over half of the deaths occurred within 1 year and most of the others within 2 years. Patients who lived over 2 years usually did so in a vegetative state. Many appeared to gradually improve after about 1–1½ years of illness. Often exacerbations followed acute respiratory infections. All 81 patients with a positive history of measles contracted it in infancy or childhood before the onset of SSPE. The age at the time of measles infection is shown in Figure 17.

Fig 17.–Age at time of measles infection. Cross-correlation with age of onset of SSPE symptoms shows shift in age at time of measles infection after 1970. (Courtesy of Haddad, F. S., et al.: Ann. Neurol. 1:211–217, March, 1977.)

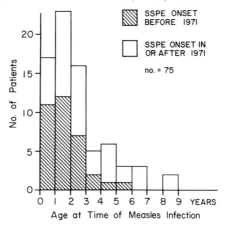

(6) Ann. Neurol. 1:211–217, March, 1977.

This study confirms earlier observations of the high incidence of SSPE in the Middle East. Virtually all the patients developed patterned myoclonic movements at some time during the illness, permitting an almost immediate diagnosis for many patients. The claim that most patients die within 1 year has not been substantiated.

▶ [Statistical and epidemiologic studies of this type are of value only if one can be certain that the thoroughness of the reporting is fairly complete and the criteria for diagnosis are strictly adhered to. To draw conclusions on incidence and prevalence of a certain disease on the basis of so few cases is of questionable value. The only conclusions that we can draw are that subacute sclerosing panencephalitis does occur in the Middle East as well as in the United States and that it seems to develop in children and adolescents who have had measles in early childhood. – Ed.] ◀

Miscellaneous Neurologic Problems

Wernicke's Encephalopathy Following Prolonged Intravenous Therapy. Thiamine administration may be omitted in hospitalized nonalcoholic patients who are liable to thiamine deficiency and Wernicke's encephalopathy if their nutrition depends solely on clear liquids or parenteral fluids. Alan M. Nadel and Peter C. Burger[7] (Duke Univ.) describe 2 nonalcoholic patients with Wernicke's encephalopathy after having parenteral nutrition.

CASE 1.—Woman, 78, was hospitalized with dehydration and obtundation 3 months after a cerebral infarction, which had caused a left-sided hemiparesis. She was lethargic and confused after rehydration and required parenteral fluids. After 4 weeks, she was placed in a nursing home and was given only clear oral fluids and infusions of 5% aqueous dextrose and 0.45% saline. She became severely obtunded 2 months after transfer and was cachectic and responsive only to pain. There were no new localizing neurologic signs. The patient died despite treatment for dehydration and sepsis. Autopsy showed bilateral pulmonary emboli, a parathyroid adenoma, chronic pyelonephritis, an old cystic infarct transecting the right internal capsule of the brain and punctate hemorrhages in several sites in the brain. Microscopy showed typical features of acute Wernicke's encephalopathy.

CASE 2.—Woman, 61, with suspected parathyroid adenoma, had had two cerebral infarctions during the past year and had hemiplegia and mild aphasia. A parathyroid adenoma was resected but persistent nausea and vomiting occurred postoperatively, necessitating administration of clear oral fluids and intravenous 5% aqueous dextrose without vitamins. She became unresponsive 6 days postoperatively without localizing signs. Thrombocytopenia and petechiae developed. The patient died 25 days postoperatively after upper gastrointestinal bleeding. Autopsy showed pulmonary edema and bronchopneumonia, gastrointestinal ulcerations, an old cortical infarction and recent hemorrhagic softening in the left

(7) J.A.M.A. 235:2403–2405, May 31, 1976.

parieto-occipital region. Fresh hemorrhages involved the mammillary bodies bilaterally.

Both patients had pathologic changes of Wernicke's encephalopathy, which was unsuspected clinically. Nystagmus was not seen in these cases. The encephalopathy could have been prevented by thiamine administration. A carbohydrate load can lead to Wernicke's disease in the thiamine-deficient person. Thiamine supplementation is necessary during prolonged intravenous fluid administration.

▶ [These cases call attention to complications accompanying the prolonged use of intravenous fluids without concurrent administration of thiamine. Thiamine depletion and its consequences can develop rapidly. – Ed.] ◀

Progressive Dialytic Encephalopathy. S. Chokroverty, M. E. Bruetman, V. Berger and M. G. Reyes[8] (Mt. Sinai Hosp. Med. Center, Chicago) report data on 11 patients in whom a characteristic clinical picture accompanied by distinctive EEG abnormalities emerged during long-term hemodialysis for chronic renal failure. The patients had been on maintenance hemodialysis 3 times weekly for 6 hours each time. A commercial dialysate was utilized. The subacute, progressive encephalopathy developed after 14 – 36 months of dialysis and lasted 3 – 15 months. It was characterized by dementia, language disorder, myoclonic jerks and behavioral disturbance. No significant changes in blood urea nitrogen or electrolytes were observed. The cerebrospinal fluid protein was slightly low in 3 cases. Brain scans and cerebral angiograms gave normal results. The EEGs showed excessive theta rhythm, bisynchronous intermittent delta waves and frontocentral spike-and-slow wave complexes, usually symmetrical. No significant differences were found in pre- and postdialysis EEGs.

Autopsies performed on 7 patients showed left ventricular hypertrophy and hepatic congestion. Four patients had bilateral end-stage kidneys. One patient had multiple lacunae at several brain sites and anoxic-ischemic changes in the cerebrum and cerebellum. One patient had an old lacunar infarction in the putamen and another had lacunar infarcts bilaterally in the putamen and in the periaqueductal gray of

(8)   J. Neurol. Neurosurg. Psychiatry 39:411 – 419, May, 1976.

the midbrain. Four patients had normal central nervous system findings.

The absence of morphological correlates for the clinical findings in these cases favors a possible metabolic cerebral dysfunction but no overall changes in systemic biochemical parameters were noted. The cause of progressive dialytic encephalopathy is unknown at present. Future studies might assess the possibilities of dopamine or asparagine deficiency or other cerebral neurochemical defects.

▶ [Since the introduction of successful extracorporeal dialysis and maintenance hemodialysis, the prognosis in terms of longevity of patients with end-stage renal failure has improved considerably. Dialysis, however, cannot be used for extended periods without certain dangers, and this article describes the development of progressive encephalopathy during long-term dialysis. — Ed.] ◀

Man in Transit: Biochemical and Physiologic Changes during Intercontinental Flights. There is little objective evidence to support the claim that persons traveling on supersonic aircraft will arrive fresher and more alert at their destination.

Malcolm Carruthers (St. Mary's Hosp., London), A. E. Arguelles and Abraham Mosovich[9] (Buenos Aires) did a pilot study of responses to one of the longest south-to-north transits in the world; a flight from Buenos Aires to London, a trip over 7,000 miles long and halfway around the world latitudinally. The flight was made in January to maximize the climatic change and minimize the time-zone change. Fifteen subjects, the crew of the plane and 2 passengers, were studied. The flight was routine, made under standard operating conditions. There was a 30 C drop in air temperature between Buenos Aires and London. Cruising altitudes ranged from 7,000 to 11,000 m.

Cholesterol and free fatty acid levels were unchanged during the 4-day study; triglyceride and glucose levels increased during the flight and returned to preflight levels the next day. Cortisol levels were reduced on days 3 and 4 compared to preflight values. Urinary noradrenaline was greatly elevated early in the flight and for 2 days afterward in the morning. Urinary adrenaline was greatly elevated on the 2d postflight day. Urine volumes were reduced during the

(9) Lancet 1:977 – 981, May 8, 1976.

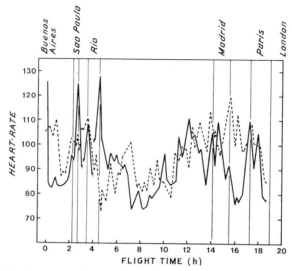

Fig 18. – Heart rates of 3 pilots *(solid line)* and 1 passenger *(broken line)* during flight from Buenos Aires to London. (Courtesy of Carruthers, M., et al.: Lancet 1: 977–981, May 8, 1976.)

flight. Heart rate changes are shown in Figure 18. The EEGs showed evidence of considerable fatigue in the crew during the quiet part of the flight, an overnight period when the plane was on "Autopilot."

Climatic conditions can cause stress in an aircrew before a flight and lead to impaired adaptation to the added strains of exacting work in rapidly changing conditions of temperature, humidity and time. Improved EEG equipment will allow assessment of the effects of stress on man in transit and may be used to show ways that the Concorde may lessen the impact of abrupt changes in time zones and climatic conditions.

► [One of the claims made with the introduction of routine supersonic services with the Concorde airplane is that the passengers and crew "will arrive at their destination fresher and more alert." This study shows that biochemical and physiologic changes do occur during such flights and that climatic conditions can prestress an aircrew before flight and lead to impaired adaptation to the additional strains of exacting work in rapidly changing surroundings of temperature, humidity and time. – Ed.] ◄

Familial Neurologic Disease Associated with Spongiform Encephalopathy. Creutzfeldt-Jakob disease is an uncommon disorder of adults characterized by progressive neurologic deterioration over several weeks to months and a protean clinical picture. The disease usually occurs sporadically; it has been transmitted experimentally to primates, and several families with affected members have been described. N. Paul Rosenthal, John Keesey, Barbara Crandall and W. Jann Brown[1] (Univ. of California, Los Angeles) describe the "W" family of Bedfordshire, England, whose remarkable frequency of heterogeneous neurologic diseases was manifested by a member having Creutzfeldt-Jakob disease.

Man, 42, presented with judgmental errors, ocular pain and poor balance. His condition deteriorated progressively over 4 weeks, with frequent limb jerks, rigidity, reduced tendon reflexes and diffuse EEG slowing with occasional spikes and spike-and-wave discharges. Administration of amantadine, 200–600 mg daily, gave no improvement and the patient died from pneumonia 13 months after onset of symptoms.

Neurologic disease was transmitted in an autosomal dominant manner in this family. The diseases ranged from subacute and chronic dementias to various motor system abnormalities without dementia. A cortical biopsy specimen from the propositus showed spongiform encephalopathy. A first cousin had a chronic dementia but no spongiform changes were seen at autopsy. Both patients had PAS-positive, eosinophilic plaques throughout the brain. A muscle biopsy specimen of the propositus showed changes suggestive of "ragged red" myopathy.

The general neuropathologic findings were typical of previously reported cases of Creutzfeldt-Jakob disease. Both pathologic studies showed neuronal loss and intense gliosis; neither patient had neurofibrillary tangles. Examination of the pedigree suggested autosomal dominant transmission of a factor associated with susceptibility to neurologic disease. The neurologic diseases in this family were remarkably heterogeneous. The family members may inherit either a metabolic abnormality having a variable neurologic expression or merely an increased susceptibility to acquired neurologic disease. Because there is no indication that Creutzfeldt-Jakob disease is related metabolically to the other neuro-

(1)   Arch. Neurol. 33:252–259, April, 1976.

logic conditions in the family, the presence of a genetically increased susceptibility to acquired disease is more likely.

► [The inheritance pattern for neurologic disease in this family suggests that the general susceptibility to such disease is a genetic trait, transmitted in an autosomal dominant fashion. There was marked heterogenicity of disease manifestations, however, and in only 1 person was a diagnosis of Creutzfeldt-Jakob disease made. It must be borne in mind that instances of Creutzfeldt-Jakob disease that appear to be inherited as an autosomal dominant trait have been reported. In the editor's experience envolving 3 sisters with Creutzfeldt-Jakob disease whose father presumably had had it also, the son of one of the sisters has died of the disease in his early 30s and the son of another sister presumably also was affected. — Ed.] ◄

Ménière's Disease and Cerebral Impairment. Patients with Ménière's disease exhibit psychologic test patterns characteristic of cerebral impairment. Löchen (1970) found neuropsychologic results comparable with those in patients with severe cerebral atrophy, but his research design made interpretation of the data difficult. William G. Crary, Murray Wexler (Los Angeles) and Mary Anna Riley[2] (Torrance, Calif.) determined whether a randomly selected group of patients with Ménière's disease differed on measures of organic impairment from other types of patients with otologic disorders, matched for such variables as age, sex and educational level. Study was made of 18 women with Ménière's disease, 14 female patients with various otologic disorders causing vertigo and 9 nonvertiginous female patients with otologic diagnoses. The Quick Test, Wechsler Adult Intelligence Scales digit symbol and digit span subtests, Trail-Making test and Kendall-Graham Memory for Designs (MFD) test were administered.

On criterion measures the only significant difference between groups was on the digits forward test, on which the Ménière patients performed significantly better than the nonvertiginous group. No more organic impairment was seen in the Ménière group than in the other groups on the MFD or Trail-Making tests. No comparisons reached significance after matching of persons from the different groups for age and educational level. In general, the tendency to organic impairment was less in the Ménière group than in the control groups.

Organic factors seem an unlikely source for the behav-

(2) Arch. Otolaryngol. 102:368–370, June, 1976.

ioral difficulties often noted in patients with Ménière's disease. The behavioral problems are most likely the consequence of the impact of this disease on the individual. The present psychologic studies indicate that there is no demonstrable evidence of organic cerebral impairment in patients with Ménière's disease.

▶ [One wonders why it would ever be assumed that a disease whose manifestations are the result of dysfunction of the labyrinth would cause cerebral impairment as well. This study refutes this point of view. Too many assumptions are made on the basis of psychologic tests, the reliability of which depends on the interpretations of the examiner, who may be prejudiced from the start. — Ed.] ◀

Sympathetic Nervous System Defect in Primary Orthostatic Hypotension was investigated by Michael G. Ziegler, C. Raymond Lake and Irwin J. Kopin[3] (Natl. Inst. of Health). Altered norepinephrine release might be expected to attend orthostatic hypotension of neurogenic origin. Failure to adapt to the upright position should be reflected in a reduction in the normal norepinephrine response to standing. Study was made of 10 patients with a diagnosis of Shy-Drager syndrome who had consistent orthostatic hypotension and had no disorder associated with secondary orthostatic hypotension. The 8 men and 2 women had a mean age of 56 years. Ten controls with a mean age of 53 years also were studied.

All study patients had evidence of peripheral autonomic dysfunction and 6 had symptoms of parkinsonism, signs of cerebellar dysfunction and such abnormalities as a Babinski sign and cranial nerve defects. These patients had normal plasma catecholamine levels while recumbent, whereas those without notable central nervous system dysfunction had low levels of circulating norepinephrine. No patient had a rise in plasma norepinephrine level on standing or after exertion. The mean blood pressure level fell by at least 35 torr 10 minutes after standing; responses were similar in the patients with normal and those with low plasma catecholamine levels. Patients with evidence of central nervous system disorder had some increase in heart rate in response to exertion but this was much less than that seen in controls. Plasma levels of dopamine-β-hydroxylase were significantly lower in reclining patients with orthostatic hypotension than in controls.

(3) N. Engl. J. Med. 296:293–297, Feb. 10, 1977.

Patients with central nervous system disease apparently cannot appropriately activate an otherwise intact sympathetic nervous system, whereas in those without signs of central nervous system disease, the deficit affects peripheral sympathetic nerves. In the latter group, plasma norepinephrine levels are low even at rest, indirectly acting sympathomimetic amines are ineffective and there is supersensitivity to exogenous norepinephrine.

► [These findings are consistent with other pathologic and pharmacologic observations suggesting that patients with orthostatic hypotension who also have central nervous system disease are unable to activate appropriately an otherwise intact sympathetic nervous system. In patients without signs of central nervous system disease, the deficit affects only peripheral sympathetic nerves. – Ed.] ◄

Treatment of Neurogenic Orthostatic Hypotension with a Monoamine Oxidase Inhibitor and Tyramine. Disabling neurogenic orthostatic hypotension may occur in many diseases and may result from degenerative nervous system disorder. It is due to dysfunction in autonomic pathways. Treatment successes have often been only partial or short lived. R. N. Nanda, R. H. Johnson and H. J. Keogh[4] (Glasgow) used a chemical preparation of tyramine in capsules combined with a monoamine oxidase inhibitor (tranylcypromine) to treat 4 men and 2 women, aged 25 – 72 years, for marked neurogenic orthostatic hypotension. They had had dizziness and syncope for 3 – 21 years. Two had other neurologic defects, parkinsonism and corticospinal dysfunction, respectively. Tranylcypromine was given in a dosage of 10 mg 3 times daily for a week and then as 20 mg 3 times daily for another week. Five patients who had pressor responses then received capsules of 5 or 10 mg tyramine with tranylcypromine. All patients continued taking fludrocortisone acetate. Three patients continued to use elastic stockings.

In supine patients receiving tranylcypromine, intravenous tyramine produced marked rises in blood pressure and heart rate. Blood pressure fell on standing but remained high and was sustained for over 90 minutes in 5 of the 6 patients. Moderate increases in supine pressure followed oral tyramine, and the rise was maintained while patients were standing and walking for 2 – 4 hours. Plasma norepineph-

(4) Lancet 2:1164 – 1167, Nov. 27, 1976.

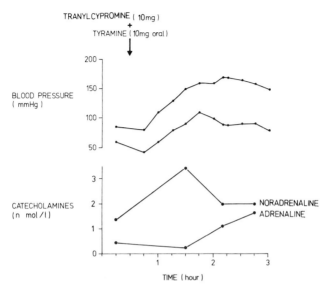

Fig 19. — Blood pressure and plasma catecholamines after combined oral dose of tranylcypromine and tyramine in man, aged 55, with orthostatic hypotension. Blood pressure increased as concentrations of norepinephrine rose. (Courtesy of Nanda, R. N., et al.: Lancet 2:1164–1167, Nov. 27, 1976.)

rine was increased 30 minutes after a dose of tyramine, and epinephrine concentrations were increased at 2 hours (Fig 19). Three patients have shown marked, continuous improvement for 8–30 months and now lead relatively normal lives. Another patient has improved, but his mobility is restricted by cerebellar ataxia. One patient became confused during treatment, and another had no pressor response to oral or intravenous tyramine before or after tranylcypromine administration.

Tyramine and tranylcypromine are useful in treating patients with neurogenic orthostatic hypotension. Those in whom there is failure of catecholamine release may not respond to this therapy. The treatment must be monitored because tyramine may cause hypertensive crises in patients receiving a monoamine oxidase inhibitor.

► [It is suggested that the pressor response to a monoamine oxidase inhibitor and tyramine should be investigated in patients with neurogenic orthostatic hypotension and that this treatment should be tried in those who respond. — Ed.] ◄

Long Survival in Orthostatic Hypotension: Case Report and a Review of the Literature. C. Davidson (Leeds Genl. Infirm., England) and D. B. Morgan[5] (Univ. of Leeds) describe a patient with idiopathic orthostatic hypotension who had no clinical evidence of generalized neurologic disease but had a history suggesting that autonomic dysfunction had been present for more than 30 years.

Woman, 65, had chest pain, dizziness on exertion and frequent faints. Syncope had occurred during a pregnancy at age 32 and had made the patient housebound, persisting to term. Syncope resumed 33 years later and increased to 4 – 6 times daily. Dim vision preceded syncope but there were no epileptic features. Findings on physical examination were normal and anticoagulant therapy gave little benefit. Saventrine was then given for orthostatic hypotension with some improvement initially, but the patient's condition gradually deteriorated and she spent most of her time in a chair. Cerebral function was normal and there was no clinical evidence of arterial disease. The patient responded well to treatment with fludrocortisone. The blood pressure level still falls 30 – 60 mm Hg on standing but the systolic blood pressure level does not fall below 110 mm Hg. The patient has been active during treatment for more than 2 years, with only occasional faints.

Grossly impaired baroreceptor-mediated reflexes were shown in this patient on tilt-table studies. Reflex sweating was absent and reflex vasodilation was absent on waterbath testing. Extensive autonomic dysfunction was documented but the patient may have first had symptoms of autonomic dysfunction 30 years before.

Most patients with idiopathic orthostatic hypotension have no obvious neurologic involvement at onset. Few patients live 10 years or longer from onset of symptoms. There is a wide prognostic range for patients with this disorder. About 1 patient in 3 will be free of neurologic complications for many years and perhaps indefinitely. Active, carefully controlled treatment of the hypotension is worthwhile. ·

▶ [These investigators suggest that the prognosis in patients with orthostatic hypotension who do not develop generalized neurologic disease is better than usually is recognized. Such patients respond well to symptomatic treatment. – Ed.] ◀

Two Hundred Thirty-Five Cases of Excessive Daytime Sleepiness: Diagnosis and Tentative Classification are discussed by Christian Guilleminault and William

(5) J. Chronic Dis. 29:733 – 742, November, 1976.

C. Dement[6] (Stanford Univ.). Currently, there is no adequate classification of disease entities manifested by complaints about sleep in otherwise apparently healthy persons. Excessive daytime sleepiness or too much sleep, or both, may be distinguished from too little sleep at night, from such disorders as sleepwalking and bed wetting and from sleep complaints clearly resulting from other illness.

Study was made of 235 consecutive patients with excessive daytime sleepiness (EDS), drawn from among nearly 600 referrals to a sleep clinic over five years. The mean age was 41.2 years and the age range, 5–66 years. Eleven patients were children. Males constituted 60% of the series. The final diagnosis was narcolepsy in 145 cases, upper airway sleep apnea in 33 adults and 11 children, narcolepsy with sleep apnea in 10 cases, drug dependency in 8, hypersomnia with abnormal cerebrospinal fluid 5-hydroxyindoleacetic acid in 7 and EDS with automatic behavior and

SCHEMA FOR DIAGNOSING
EDS SYNDROMES

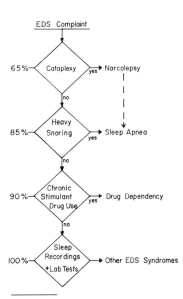

Fig 20. – Schema for diagnosing EDS syndromes shows that diagnosis can be made in about 90% of patients on the basis of clinical symptoms and history. (Courtesy of Guilleminault, C., and Dement, W. C.: J. Neurol. Sci. 31:13–27, Jan.–Feb., 1977.)

(6)   J. Neurol. Sci. 31:13–27, Jan.–Feb., 1977.

abnormal nocturnal sleep (neutral state syndrome) in 5. Seven patients were unclassified. Less common diagnoses included EDS associated with depression and periodic hypersomnia associated with menstruation.

A diagnostic scheme for EDS is shown in Figure 20. An effective diagnosis can be made in most cases without polygraphic sleep recordings or other laboratory tests. The first step is to elicit a history of cataplexy and the second concerns heavy snoring. Drug ingestion should be investigated subsequently. Patients who cannot be diagnosed by these investigations probably have a disorder requiring extensive laboratory testing, but only about 1 in 9 patients in this series had such disorders. If a presumptive diagnosis of sleep apnea is made, the patient should be referred to a sleep laboratory for quantitative evaluation of the syndrome unless the EDS is completely disabling and hemodynamic abnormalities are present.

The distinction between primary and secondary disorders is somewhat arbitrary. The EDS complaint always must be taken seriously; it is no longer acceptable that a long period should elapse before an accurate diagnosis is made.

► [In most patients who complain of excessive daytime sleepiness, the etiologic diagnosis can be made on the basis of clinical symptoms and history. Only a small percentage of patients require sleep recordings and extensive laboratory diagnostic procedures. — Ed.] ◄

Lumping or Splitting? "Ophthalmoplegia-Plus" or Kearns-Sayre Syndrome? It is unclear whether progressive ophthalmoplegia is a neurogenic or myopathic disorder and whether specific syndromes can be delineated. R. A. Berenberg, J. M. Pellock, S. DiMauro, D. L. Schotland, E. Bonilla, A. Eastwood, A. Hays, C. T. Vicale, M. Behrens, A. Chutorian and L. P. Rowland[7] reviewed 5 new cases and 30 from the literature. All patients had progressive external ophthalmoplegia, pigmentary degeneration of the retina, heart block and an onset before age 20 years. Ptosis or ophthalmoplegia was the first diagnostic feature in 31 patients. Pigmentary retinal degeneration was the sole presenting feature or occurred with ophthalmoplegia in 8 patients. Ophthalmoplegia was almost always preceded by ptosis. The retinal degeneration was almost always "atypi-

(7)   Ann. Neurol. 1:37–54, January, 1977.

cal," in contrast to "typical" retinitis pigmentosa. Cardiac conduction defects ranged from prolonged intraventricular conduction time to complete atrioventricular block; the severity of conduction disturbances increased progressively.

Short stature was recorded in 63% of patients, cerebellar signs in 69%, neurosensory hearing loss in 54%, mental retardation in 40%, vestibular dysfunction in 33% and delayed puberty in 33%. Eleven of the 21 patients examined had a myopathic electromyographic pattern.

The manifestations in these cases implicate the retina, brain stem, auditory and vestibular systems, cerebellum, pyramidal tract, skeletal muscle (Fig 20A), hypothalamus and myocardium. Some manifestations may be lacking when the patient is first seen.

When progressive external ophthalmoplegia has its onset in childhood or adolescence and is associated with atypical retinal degeneration and a cardiac conduction defect, the

Fig 20A. – Light micrograph showing increased oxidative enzyme activity in the subsarcolemmal and intermyofibrillar regions of two muscle fibers *(arrows)*. Diphosphopyridine nucleotide-trichrome stain; reduced from ×100. (Courtesy of Berenberg, R.A., et al.: Ann. Neurol. 1:37–54, January, 1977.)

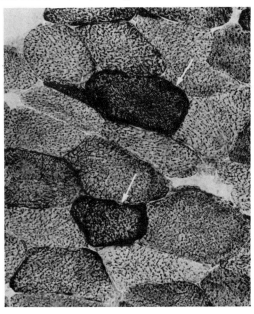

term "Kearns-Sayre syndrome" may be applied. The authors express the belief that the Kearns-Sayre syndrome is a distinct entity within the group of progressive ophthalmoplegias. There is no evidence of genetic abnormality or metabolic defect in the Kearns-Sayre syndrome. The significance of the mitochondrial abnormalities found in muscle is unclear, because they have appeared in many different clinical syndromes and because there is no characteristic biochemical abnormality of isolated mitochondria. The mitochondrial abnormalities are probably secondary and occur as a result of more than one unknown primary defect in the different syndromes.

▶ [Several different neurologic and muscular syndromes may occur in association with chronic progressive ophthalmoplegia. This article deals with a specific syndrome in which progressive external ophthalmoplegia is one manifestation. It does not assert, as one might infer from its title, that the eponym "Kearns-Sayre syndrome" is a synonym for that inaptly named condition "ophthalmoplegia-plus." If progressive external ophthalmoplegia occurs in association with other myopathic, neuromuscular or neural changes, these should be included in the diagnostic term used. In another recent report by I. J. Butler and N. Gadoth (Arch. Intern. Med. 136:1290, 1976), the Kearns-Sayre syndrome is referred to as a multisystem disorder of children and young adults. – Ed.] ◀

Central Pontine Myelinolysis: Clinical Reappraisal is presented by W. C. Wiederholt, Ronald M. Kobayashi, James J. Stockard and Valerie S. Rossiter[8] (Univ. of California, San Diego). The diagnosis of central pontine myelinolysis (CPM) is almost exclusively made at autopsy. Recently 2 patients with the clinical picture of CPM survived. Their time course of recovery was compatible with at least partial pontine remyelination. A third patient died of cardiac arrest while improving neurologically. The 3 men were chronic alcoholics aged 48–59. They had facial weakness, quadriparesis, hyperreflexia and Babinski signs over 1–2 weeks. Two had eye movement abnormalities with preservation of vertical gaze and sensory changes different from those associated with the preexisting alcoholic peripheral neuropathy. Consciousness and higher cerebral functions remained intact throughout the illness. The maximal neurologic deficit lasted 2–4 weeks; improvement continued over many months. The clinical features were indicative of a lesion in the basis pontis and ventral pontine tegmentum.

(8) Arch. Neurol. 34:220–223, April, 1977.

Autopsy examination of the patient who died showed marked softening of the central pons, with gross demyelination, no remyelination, a marked decrease in oligodendroglia, preserved axis cylinders and neurons and debris-laden macrophages. Serial brain stem auditory evoked potential studies in 2 patients provided further evidence that pontine involvement was present in the survivors. Prolonged latencies returned to normal in 6–12 weeks. The patient who died was considerably improved neurologically at the time of death.

Central pontine myelinolysis can be diagnosed clinically and patients may recover if intercurrent illnesses are vigorously treated. Edema may contribute to impaired function before demyelination occurs; intramyelinic edema may have a role in the pathogenesis of CPM. It is possible that early clinical improvement is due to clearing of edema. The continuing improvement seen over 15 months in 1 of the present patients suggests that remyelination probably occurs.

► [The postmortem clinical diagnosis of central pontine myelinosis has been reported in only a very few instances. These authors describe 3 patients, 2 of whom survived with only minimal neurologic deficits. They conclude that patients with this disorder may survive if intercurrent illnesses are treated vigorously.—Ed.] ◄

Neurologic and Psychologic Manifestations of Decompression Illness in Divers. Bruce H. Peters, Harvey S. Levin and Patrick J. Kelly[9] (Univ. of Texas, Galveston) evaluated the neurologic and psychologic status of divers after decompression illness in 20 patients seen for neurologic complaints related to diving. Nineteen were male commercial divers and 1 was a female recreational diver. Ten gave a definite history of at least one episode of decompression illness involving the central nervous system and some reported multiple traumatic decompressions. The interval from the event to examination ranged from 1 day to 2 years. The test battery included the Wechsler scales, the Reitan Trail Making test, the Reitan Finger-Tapping test, a digit storage test and the Minnesota Multiphasic Personality Inventory (MMPI).

Eight divers were neurologically abnormal. Six had cerebral defects on mental status testing. Cerebellar abnormalities and brain stem dysfunction also were observed. Seven of

(9)   Neurology (Minneap.) 27:125–127, February, 1977.

19 divers exhibited deficits of cerebral dysfunction on neuropsychologic assessment. The findings were equivocal in 4 patients. Impaired divers scored below normal on both verbal and relatively nonverbal subtests of the Wechsler scales. They exhibited a marked disruption of storage of new information and were significantly slow on the Reitan test. The MMPI showed greater acute distress, depression, anxiety and somatic concern in impaired divers. All 7 divers with abnormal neurologic findings who had neuropsychologic testing were impaired. Nine of 10 divers whose histories suggested central nervous system decompression illness had abnormalities on either neurologic or neuropsychology testing.

These findings contrast with the widely held view that diving-related central nervous system decompression illness is largely confined to the spinal cord. Most affected divers had neurologic findings compatible with multiple lesions, usually affecting more than one area of the nervous system. Decompression illness of the central nervous system in divers probably does not differ materially from that described in caisson workers or in high altitude flyers. Baseline neurobehavioral studies of professional divers at the time of initial employment would help clarify the extent of central nervous system dysfunction after subsequent real or alleged episodes of central nervous system decompression illness. Such testing might help predict accident-proneness, psychosomatic illness or the potential for symptom accentuation due to emotional instability.

► [This study shows that diffuse and multiple central nervous system abnormalities may result from decompression illness. The importance of thorough neurologic and neuropsychologic evaluation of patients after diving accidents is stressed. – Ed.] ◄

Neocortical Cholinergic Neurons in Elderly People. Choline acetyltransferase (CAT) activity, a potential marker of the presynaptic cholinergic system, appears to be reduced in neocortex from patients with Alzheimer's disease or senile dementia. Senile degeneration and neocortical neuronal loss can be as intense in elderly demented persons with appreciable cerebrovascular disease as in Alzheimer's disease. P. White, C. R. Hiley, M. J. Goodhardt, L. H. Carrasco, J. P. Keet, I. E. I. Williams and D. M. Bowen[1]

(1) Lancet 1:668–671, Mar. 26, 1977.

(London, England) measured CAT activity and muscarinic receptor binding sites in brain tissue taken at autopsy from both mentally normal and demented old persons. Study was made of 14 normal brains, 8 cases of Alzheimer's disease, 7 of mixed senile and vascular dementia and 9 "psychiatric" control cases. The age range was 65 – 93.

Receptor binding sites declined with advancing age in control cases, independent of mental state. The CAT activity was not significantly correlated with age at death. The CAT activity was 64% of the age-matched control value for cortex in cases of organic "senile-type" dementia without appreciable senile degeneration. In Alzheimer's disease, CAT activity was 50% of normal, whereas receptor binding was unchanged. The cholinergic markers were not significantly reduced in mixed senile and vascular dementia.

Apart from the age at onset, there is no good reason on neuropathologic grounds to separate Alzheimer's disease from senile dementia. The presynaptic cholinergic system is probably important in Alzheimer's disease; the neurofibrillary change is probably related to this biochemical defect. The intraneuronal deposition of tangles may reduce neuronal activity and metabolism, with a decrease in the amount of CAT apoenzyme per neuron resulting. Alternatively, reduced CAT activity and essentially normal receptor binding may reflect the balance between changes due to "denervation supersensitivity" and the selective loss of cholinergic neurons. Because the density of receptor binding sites appears to be nearly normal in Alzheimer's disease, treatment with central acting anticholinesterases may be beneficial, particularly before neuronal loss is advanced.

► [Although the cause of Alzheimer's disease is unknown, it has been suggested that the presynaptic cholinergic system is important in development of the disease. The neurofibrillary changes present in the disease may be due to this biochemical defect. On the basis of the biochemical studies presented by these authors, it is suggested that treatment with centrally acting anticholinesterase agents may be beneficial in this disease, particularly if they can be administered before neuronal loss becomes advanced. – Ed.] ◄

Multiple Sclerosis

Cerebrospinal Fluid T and B Lymphocyte Kinetics Related to Exacerbations of Multiple Sclerosis. Cellular immune responses have been implicated in the pathogenesis of multiple sclerosis. Jeffrey C. Allen, William Sheremata, J. B. R. Cosgrove, Kirk Osterland and Mary Shea[2] (Royal Victoria Hosp., Montreal) used the E-rosette assay to enumerate thymus-derived or T cells and the fluoresceinated rabbit antihuman immunoglobulin assay to enumerate bone marrow-derived or B cells in specimens of cerebrospinal fluid and blood from patients with multiple sclerosis. Patients with optic neuritis only and those with neuromyelitis optica or who had received steroid or other immunosuppressive therapy were excluded from study. Cerebrospinal fluid was sampled randomly from patients with stable disease and at intervals after the onset of a new attack in those with relapsing disease.

Twenty-one patients had a relapsing course and 10 had a stable course. Age at onset and mean cerebrospinal fluid protein measurements were similar in both groups. The respective mean ages were 30.4 and 45.7 years and the respective mean duration of illness was 3.2 and 15.6 years. The T cells in cerebrospinal fluid varied significantly after onset of an attack in the relapsing group; peak values were found in the 1st week. The B cells tended to increase by the 3d week. Patients with a stable course had a lower percentage of T cells and more nonreacting cells compared to those in the 1st week of relapse; B cells did not vary significantly in this group. Blood T cells were reduced in number in the relapsing group. The cerebrospinal fluid B cell number was significantly lower than the blood count. Sequential cerebrospinal fluid cell assays in a patient having a prolonged relapse are shown in Figure 21.

Patients with long-standing, relatively inactive multiple

(2) Neurology (Minneap.) 26:579–583, June, 1976.

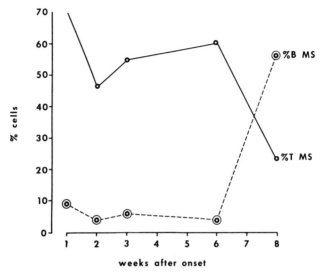

Fig 21.—Sequential cerebrospinal fluid and B cell assays in 1 patient with a prolonged multiple sclerosis relapse. (Courtesy of Allen, J. C., et al.: Neurology (Minneap.) 26:579–583, June, 1976.)

sclerosis in this preliminary study had reduced T cells and increased null cells in the cerebrospinal fluid, whereas patients with acute relapsing disease had the highest proportion of T cells. These observations further implicate cellular immune responses in the pathogenesis of multiple sclerosis.

► [These findings give further evidence of the presence of cellular immune mechanisms in the pathogenesis of multiple sclerosis. – Ed.] ◄

Histocompatibility Studies and Multiple Sclerosis are discussed by Dale E. McFarlin and Henry F. McFarland[3] (Natl. Inst. of Health). Most studies have reported an increased frequency of HL-A7 and, to a lesser extent, of HL-A3 in multiple sclerosis, and increases or decreases in other HL-A antigens also have been described. Although significant, the association between serologically detectable (SD) determinants and multiple sclerosis is not strong. A more marked correlation with a lymphocyte-detected (LD) determinant has been identified. About 60% of multiple sclerosis patients express the LD-7a antigen, which is strongly asso-

(3)　Arch. Neurol. 33:395–398, June, 1976.

ciated with the HL-A7 antigen of the Four locus. An even more striking correlation has been reported with respect to a proposed HL-B antigen, Ag-7a, which is found in about 33% of normal LD-7a persons and in 18% of normal non-LD-7a persons.

Studies in familial multiple sclerosis have been interpreted as generally supporting the view that a histocompatibility-linked gene or genes are related to the occurrence of multiple sclerosis. There is an increase in the frequency of HL-A7 in family studies, but the incidence in affected compared to unaffected family members is more difficult to assess. Studies of the relationship between the magnitude of the humoral immune responses to measles virus and HL-A antigens have given conflicting results. It is not possible at present to reconcile the discrepancies between various studies. The relationship of histocompatibility type to immune response has been studied only with respect to humoral responses in multiple sclerosis. Because Ir genes are related to T cell responsiveness, the cell-mediated immune response may be of considerable importance and may have a direct or inverse relationship with the humoral response.

It remains likely that studies of histocompatibility antigens in relationship to specific humoral and cellular immune mechanisms will contribute to the understanding of multiple sclerosis. Studies of familial cases may be of value in delineating the role of genetic factors. The full understanding of these variables awaits a clearer definition of the histocompatibility-linked genes in man and the development of reliable and reproducible tests for T and B cell responsiveness to particular antigens.

▶ [The various histocompatibility studies taken together point to a multifactorial etiology in multiple sclerosis. Whereas individual genetic factors may relate to the degree of susceptibility to the disease, geographic studies suggest an environmental element as a causative factor. Numerous related articles are published in Volume 33 of *Archives of Neurology* June, 1976. Among these are "Immunogenetic Analysis and Serum Viral Antibody Titers in Multiple Sclerosis, by J. N. Whitaker et al. (pp. 399–403); "Histocompatibility Types and Viral Antibodies" by J. R. Lehrich and B. G. W. Aranason (pp. 404–405); "Histocompatibility (HL-A) Factors in Familial Multiple Sclerosis," by D. A. Drachman et al. (pp. 406–413); "Antibodies to Vaccinia and Measles Viruses in Multiple Sclerosis," by H. Miyamoto et al. (pp. 414–417); and "Neuroelectric Blocking Factors in Multiple Sclerosis and Normal Human Serums," by F. J. Seil et al. (pp. 418–422).—Ed.] ◀

Disease Markers in Acute Multiple Sclerosis. Peter C. Dowling (VA Hosp., East Orange, N. J.) and Stuart D. Cook[4] (College of Medicine and Dentistry of New Jersey, Newark) have conducted a series of studies to find a simple serologic method of determining disease activity in multiple sclerosis (MS). Review was made of the serologic findings in 13 acutely ill patients with MS; all had findings of active demyelinating disease of central origin and none had secondary complications. Multiple sclerosis was proved by tissue study or autopsy in 3 cases. Twelve patients were ambulatory after discharge and during the study.

Positive C-reactive protein tests were obtained in 70% of cases. Serum levels of two other acute-phase reactants, C3PA (C3 proactivator) and orosomucoid, substantially were elevated in over half the patients. Serum IgM levels also were increased in nearly half the patients. In 2 sequentially studied patients, clinical recovery was associated with a substantial decline in the levels of these serum proteins. In 1 case, initial serum levels were in the high-normal range, while subsequent levels were higher and then lower levels returned, emphasizing the importance of obtaining serum over a long period at weekly intervals.

The peripheral blood of acutely ill MS patients often contains substantially elevated levels of C-reactive protein, orosomucoid, C3PA and IgM, which may show close correlation with disease activity. Further studies are needed to document the relationship between these circulating substances and disease activity. A more rational approach to therapy, cause and pathogenesis may result.

► [The findings suggest that measurement of these serum proteins may be of value in assessing the progress of disease activity in multiple sclerosis. —Ed.] ◄

Multiple Sclerosis and Cell-Mediated Hypersensitivity to Myelin A_1 Protein. Multiple sclerosis (MS) has long been considered an autoimmune disease but few studies have provided direct support for this hypothesis. Sheremata et al. showed that macrophage migration inhibition factor (MIF) production regularly could be found within 3 weeks of an attack. William Sheremata, J. B. R. Cosgrove and E. H.

(4) Arch. Neurol. 33:668–670, October, 1976.

Eylar[5] (McGill Univ.) have now determined the frequency with which cell-mediated hypersensitivity to myelin basic (A_1) protein is found in MS.

Studies were done in 246 patients, including 100 with suspected or probable MS, 48 with other central nervous system disease, 48 with peripheral nervous system disease and 50 normal subjects. There were 79 patients with "probable" MS and 21 with "suspect" MS. Studies were done using human A_1 protein of high purity and the macrophage MIF assay.

The results are shown in Figure 22. The mean migration index was 59% within 4 weeks of an acute attack and 86% in the convalescent group. The mean index in "chronic" patients studied 6 months or more after an attack was 91%.

Fig 22. – Results in acute group (up to 4 weeks after onset of attack) compared with convalescent (5 – 12 weeks after onset) and chronic groups (24 or more weeks after onset) and suspect MS patients. Solid line represents 2 SD below mean migration in controls. Values below this line are considered significant. Mean migrations in each column are indicated by dotted line. (Courtesy of Sheremata, W., et al.: J. Neurol. Sci. 27:413–425, April, 1976.)

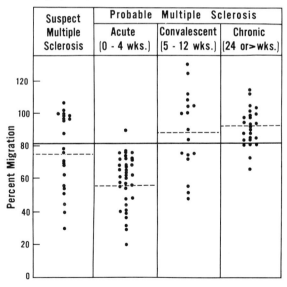

(5)   J. Neurol. Sci. 27:413–425, April, 1976.

The overall mean index for MS patients was 75%, compared to 91% for 15 patients with cerebral infarction. A few patients with postinfectious encephalomyelitis or spinocerebellar degenerations had positive results as did 3 of 22 with the Guillain-Barré syndrome. Eight of 44 patients with peripheral nervous system disease showed evidence of cell-mediated hypersensitivity to human A_1 protein.

Cell-mediated hypersensitivity to myelin basic protein is present at the onset of acute exacerbations of MS. A temporal relationship has been found between acute attacks of MS and in vitro evidence of cellular hypersensitivity to this central nervous system antigen. The findings support the concept but do not prove that MS is the result of such hypersensitization. It remains to be shown that sensitization in MS is directed toward the encephalitogenic portions of the basic protein molecule.

► [The results of this study clearly establish a temporal relationship between in vitro evidence of hypersensitivity to A_1 protein in patients with multiple sclerosis and the clinical expression of the disease. Whereas these results give support to the hypothesis that multiple sclerosis is an autoimmune disease, it must be borne in mind that similar results were found in other diseases of the nervous system, some of which, like cerebral infarction, obviously are not autoimmune disorders. The genetic, environmental and other factors that result in the emergence of cellular hypersensitivity to this encephalitogenic antigen await elucidation. — Ed.]

Blood Test for Multiple Sclerosis Based on Adherence of Lymphocytes to Measles-Infected Cells. The initial diagnosis of multiple sclerosis (MS) is usually difficult. The increased capacity of lymphocytes from these patients to adhere to human epithelial cells persistently infected with measles virus has provided an accurate blood test for MS. Nelson L. Levy, Paul S. Auerbach and Edward C. Hayes[6] (Duke Univ.) examined the potential of the measles-adherent lymphocyte test on peripheral blood as a diagnostic test for MS.

Studies were done in 27 patients with unequivocal MS, 19 of them women. The age range was 22–57. Ten patients were in remission, 9 had active disease and 8 had slowly progressive disease but had had no new lesions in the past 6 months. Twenty-six patients with various other neurologic diseases and 10 healthy controls were also evaluated. Hu-

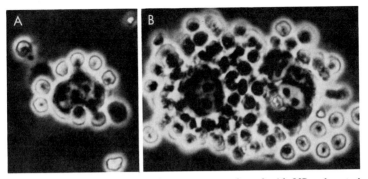

Fig 23. — Qualitative difference between rosettes formed with MS and control lymphocytes in phase contrast photomicrographs. **A,** typical rosette formed between measles-infected HEp-2 cells and control lymphocytes. **B,** aggregated rosettes that formed between measles-infected HEp-2 cells and lymphocytes from patients with MS, in whom both single and aggregated rosettes were seen. Only single rosettes were seen in controls; reduced from ×300. (Courtesy of Levy, N. L., et al.: N. Engl. J. Med. 294:1423–1427, June 24, 1976.)

man epithelial (HEp-2) cells persistently infected with Edmonston measles virus were used in the assay for measles-adherent lymphocytes. The E rosette-forming lymphocytes were also assayed.

The mean proportion of measles-infected cells that formed rosettes with lymphocytes from study patients was over twice that from controls. There was a complete lack of overlap between the MS and control groups. No differences were found between study patients in the active stage and those in remission or with slowly progressive disease. The rosettes formed with lymphocytes from study patients often aggregated into large masses (Fig 23). There was no significant difference in percentages of E rosette-forming cells in the peripheral blood of patients with MS and controls.

This study indicates the diagnostic potential of the test for adherence of lymphocytes to measles-infected cells in MS. The degree of rosette formation was unaffected by the severity, duration or activity of the disease. Possibly measles infection alters normal cell surface structures and provides a general recognition site for a T cell subpopulation, or measles-associated determinants themselves are cross-reactive with such recognition structures.

▶ [The authors state that the increased capacity of lymphocytes from patients with multiple sclerosis to adhere to human epithelial cells persistently infected with measles virus has provided an accurate blood test for multiple sclerosis. The severity, duration and activity of the disease do not influence the activity of the test. Further studies are necessary, however, to isolate and characterize the lymphocyte and measles cell receptors and to investigate the role of the receptors in various immunologic functions.

In a letter to the editor, H. Offner et al. (N. Engl. J. Med. 296:451, 1977), using the same method and cell line as Levy et al., obtained the same positive results as did the original observers, but found further that the values of patients with multiple sclerosis overlapped with those of patients with other neurologic diseases. This was contrary to the findings of Levy et al. Offner et al. express the belief that the final conclusion of these experiments must await confirmation from other laboratories using standardized conditions of the rosetting test. — Ed.] ◄

Acute Optic Neuritis and Prognosis for Multiple Sclerosis. There is wide variation in the reported incidence of multiple sclerosis (MS) after optic neuritis. W. M. Hutchinson[7] (Royal Victoria Hosp., Belfast) reviewed data on all patients with a diagnosis of acute optic neuritis or MS initiated by acute optic neuritis during 1960–74 at major hospitals in Northern Ireland.

Among the 152 patients, 8 children under age 12 were excluded, 5 had died of causes related to MS and 12 were lost to follow-up. Attacks of optic neuritis had been unilateral in 57% of the patients, recurrent in 24% and bilateral in 19%. Women constituted 73% of the entire series. Three fourths of the patients were aged 20–50; the median age of onset of acute optic neuritis was 29. Attack rates were highest in April to July and low in August to November.

The onset of visual symptoms was sudden in 20% of the patients. Pain was present in 77% of the patients and papillitis was described in 17%. Acuity at follow-up was poorer in patients with recurrent attacks than in the others but only 2 patients were left with severe visual disability. The cerebrospinal fluid was abnormal in 11 of 31 patients evaluated during the acute attack. Further features of MS developed in 51% of the patients followed and in 65% of patients with bilateral neuritis. The mean follow-up period was about 90 months. The follow-up findings are shown in Figure 24.

The probability of developing MS after an attack of optic neuritis increases steadily with time. Over 75% of the patients may be so affected after 15 years. The likelihood of MS developing soon after acute optic neuritis varies according

(7) J. Neurol. Neurosurg. Psychiatry 39:283–289, March, 1976.

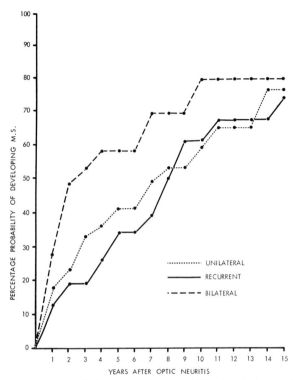

Fig 24. – Percentage probability of developing multiple sclerosis for up to 15 years after attack of unilateral, recurrent or bilateral optic neuritis. (Courtesy of Hutchinson, W. M.: J. Neurol. Neurosurg. Psychiatry 39:283 – 289, March, 1976.)

to the type of initial attack but the risk is not related to the presence or absence of a cerebrospinal fluid abnormality. Bilateral optic neuritis in adults appears to have a worse prognosis than either unilateral or recurrent optic neuritis for the development of earlier and more disabling MS.

▶ [Earlier investigators, including McAlpine (Brain 84:186, 1961), stated that up to 85% of patients who had optic neuritis and were studied for up to 5 years acquired manifestations of multiple sclerosis. In contrast, Kurland et al. (Acta Neurol Scand. [Suppl 19] p. 157, 1966), observing United States Army servicemen for 12– 18 years, stated that only 13% developed multiple sclerosis. This study by Hutchinson leads us back to the former concept in that 78% of patients with optic neuritis have the probability of developing multiple sclerosis. It is of interest, however, that in three

Multiple Sclerosis Cerebrospinal Fluid Produces Myelin Lesions in Tadpole Optic Nerves. Demyelinating factors have not been identified in unconcentrated cerebrospinal fluid from patients with multiple sclerosis (MS) by tissue-culture techniques. Takeshi Tabira, Henry deF. Webster and Shirley H. Wray[8] report the use of an in vivo model system, the optic nerves of xenopus tadpoles, for double-blind tests of human cerebrospinal fluid myelinotoxic activity. The test requires only 0.5 ml cerebrospinal fluid, and the results are known in 5 days.

Cerebrospinal fluid was obtained from 46 patients, including 19 with MS, 7 with acute idiopathic optic neuritis and 20 control subjects with other neurologic diseases. None was receiving steroids, other drugs or irradiation. Double-blind tests for cerebrospinal fluid myelinotoxic activity were carried out by injecting cerebrospinal fluid near the optic nerve in tadpoles and preparing whole mounts of optic nerves 48 hours later. A differential interference microscope was used to count myelin lesions.

Cerebrospinal fluid samples from 60% of the patients with acute, definite MS had myelinotoxic activity. This activity correlated best with the severity and duration of the disease, rather than with γ-globulin or total protein concentrations. Activity was absent in 85% of samples from control subjects. The most common abnormality was the presence of small ovoids scattered along myelin internodes. Generally the axons remained normal. One of 9 samples from patients with possible MS was positive, and 1 was borderline. No sample from a patient with acute optic neuritis had significant myelinotoxic activity. Heating cerebrospinal fluid samples at 56 C for 30 minutes destroyed the myelinotoxic activity.

These data may be consistent with the results of tests of concentrated cerebrospinal fluid in tissue cultures. Although the mechanisms responsible for the effect are not defined and may be complex, this in vivo test appears to be a useful means of investigating cerebrospinal fluid myelinotoxic factors in MS. The relationship of positive activity to

(8) N. Engl. J. Med. 295:644–649, Sept. 16, 1976.

the clinical course of MS remains to be explored, and fractions of positive cerebrospinal fluids should be prepared and tested for their myelinotoxic effects.

▶ [Many years ago, attempts were made to demonstrate myelinolytic activity in the cerebrospinal fluid and serum of patients with multiple sclerosis, but the studies were made on human spinal cord without tissue culture. Methods were not as well developed as they are at this time. Positive results were produced in this study, but the authors believe that although the test is useful in investigating myelinotoxic factors in cerebrospinal fluid of patients with multiple sclerosis, it may not be helpful in diagnosis. — Ed.] ◀

Changes in Nystagmus on Raising Body Temperature in Clinically Suspected and Proved Multiple Sclerosis. An increase in body temperature in multiple sclerosis often causes a transient deterioration in clinical status. The inconvenient "hot bath" test has been widely used in diagnosis in cases of suspected multiple sclerosis. J. V. Jestico and P. D. M. Ellis[9] (London) devised a simple, quantitative method of studying the appearance or alteration of nystagmus induced by changes in body temperature. Studies were done in 15 patients with definite and 12 with suspected multiple sclerosis, 12 with other neurologic diseases and 10 normal subjects. Horizontal eye movements were recorded as body temperature was raised by 1 C with a standard heat

Fig 25. — Electronystagmogram from patient with clinically definite multiple sclerosis, showing increased nystagmus after body temperature was raised. (Courtesy of Jestico, J. V., and Ellis, P. D. M.: Br. Med. J. 2:970–972, Oct. 23, 1976.)

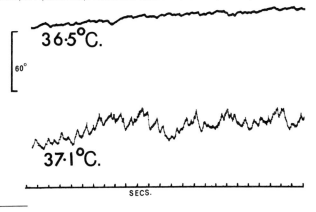

cradle operated by electric lamps. The patients lay on a couch and were covered by blankets.

Seven patients with definite multiple sclerosis had nystagmus at normal body temperature, and in all of them it was increased by heating (Fig 25). Six other patients developed nystagmus after heating. Five patients with suspected multiple sclerosis had nystagmus basally, and in all it was increased by heating. Three others in this group developed nystagmus after heating. Six patients with other neurologic diseases had nystagmus at normal body temperature, and 3 other patients had nystagmus after stapedectomy. None had an increase in nystagmus on body heating. Three patients in this group had no nystagmus either before or after heating. No control subject had nystagmus before or after heating.

Multiple sclerosis patients with nystagmus show an increase in nystagmus on body heating, and many patients without nystagmus basally develop it on body heating. Similar phenomena are seen in patients with suspected multiple sclerosis. This technique may be a practicable diagnostic procedure, especially in cases of spastic paraparesis in which a definite level below the brain stem can be identified. The necessary equipment is in current use. The technique is simple, causes little patient disconfort and may be performed in the outpatient clinic. It is expected to provide useful further information in patients suspected of having multiple sclerosis.

► [This test is an amplification of the observation originally made by Uhthoff that raising the body temperature causes a transient increase in the clinical manifestations of multiple sclerosis, although these authors fail to give credit to the original observer. The technique is simple to use and may have a role in the diagnosis of multiple sclerosis. – Ed.] ◄

Mental Change as an Early Feature of Multiple Sclerosis. It is recognized that mental and emotional changes occur in patients with multiple sclerosis, but mental changes are considered to be rare in the early stages of the disease. A. C. Young, J. Saunders and J. R. Ponsford[1] (Oxford, England) describe 5 patients who had mental change as a prominent and early feature of an illness that appeared to be multiple sclerosis. All also had clinical signs of pre-

(1) J. Neurol. Neurosurg. Psychiatry 39:1008–1013, October, 1976.

dominant brain stem involvement, and the cerebrospinal fluid findings were similar.

Woman, 30, had begun neglecting her housework 4 years earlier and had become nervous and inactive. Diplopia developed about a year later, and examination had shown ptosis, disorganized eye movements, vertical nystagmus and hyperreflexia. The full-scale Wechsler IQ was 97 at this time, representing a fall-off in the premorbid level. Steroids produced apparent improvement, but next year the mental state deteriorated and the patient became ataxic and dysarthric. An air study showed ventricular dilatation and the right optic disc was pale. The IQ was 76 at this time. At current admission the patient exhibited dysphagia, occasional urinary incontinence and intermittent diplopia. She was disoriented for place and performed intellectual tasks poorly. Examination showed nystagmus, a left lower motor neuron facial palsy, dysarthria, a dystonic neck posture and ataxia of all limbs. Plantar responses were extensor. An EEG showed a moderately severe, diffuse abnormality. The cerebrospinal fluid contained 0.3 gm protein per L and had a Lange curve of 4433221.

All the patients had evidence of intellectual impairment on simple bedside testing, confirmed by more detailed psychologic testing. A change in affect or deterioration in intellect had been noticed at or soon after onset of illness. Four patients presented with behavioral or intellectual change. In each case the clinical picture ultimately suggested multiple sclerosis. Three patients had extremely high cerebrospinal fluid IgG levels and paretic Lange curves.

Early mental changes in multiple sclerosis are invariably associated with widespread plaques of demyelination not confined to the brain stem. Diffuse cerebral hemispheric damage probably accounts for the mental changes even in patients in whom clinically the brain stem is predominantly affected. Multiple sclerosis deserves to be considered more frequently in the differential diagnosis of behavioral and mental change in the young patient, even in the absence of neurologic signs.

▶ [Intellectual deterioration and other mental changes may be early features of multiple sclerosis, even in those patients in whom the onset of the disease is insidious. — Ed.] ◀

Transfer-Factor Therapy in Multiple Sclerosis. There is circumstantial evidence suggesting an abnormal immunologic process in multiple sclerosis (MS) and stronger evidence implicating a viral infection. The two mechanisms are not mutually exclusive. Transfer factor has been used beneficially in the immunotherapy of viral infections. Peter O. Behan, Ian D. Melville, William F. Durward, Anne P. McGeorge and Wilhelmina M. H. Behan[2] (Glasgow) studied the effect of transfer factor, prepared from relatives of MS patients and from unrelated donors, on the course of MS in 15 patients of each sex with the disease. The mean age of men was 30 years and of women, 34 years. The respective average durations of disease were 4 and 7 years. Forty-five donors aged 18–60 years, 30 relatives and 15 unrelated donors, were used; all had been in good health. Either transfer factor or placebo was given intramuscularly and two additional injections followed at monthly intervals. After 3 months, the procedures were repeated. Fifteen patients in the trial received transfer factor and 15 received placebo.

No adverse reactions to transfer factor were noted. One patient left the trial because of a lack of progress. No clinical difference between transfer factor and placebo was found and no EEG differences were seen. The abnormal visual evoked potentials found in some patients before the trial were unchanged afterward. No change in the cerebrospinal fluid cell content was found in either group. Variations in total cerebrospinal fluid protein and IgG were comparable in the transfer factor-treated and placebo patients.

Transfer factor was ineffective in this trial of patients with MS. The putative specific MS antigen is unknown and the transfer factor may not have transferred sensitivity to this. Exquisite sensitization is necessary in the donor before successful transfer can be done. Blocking factors in the recipient may also account for the failure. Further trials of transfer factor in MS seem unnecessary until more is known of the causal agent and of the pathogenesis of MS.

► [Patients with multiple sclerosis and their families follow the news media carefully and discuss with friends and acquaintances any possible leads regarding the treatment of the disorder. The use of transfer factor is one such therapeutic regimen about which questions are often asked. This study indicates that it appears to have no therapeutic value. – Ed.] ◄

Chronic Relapsing Experimental Allergic Encephalomyelitis: Experimental Model of Multiple Sclerosis.

(2)   Lancet 1:988–990, May 8, 1976.

H. M. Wiśniewski and A. B. Keith[3] (Genl. Hosp., Newcastle upon Tyne, England) induced a chronic relapsing form of experimental allergic encephalomyelitis (EAE) by single sensitization of immature strain-13 and Hartley strain guinea pigs. Antigen was prepared by homogenizing guinea pig spinal cord in saline with Freund's adjuvant. Antigen was injected into the dorsa of the feet or into the nuchal area.

Acute monophasic EAE developed in 30 of 52 Hartley animals inoculated in all 4 feet. It was characterized by weight loss and varying degrees of paraparesis or tetraparesis. The disease began an average of 18 days after sensitization and animals survived for 1 – 11 days more. Twelve animals acquired chronic relapsing EAE. The second episode resembled the first clinically but the neurologic signs lasted 7 – 14 days. Remissions after second attacks lasted 30 – 60 days in most animals. No animal recovered completely after a third episode. Relapsing disease also developed in some animals sensitized by nuchal injections or into the dorsa of 2 feet.

Fig 26. – Low-magnification view of two plaques, recent one on right and old one on left. Recent plaque contains dark, scattered dots aggregated in cuff form around vessels. (Courtesy of Wiśniewski, H. M., and Keith, A. B.: Ann. Neurol. 1:144 – 148, February, 1977.)

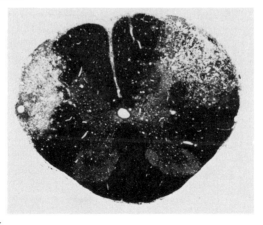

---

(3) Ann. Neurol. 1:144 – 148, February, 1977.

Chronic relapsing EAE was characterized histologically by the presence of old and recent demyelinating plaques (Fig 26). Plaques were present in the cord of Hartley guinea pigs and in the cord, brain and cerebellum of strain-13 animals. The thoracic and lumbosacral segments of the cord were the areas most affected. The old lesions were generally free of inflammatory cells. Remyelination was common in old plaques.

A chronic relapsing form of EAE has been developed in guinea pigs. Substantial morphologic differences were found between the two strains of guinea pigs used in the present study. The sequence of events leading to demyelination in multiple sclerosis appears to be similar to that observed in EAE. If this is so, the chronic relapsing form of EAE will permit study of the immunologic mechanism involved in the pathogenesis of multiple sclerosis. Relapsing EAE also appears to be the best laboratory model for evaluating drugs used to treat multiple sclerosis.

► [At present, the closest approach to an experimental model of multiple sclerosis is experimental allergic encephalomyelitis. Its normal course, however, is not marked by unpredictable cycles of exacerbation and remission, so characteristic of multiple sclerosis. The relapsing experimental encephalomyelitis produced by these investigators shows more resemblance clinically to multiple sclerosis; thus, it may be a medium for studying the immunologic mechanisms underlying the course of multiple sclerosis and may offer new opportunities for evaluating the effects of drugs in its treatment. — Ed.] ◄

Myasthenia Gravis

Myasthenia Gravis: Study of Humoral Immune Mechanisms by Passive Transfer to Mice. The site of the defect in myasthenia gravis was identified recently as the acetylcholine receptor. The finding of myasthenic features in rabbits immunized with acetylcholine receptor suggested that a similar autoimmune process might occur in man. Klaus V. Toyka, Daniel B. Drachman, Diane E. Griffin, Alan Pestronk, Jerry A. Winkelstein, Kenneth H. Fischbeck, Jr., and Ing Kao[4] (Johns Hopkins Univ.) found that passive transfer of a serum immunoglobulin fraction from myasthenic patients reproduces typical features of the disease in mice and used this model to study the nature of myasthenia-producing factor and its mode of action. Study was made of 16 patients. A decrement of more than 15% on repetitive nerve stimulation at 2 or 5 Hz was demonstrated in 15 patients. Immunoglobulins were injected into mice daily for 1–14 days.

Typical myasthenic features of reduction in amplitude of miniature end-plate potentials or a reduction in acetylcholine receptors at neuromuscular junctions were produced by immunoglobulin from 15 of the 16 study patients. The mean reduction in end-plate potential amplitude was more than 50%, and the mean reduction in receptors was more than 50%. Some mice also showed weakness or decremental responses to repetitive nerve stimulation. The active fraction was identified as IgG by three different purification methods. Its effect was enhanced by C3, but C5 had no effect. A loose correlation was found between the clinical state of patients and the myasthenia-producing activity in mice; immunoglobulin from the most severely affected patients produced unequivocal myasthenic effects in all recipient mice.

The serums of most myasthenic patients contain an im-

(4) N. Engl. J. Med. 296:125–131, Jan. 20, 1977.

munoglobulin factor capable of producing typical features of myasthenia gravis in mice. The action of the myasthenic IgG in the recipient animal is influenced by the complement system. The transfer appears to be a truly passive effect. The present findings are consistent with the concept of myasthenia gravis as an autoimmune disorder. The data strongly suggest that the pathogenesis of myasthenia gravis commonly involves an antibody-mediated autoimmune attack directed against the acetylcholine receptors of the neuromuscular junction.

Myasthenia: Recent Immunologic Data were reviewed by O. Meyer[5] (Paris). The immunologic approach in myasthenia rests on clinical and laboratory observations in the human being. Experimental studies in animals have reproduced the human disease and have led to evidence in favor of an autoimmune pathogenesis.

The exact pathogenic mechanism, however, is still unknown. But two schemata are hereby proposed, and a compromise is probable between a thymus hormone (a polypeptide substance of the thymus or thymopoietin) and antiacetylcholine receptor (anti-AChR) antibodies:

$$1. \text{ Etiologic agent(s)} \rightarrow \text{autoimmune reaction} \begin{array}{l} \nearrow \text{thymitis} \\ \\ \searrow \text{block} \end{array}$$
$$\text{against AChR}$$

$$2. \text{ Etiologic agent(s)} \rightarrow \text{thymitis} \rightarrow \text{thymopoietin} \rightarrow \text{autoimmune block}$$

Modern immunologic data have little application at present. It is important to search for a thymoma of the HL-A3 or HL-A2 tissue group in myasthenic persons. In effect, treatment for human myasthenia remains empirical and palliative because it rests on anticholinesterases and, in certain cases, thymectomy. The beneficial effect of corticosteroid therapy in certain forms cannot be ascribed to an immunosuppressant action because the doses used are too small to maintain this action regularly. Corticoids could, however, diminish the sensitivity of lymphocytes to AChR.

(5) Nouv. Presse Med. 5:2459–2463, Nov. 6, 1976.

Treatments based directly on autoimmune pathogenesis, such as use of immunosuppressants, antilymphocytic serum or cannulation of the thoracic canal, are too recent and the results too fragmented for reasonable evaluation of their effectiveness.

► [The data in this article and the preceding one suggest that the pathogenesis of myasthenia gravis often involves an antibody-mediated autoimmune attack on the acetylcholine receptors at the neuromuscular junction. — Ed.] ◄

Antibody to Acetylcholine Receptor in Myasthenia Gravis: Prevalence, Clinical Correlates and Diagnostic Value. Animals immunized with acetylcholine receptor exhibit striking similarities to patients with myasthenia gravis. Animals with experimental autoimmune myasthenia gravis acquire antibodies to acetylcholine receptor. Jon M. Lindstrom, Marjorie E. Seybold, Vanda A. Lennon, Senga Whittingham and Drake D. Duane[6] correlated antibody titers with clinical parameters of myasthenia gravis in 71 patients. Studies were also done of 175 patients without myasthenia, including some with other neurologic or autoimmune diseases. Myasthenia was confirmed by tests with edrophonium, neostigmine or curare in all but 2 cases. Serums were assayed for antibodies to human muscle acetylcholine receptor by immunoprecipitation.

The findings are shown in Figure 27. Only serums from patients with myasthenia gravis caused precipitation of large amounts of ^{125}I-toxin-labeled acetylcholine receptor. Serums from nonmyasthenic patients caused precipitation differing only slightly from that present nonspecifically in control samples. Significant titers were found in 87% of patients with myasthenia gravis. Patients with thymoma had higher titers than thymectomized patients, and those with ocular myasthenia had lower titers than those with mild or moderate generalized disease. Only 6 of 16 serums from myasthenic patients inhibited toxin binding to acetylcholine receptor preincubated with serum to a greater extent than any normal serum.

Antireceptor antibody similar to that found in animals with experimental autoimmune myasthenia gravis is detectable in patients with myasthenia gravis. Antireceptor,

---

(6) Neurology (Minneap.) 26:1054–1059, November, 1976.

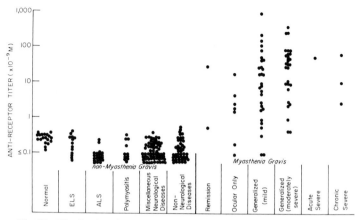

Fig 27.—Distribution of antireceptor antibody titers in subjects with and without myasthenia gravis. *ELS,* Eaton-Lambert syndrome; *ALS,* amyotrophic lateral sclerosis. (Courtesy of Lindstrom, J. M., et al.: Neurology [Minneap.] 26:1054–1059, November, 1976.)

but not antiacetylcholine site, antibody is found in most myasthenic patients but not in patients without myasthenia gravis. Assay of antireceptor antibody may prove to be a useful test in the diagnosis of myasthenia gravis.

▶ [Assay of antireceptor antibody should prove to be a useful test in the diagnosis of myasthenia gravis.—Ed.] ◄

Long-Term Administration of Corticosteroids in Myasthenia Gravis. J. Douglas Mann, T. R. Johns and Justiniano F. Campa[7] (Univ. of Virginia Med. Center) report experience with high- and, subsequently, lower-dose prednisone therapy in 30 consecutive patients with myasthenia gravis. The 16 female and 14 male patients, aged 13–81 years, had 45 incidents of prednisone therapy for myasthenia gravis. The mean duration of illness before the first treatment with prednisone was 4 years. Three patients had polymyositis, 2 had benign thymomas, 1 had a malignant thymoma and 1 each had thymic vein thrombosis, rheumatoid arthritis, hepatic dysfunction and scleroderma. Treatment was begun with a mean dose of 59 mg prednisone daily, continued for a mean of 29 days until untoward side effects occurred or improvement was sustained for 4–5 days.

(7) Neurology (Minneap.) 26:729–740, August, 1976.

Steroids were then gradually reduced and usually given on alternate days.

Sustained improvement began a mean of 13 days after the start of prednisone therapy and most patients were markedly improved within 6–8 weeks. After an alternate-day dose of 60 mg was reached, reductions to maintenance levels were made more slowly in 5-mg increments. Reduction to the smallest adequate dose required an average of 4.1 months. In 62% of treatment courses, a mean maintenance dose of about 35 mg on alternate days was given. Marked reduction in requirements for cholinesterase inhibitors was common in early therapy. Exacerbation of myasthenic weakness occurred in nearly half the treatment courses. Other side effects were not a major problem in most patients.

Nineteen patients underwent thymectomy after improving or remitting on steroid therapy. No patient with a normal or involuted thymus failed to achieve remission on prednisone therapy. Improvement induced by thymectomy may not occur for up to 10 years. Attempts have been made to discontinue steroids about a year after thymectomy, and 4 patients have sustained prolonged remissions to date.

Complete remission occurred on steroid therapy in about two thirds of the treatment courses in these patients and marked improvement in another 20%. Thymectomy remains the treatment of choice for patients who do not respond favorably to steroid therapy. Antimetabolites or antithymocyte serum have not had to be used in myasthenia gravis patients who are refractory to steroids.

► [This is a long-term study by investigators who have had much experience with the treatment of myasthenia gravis. The results of this study make one optimistic about advances in the treatment of this often disabling disorder. – Ed.] ◄

Myopathies

Are Muscle Fibers Denervated in Myotonic Dystrophy? Recently it has been suggested that abnormalities of the motor nerves might be fundamental to the pathogenesis of the muscular dystrophies. Daniel B. Drachman (Johns Hopkins Univ.) and Douglas M. Fambrough[8] (Carnegie Inst. of Washington, Baltimore) tested the denervation hypothesis by applying to human dystrophic muscle a widely accepted criterion of denervation, an increase in the density of extrajunctional acetylcholine (ACh) receptor sites. The extrajunctional receptors were measured with the use of ^{125}I-labeled α-bungarotoxin, a purified fraction of snake venom that binds specifically and quantitatively to ACh receptors. Studies were done in 9 patients, aged 19–58, with typical myotonic dystrophy and 3 patients with amyotrophic lateral sclerosis (ALS). All the former patients had family histories consistent with autosomal dominant inheritance and typical clinical features of the disorder. Junctional and extrajunctional ACh receptor sites were measured quantitatively in muscle biopsy specimens. Acetylcholine receptor sites were analyzed autoradiographically.

The density of extrajunctional receptor sites in myotonic dystrophy muscles was comparable to that in other normally innervated mammalian muscles. The mean number of ACh receptor sites per neuromuscular junction was within normal limits. Autoradiographs showed a normal pattern of ACh receptor sites on muscle fibers of patients with myotonic dystrophy. Autoradiographs of denervated muscle fibers show a high density of extrajunctional ACh receptors. Even very small fibers from myotonic dystrophy patients had a normal grain distribution. High grain densities were seen in both 14-day denervated rat skeletal muscle and in ALS denervated fibers. Muscles from myotonic dystrophy patients

(8)   Arch. Neurol. 33:485–488, July, 1976.

did not contain any fibers that displayed large numbers of extrajunctional silver grains.

These findings suggest that there is not a population of denervated muscle fibers in myotonic dystrophy. The possibility of a selective abnormality in neurotropic function existing in myotonic dystrophy cannot be excluded, but there is no precedent for denervation occurring without an increase in extrajunctional receptors. By the criterion of denervation applied, the present findings do not support the hypothesis of a neurogenic defect in myotonic dystrophy.

▶ [These studies indicate that there is no evidence of motor nerve abnormality or of muscle denervation in myotonic dystrophy. — Ed.] ◀

Adenyl Cyclase Abnormality in Duchenne Muscular Dystrophy: Muscle Cells in Culture. Whether the fundamental disorder of Duchenne muscular dystrophy is in the motor neuron or in the muscle cell has been debated. The nature of the inherited biochemical defect is unknown. Shiro Mawatari, Armand Miranda and Lewis P. Rowland[9] cultured biopsy specimens of muscle in Eagle's minimal essential medium enriched with amino acids, pyruvate, vitamins and 15% fetal calf serum in the presence of antibiotics. Cultures were assayed $3-5$ days after initiation of fusion. A ^3H assay method was used.

No morphologic abnormality of the cells in culture was observed by phase microscopy or growth pattern before or after fusion. After fusion, cells from 5 patients with Duchenne dystrophy showed a significantly elevated basal adenyl cyclase activity, a lack of significant enzyme stimulation by $10^{-4}M$ epinephrine or isoproterenol and less stimulation of enzyme activity by sodium fluoride than in control cells. The abnormal responses of Duchenne myotubules could not be attributed to contamination by fibroblasts. Before fusion, the basal adenyl cyclase activity of control cells was $1\frac{1}{2}-3$ times greater than in fused cells. The enzyme of unfused human myoblasts was not stimulated by catecholamines and the response to sodium fluoride was proportionately much less than after fusion.

These observations suggest that responsiveness to catecholamines in human muscle cells is acquired at fusion, with a concomitant decrease in basal adenyl cyclase activity

(9) Neurology (Minneap.) 26:1021–1026, November, 1976.

relative to total protein content. If Duchenne dystrophy is a membrane disease, this would be a new category of heritable human disorder; similar suspicions have been expressed for myotonic dystrophy. The precise nature of the presumed muscle membrane abnormality in Duchenne dystrophy and its relationship to the clinical manifestations of the disease or to the progressive degeneration of muscle are unknown.

▶ [The genetic defect in Duchenne muscular dystrophy may be an abnormality of the surface membrane of muscle. — Ed.] ◀

Pathogenesis of Muscular Dystrophies is discussed by Lewis P. Rowland (Columbia Univ.). The heritable etiology of the muscular dystrophies is clear enough but their pathogenesis is elusive. Both vascular and neurogenic theories have been proposed. Interest in the neurogenic theory seems to be fading but the issue is open. These theories derive primarily from observations made with a special technique, whereas the membrane theory evolved from concepts of biochemical genetics. The interrelations between nerve and muscle are so close that a genetic fault in motor neurons could be reflected in altered muscle function.

Increased creatine excretion has been found in wasting conditions other than Duchenne dystrophy and the mechanism of the abnormality has not been fully revealed. Serum aldolase activity is increased in patients with Duchenne dystrophy. It has been assumed that the serum enzyme proteins arise from muscle but this has not been proved. A structural abnormality of muscle surface membrane, supporting the leaky membrane hypothesis, has not been demonstrated in any species. Studies on the effect of ouabain on (Na, K)-adenosine triphosphatase of red blood cell ghosts have suggested membrane abnormality in Duchenne dystrophy. Physiologic studies have suggested involvement of the surface membrane of muscle in myotonic dystrophy. There is increasing evidence of abnormal muscle surface membranes in myotonic disorders. The muscle membrane seems to be unstable and tends to fire repetitively. As in Duchenne dystrophy, several abnormalities of red blood cell membranes have been described in myotonic dystrophy. The red blood cell abnormalities have no clinical counterparts in disordered erythrocyte function and the specific biochemical abnormality is unclear.

(1)   Arch. Neurol. 33:315–320, May, 1976.

Increased attention is being paid to surface cell membranes in several areas of medicine and biology. Increased emphasis on the surface membrane in muscular dystrophy research is likely.

► [The cumulative evidence suggests that an abnormal muscle surface membrane is the most likely cause of muscular dystrophy. The author does state, however, that this is still to be proved. — Ed.] ◄

Congenital Muscular Dystrophy as a Disease of the Central Nervous System. Congenital muscular dystrophy is a unique type of muscular dystrophy and is characterized by early-onset hypotonia, facial muscle involvement, joint contracture, severe mental retardation with occasional convulsions and a slowly progressive course. Autosomal recessive inheritance is probable. In Japan this is one of the most common causes of the floppy infant syndrome. Shigehiko Kamoshita (Tochigi-Ken, Japan), Yumiko Konishi, Masaya Segawa and Yukio Fukuyama[2] (Tokyo) report on an autopsy study of a typical case of congenital muscular dystrophy in which striking dysplastic abnormalities were found in the brain.

Japanese boy, born at term to a mother who had had a spontaneous abortion and another child who had died shortly after premature birth, had poor head control at age 1 year, was always bedridden and lacked meaningful speech. He was institutionalized until his death at age 6½ years. Examination showed short stature and marked hypotonia and evidence of undernourishment. A masklike facies and convergent strabismus were noted. Only occasional spontaneous finger movements were seen. There were flexion contractures at the knees. Postural, tendon and skin reflexes were not elicited. Slight to moderate increases in enzymes were found. An EEG showed slight slowing and an electromyogram showed generalized low voltage without denervation potentials. Frequent respiratory infections occurred after age 5 and the patient eventually died of bronchopneumonia.

Autopsy showed emaciation and muscle wasting, gastrointestinal erosions and bronchopneumonia with microabscess formation. The muscles showed variation in fiber size and replacement by fat tissue, with no group atrophy. The brain exhibited diffuse micropolygyria with loss of the normal cortical architecture, mostly in the cerebellum, and its replacement by fibrous tissue. The pyramidal tract pattern appeared abnormal in the pons, but otherwise the brain stem architecture was unremarkable. The anterior

(2) Arch. Neurol. 33:513–516, July, 1976.

horns were slightly depopulated, but the residual neurons appeared normal.

The cerebral abnormality in congenital muscular dystrophy is not dystrophic or degenerative, but apparently dysplastic or dysgenetic. A dysplastic process of this type could be acquired in utero from congenital cytomegalovirus infection, but there is no evidence of this and the absence of destructive changes makes any type of viral infection a remote possibility. There is little doubt about the heredofamilial nature of this disease, which appears to be a malformation of the brain associated with a dystrophic muscle disorder. A single gene with polymorphic effects could be responsible for both the cerebral malformation and the muscular dystrophy.

▶ [Eight autopsied cases of congenital muscular dystrophy with central nervous system alterations have been reported in Japan. Although the lesions in the brain are quantitatively different from case to case, the findings indicate that congenital muscular dystrophy is a dysplastic disease of the central nervous system with dystrophic involvement of skeletal muscles. — Ed.] ◀

Evaluation and Detection of Duchenne and Becker's Muscular Dystrophy Carriers by Manual Muscle Testing. About 10% of carriers of Duchenne muscular dystrophy are symptomatic. New mutations may account for about one third of the cases of Duchenne muscular dystrophy. Marcia Sirotkin Roses, Megan Thomas Nicholson, Cathy Scanlon Kircher and Allen David Roses[3] (Duke Univ.) believe that through specific, standardized manual muscle tests, weak proximal muscles can be demonstrated in most carriers. Review was made of the findings in the first 28 consecutive families examined at a neuromuscular research clinic. All available relatives of patients were examined. Muscles were tested unilaterally.

By the commonly used clinical classification there were 6 definite, 3 probable and 16 possible carriers among mothers of sons with Duchenne or Becker's muscular dystrophy, excluding 2 stepmothers. Most mothers reported having hamstring or calf pains at night. In 1 family, four generations of mothers had had severe thigh and calf cramps after exercise and at night. Most mothers had abnormal postural patterns but no consistent abnormal gait patterns were ob-

(3) Neurology (Minneap.) 27:20– 25, January, 1977.

served. Proximal muscles were weak most often; the iliopsoas was weak in 76% of 25 mothers and the anterior neck flexors in 68%. Weak muscles were found only occasionally in control women. Generally, the percentage of weak muscles in possible carriers was about the same as in definite and probable carriers.

The most practical approach to carrier detection is to use all available clinical and experimental tools to examine all female relatives of patients who could be possible carriers of muscular dystrophy. Manual muscle testing is a valuable adjunct. By identifying carriers in the population, Duchenne dystrophy can be eliminated by genetic counseling and prenatal diagnostic methods as they are developed.

▶ [The authors are to be congratulated on this study. It is surprising that through the many years in which methods have been devised to develop clinical and biochemical tools for the detection of carriers of Duchenne and Becker's muscular dystrophy, it has not been apparent that manual muscle testing would give valuable information. Detailed muscle testing is a much neglected part of the neurologic examination. – Ed.] ◀

Clinical Effects of Myotonic Dystrophy on Pregnancy and the Neonate. Harvey B. Sarnat, Timothy O'Connor and Paul A. Byrne[4] (St. Louis Univ.) add 5 cases of pregnancy and labor in myotonic dystrophy to the 10 well-described cases found in a review of the literature. The products of the pregnancies were 1 normal infant and 4 severely involved neonates with common clinical manifestations of generalized weakness, hypotonia, multiple contractures and often facial diplegia. Three of the 4 affected infants died by age 3 weeks of respiratory difficulties or aspiration and the fourth has respiratory and swallowing difficulties at age 4 months.

It is not clear whether fertility is reduced in women with myotonic dystrophy. Disability from weakness and myotonia either continues unchanged or increases during pregnancy; improvement may follow delivery. There is a high rate of fetal loss due to spontaneous abortion, premature delivery and neonatal death. Only 2 cases of prolonged true 1st stage of labor have been described. The 2d stage may be prolonged by maternal weakness. Four patients had postpartum hemorrhages, 3 after instrumental delivery.

The 4 infants with neonatal myotonic dystrophy were severely involved at birth and there was a family history of

(4) Arch. Neurol. 33:459–465, July, 1976.

maternal myotonic dystrophy of late onset. Predominantly proximal muscle weakness and hypotonia are noted in neonates and gradually change to a distal distribution of weakness and atrophy in midchildhood. A cardiomyopathy was found in all autopsy cases, although no infant was in heart failure and the ECG findings were inconsistent. About half of adults with myotonic dystrophy have abnormalities of cardiac conduction or rhythm.

The type of contracture found is related to the in utero position of the fetus. The most consistent clinical features of severe neonatal myotonic dystrophy are arthrogryposis multiplex congenita, pharyngeal weakness and generalized weakness and hypotonia predominating in the lower extremities. Less constant features include polyhydramnios, respiratory failure, facial diplegia, congenital cataracts and ECG abnormalities. A muscle biopsy specimen with histochemical analysis is the most specific available laboratory test. The course of labor in myotonic dystrophy is independent of fetal involvement.

► [The symptoms of myotonic dystrophy worsen during pregnancy. There also is a high rate of fetal loss due to spontaneous abortion, prematurity and neonatal involvement with the disease. Prolonged labor has been described. Although many neonates with myotonic dystrophy are asymptomatic, severely affected newborns have a recognizable disorder unrelated to the severity of the maternal disease. One must conclude that pregnancy is inadvisable in women with myotonic dystrophy. – Ed.] ◄

Muscle Pathology of Myotonia Congenita. Myotonia congenita is a rare disorder of voluntary muscle characterized by delayed relaxation. Myotonia is usually enhanced by cold and reduced by repetitive muscle activity. The uncontrollable delay in relaxation may cause the patient to fall. Both autosomal dominant and recessive inheritance have been described. Jerry Crews (VA Hosp., Dallas), Kenneth K. Kaiser (Univ. of Colorado) and Michael H. Brooke[5] (Washington Univ.) obtained muscle biopsy specimens from 8 patients with myotonia congenita. Five were from 2 families with recessive inheritance. There was 1 autosomal dominant case and 2 sporadic cases.

Five specimens were normal or showed only minor changes on routine trichrome and hematoxylin-eosin staining. There were occasional atrophic fibers and some fiber

(5)   J. Neurol. Sci. 28:449–457, August, 1976.

hypertrophy. More severe changes were found in the other 3 patients, all severely affected males, including numerous atrophic fibers, increased internal nuclei and prominent fiber hypertrophy. Oxidative enzyme reactions showed no abnormality of the intermyofibrillar network pattern in any biopsy. Type 2B fibers were absent in all cases using the myosin adenosine triphosphatase method. Histograms showed significant fiber hypertrophy in 4 cases. Over 55% of the fibers were type 2A in 4 of the 7 specimens analyzed. The percentage of type 1 fibers was always normal. A biopsy sample from the mother of 3 patients, who is presumably a normal heterozygote carrier, showed no abnormalities.

This is the first report of an entity in which there is consistent absence of a muscle fiber type. Symptoms began in infancy or early childhood in the recessive cases. Female patients were less severely involved. Responses to drug therapy for myotonia were variable; most patients were not significantly helped by phenytoin and procainamide was not effective. Quinine led to transient improvement in 3 patients.

► [The muscle pathology of myotonia congenita has received little attention, and there have been only a few isolated investigations of it since the advent of histochemical pathologic studies in muscle disease. This study indicates that there is a complete absence of type 2B muscle fibers in all patients with this disorder, regardless of whether it is inherited as an autosomal dominant or an autosomal recessive trait or whether it occurs sporadically. — Ed.] ◄

Proximal Myopathy Caused by Iatrogenic Phosphate Depletion. Effective antacid therapy to prevent secondary hyperparathyroidism may result in hypophosphatemia, which may be associated with severe proximal myopathy, osteomalacia, rheumatic manifestations, hemolytic anemia or a rapidly fatal illness. Phosphate depletion may be overlooked in patients with chronic renal failure. Mordchai Ravid and Michael Robson[6] (Tel Aviv Univ.) describe 3 patients with chronic renal failure who received aluminum hydroxide gel and had severe proximal myopathy in association with hypophosphatemia.

Man, 44, with long-term renal failure of unknown origin, had received 90 ml aluminum hydroxide daily for 3 years and had noted recent increasing weakness. Generalized muscle weakness was

(6)   J.A.M.A. 236:1380–1381, Sept. 20, 1976.

seen, especially in proximal limb groups, with intact reflexes and normal sensation. Paralysis of all limbs and severe pain on passive movement developed. The hemoglobin level was 7.3 gm/100 ml, blood urea nitrogen level was 150 mg/100 ml and the serum phosphate level, 2.2 mg/100 ml. Phosphate excretion was 250 mg/24 hours. Sodium phosphate was given in a daily dose of 15 gm; dramatic pain relief was seen within 3 days. Muscle strength improved in the next few weeks as the phosphate level rose gradually to 6 mg/100 ml. Hypocalcemia of 6.6 mg/100 ml developed, with no symptoms of tetany. The creatinine clearance fell to 4 ml/minute after another month of treatment and regular hemodialysis was begun. Muscle strength has increased since then. Phosphate supplements have been discontinued. The serum phosphate level has remained low at 3.5 mg/100 ml.

The illness in these patients initially was misdiagnosed as uremic myopathy and as an exacerbation of rheumatoid arthritis. Discontinuation of antacid therapy was followed by gradual recovery. Oral administration of sodium phosphate led to prompt relief of muscle pain and stiffness. Intravenous administration of phosphate should not be used in these cases. Hypophosphatemia may occur more often with the use of new, palatable preparations of aluminum hydroxide. The pathogenesis of this neuromuscular disturbance is unknown.

► [The medications being ingested must be considered in the diagnosis of patients with diseases of apparently unknown etiology. – Ed.] ◄

Childhood Type of Dermatomyositis. Stirling Carpenter, George Karpati, Stanley Rothman and Gordon Watters[7] (Montreal) reviewed the findings in 6 patients with childhood-type dermatomyositis. Two were aged 17 and 19 years when the disease developed but in other respects were indistinguishable from the younger patients. All patients had typical skin lesions and proximal muscle weakness with muscle pain or tenderness. Electromyograms showed small-amplitude, short-duration, readily recruitable motor unit action potentials. All patients showed definite improvement on steroid therapy. One had an intestinal perforation due to vasculitis and necrosis of the bowel wall. Biopsy specimens of the biceps or quadriceps muscles were obtained before treatment and 2 patients were restudied up to 18 months after the institution of steroid therapy. Biopsy specimens

(7) Neurology (Minneap.) 26:952–962, October, 1976.

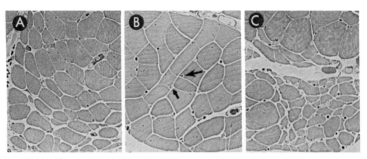

Fig 28. – **A,** paucity of capillaries toward the periphery of fascicle where abnormal fibers are found in patient aged 19. **B,** control muscle from girl aged 11 with pontine glioma, showing normal ratio of capillaries to muscle fibers. *Long arrow,* capillary containing a red blood cell; *short arrow,* capillary with empty lumen. **C,** control muscle from woman aged 40 with motor neuron disease. Severe muscle fiber atrophy resulting from denervation brought capillaries closer together without causing much diminution in their number. All sections: semithin epoxy resin; reduced from ×328. (Courtesy of Carpenter, S., et al.: Neurology (Minneap.) 26:952–962, October, 1976.)

from 8 other patients with normal or virtually normal muscle also were examined.

Capillary necrosis led to capillary loss, generally starting on the periphery of muscle fascicles (Fig 28). Electron microscopy showed undulating tubules in endothelial cells, lymphocytes, pericytes and pseudosatellite cells. The muscle fiber damage was coextensive with capillary damage. Muscle cells, before atrophying, exhibited mitochondrial elongation, Z-disk streaming, focal myofibrillary loss and, occasionally, selective thick-filament loss. Muscle cell necrosis was rare and was limited to infarct-like lesions. Inflammatory infiltrates, when present, occurred only in connective tissue septa. Undulating tubules were identified in capillary cells in all cases.

The muscle fiber damage in childhood-type dermatomyositis appears to be ischemic. Loss of capillaries appears to be a consistent finding in the muscle of patients with this disease. The process by which the capillaries are destroyed in childhood-type dermatomyositis is obscure. It seems as if the capillaries are primarily affected in this state, whereas in adults, the changes may progress to involve the muscle fibers themselves.

▶ [It appears that the type of dermatomyositis that occurs in children and young adults shows specific pathologic and electron microscopic features that differ from those seen in the adult type of the disease. – Ed.] ◀

Eosinophilic Polymyositis. Robert B. Layzer, Martin A. Shearn and Saty Satya-Murti[8] describe 3 patients with eosinophilic polymyositis accompanied by eosinophilia of the blood and involvement of other organ systems. The patients had the syndrome of disseminated eosinophilic collagen disease or hypereosinophilic syndrome (HES).

Man, 46, acquired stiff, swollen, painful calf muscles 2 years before and had a blood eosinophil count of 12%. Weakness and pain spread to the thighs, and Raynaud's phenomenon appeared in the hands. A muscle biopsy, done 8 months before hospitalization, showed marked perivascular and interstitial inflammatory infiltration by eosinophils, plasma cells and lymphocytes. Random segmental degeneration of muscle fibers was seen. Eosinophils comprised 15% of nucleated blood cells in a bone marrow aspirate. Examination showed generalized muscle atrophy and a violaceous hue of the upper eyelids. Muscle stretch reflexes were reduced or absent.

A gastric ulcer healed on dietary therapy. Prednisone was given but calf pain increased and right tibial pain and tenderness suddenly appeared. Attacks of Adams-Stokes syncope began at the same time and an ECG showed complete heart block. A pacemaker was inserted. A muscle biopsy specimen showed markedly increased muscle-fiber degeneration and abundant regenerating fibers but eosinophils were absent. The rheumatoid factor titer was 1:400. Finger ischemia worsened after prednisone was stopped because of recurrent gastric ulcer and a scaly rash appeared on the upper limbs. Dyspnea and a pericardial friction rub occurred and the patient died suddenly 3 years after the onset of symptoms.

Autopsy showed foci of old fibrosis in the myocardium, a large, scarred area in the left ventricle and a fibrinous exudate covering the heart. Skeletal muscle sections showed scattered degeneration and phagocytosis of muscle fibers, and some attempts at regeneration. There was a minimal amount of focal perivascular and interstitial infiltration with lymphocytes, but eosinophils were absent.

These patients had the usual presenting clinical features of polymyositis but the muscle infiltrates mainly consisted of eosinophils. Heart disease usually consisted of endocardial fibrosis with adherent thrombi, indistinguishable from the lesions of Löffler's endocarditis. Eosinophilic infiltration was common in the liver, spleen and lungs. Thrombosis of small vessels and numerous small areas of infarction or necrosis were found in many organs. Subungual petechiae

(8) Ann. Neurol. 1:65–71, January, 1977.

were seen in 2 patients. Responses to steroid therapy have been inconsistent.

Little is known about the role of eosinophils in immediate hypersensitivity and there is no direct evidence that eosinophils contribute to tissue damage in diseases with eosinophilia as a feature. It seems appropriate to consider use of leukophoresis for patients who do not respond to steroids, or, alternately, use of an antiserum against eosinophils.

► [Myopathy has been noted only rarely in the hypereosinophilic syndrome. This article shows, however, that it may occur; when it does, the prognosis is poor. — Ed.] ◄

Neurochemistry and Neuropathology

Frequency of Alzheimer's Neurofibrillary Tangles in Cerebral Cortex in Progressive Supranuclear Palsy (Subcortical Argyrophilic Dystrophy). H. Ishino and S. Otsuki[9] (Okayama Univ.) determined the frequency of Alzheimer's neurofibrillary tangles (ANT) in the cerebral cortex in 2 patients with progressive supranuclear palsy, using large cerebral hemispheric sections.

One patient, a man aged 71 at death, had become ill at age 69 and had nerve cell loss, gliosis and myelin loss at several brain sites at autopsy, and ANT in the cerebral cortex, globus pallidus, subthalamic nucleus, midbrain reticular formation, substantia nigra, locus ceruleus, pons and olivary nucleus. The other patient, aged 62 at death after 3 years of illness, had moderate to marked nerve cell loss and astrocytic proliferation, and ANT in several structures including the cerebral cortex, globus pallidus, subthalamic nucleus and reticular formation of the midbrain and pons.

Despite differences in the numbers of neurons with ANT, the distribution was essentially similar in these 2 patients. The ANT were most frequent in the third layer of the cortex and were present in the smaller nerve cells except in the hippocampus. The triangular type was seen in a small number of cells. Most neurons with ANT showed a well-preserved nucleus and a single or a few thickened argyrophilic neurofibrillary filaments in the cytoplasm (Fig 29). In some nerve cells, irregularly interwoven ANT were present in the cytoplasm. In still others a mass of tangles was seen filling the entire cytoplasm.

There has been considerable dispute concerning the pathologic findings in the cerebral cortex and the occurrence of ANT. Most ANT in the present patients were seen in the

(9) J. Neurol. Sci. 28:309–316, July, 1976.

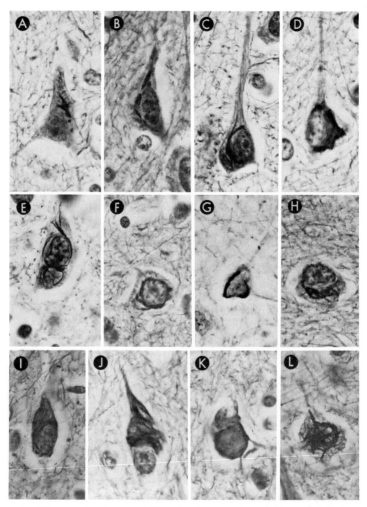

Fig 29. — Alzheimer's neurofibrillary tangles in cerebral cortex. **A,** Case 1, gyrus frontalis medius; **B,** Case 2, gyrus occipitotemporalis lateralis; **C,** Case 1, gyrus frontalis superior; **D,** Case 1, gyrus frontalis superior; **E,** Case 1, gyrus frontalis inferior; **F,** Case 2, gyrus temporalis inferior; **G,** Case 2, gyrus occipitotemporalis lateralis; **H,** Case 2, gyrus frontalis medius; **I,** Case 2, gyrus temporalis medius; **J,** Case 1, gyrus frontalis inferior; **K,** Case 2, gyrus occipitotemporalis lateralis; **L,** Case 1, gyrus temporalis inferior. Bodian; reduced from ×1000. (Courtesy of Ishino, H., and Otsuki, S.: J. Neurol. Sci. 28:309–316, July, 1976.)

smaller neurons of the third layer of the cortex. The typical triangular form found in the cortex in Alzheimer's disease or senile dementia was uncommon. Most of the ANT showed argyrophilic neurofibrillary filaments or thickened fibers that coiled around the well-preserved nucleus. In view of the absence of neuronal loss, these ANT appear to survive in this state for a long time. Their occurrence in the cortex is considered one of the morphologic manifestations of the disease process.

► [Most pathologists have stated that the major pathologic alterations in progressive supranuclear palsy appear in the globus pallidus, subthalamic nucleus, midbrain reticular formation, substantia nigra and locus ceruleus. These investigators conclude that the occurrence of neurofibrillary tangles in the cerebral cortex, especially in the hippocampus, is one of the major manifestations of the disease. — Ed.] ◄

Acetylcholine Receptor in Normal and Pathologic States: Immunoperoxidase Visualization of α-Bungarotoxin Binding at a Light and Electron Microscopic Level. Adam N. Bender, Steven P. Ringel and W. King Engel[1] (Natl. Inst. of Health) found that in muscle the acetylcholine receptor localization is changed in two diseases that each affect it in a distinct way: denervation and myasthenia gravis.

Acetylcholine receptor was visualized in the sarcolemmal membrane of the muscle by immunoperoxidase staining of α-bungarotoxin (αBT), a substance that binds specifically to the receptor. Studies were done on motor-point muscle biopsy specimens from patients with various neuromuscular diseases and subjects without neuromuscular pathology. An experimental denervation study was also done on rats; 1 phrenic nerve was resected 2–40 days before the animal was killed. The effect of myasthenic serums on normal acetylcholine receptor was tested using sections from fresh-frozen human muscle.

Positive staining indicating αBT-binding to acetylcholine receptor is shown in Figure 30. Staining was sharply localized to the neuromuscular junction in normal human and rat skeletal muscle, at and adjacent to the peaks of the post-junctional folds of the sarcolemmal membrane. Less intense staining of the presynaptic axonal membrane was seen. Sarcolemmal or "extrajunctional" staining peaked about 2

(1) Neurology (Minneap.) 26:477–483, May, 1976.

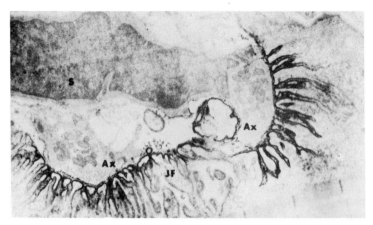

Fig 30. — Normal human neuromuscular junction, by electron micrography, showing acetylcholine receptor localized by immunoperoxidase staining (black precipitate) of αBT-binding. Two axonal tips *(Ax)* are present with an overlying Schwann cell nucleus *(S)*. Junctional folds *(JF)* are stained at and near their peaks. Some at the right are cut obliquely, giving the appearance of staining deeper than the peaks. Extrajunctional sarcolemma is unstained; reduced from ×12,000. (Courtesy of Bender, A. N., et al.: Neurology (Minneap.) 26:477–483, May, 1976.)

weeks after denervation in the rat diaphragm. Many small angular fibers in biopsy specimens from patients with lower motor neuron diseases showed diffuse staining on their rims on cross-section; such staining was not seen in biopsy specimens from patients with myasthenia gravis. Fourteen of 32 myasthenic serums blocked neuromuscular junction staining. The blocking factor was positively correlated with disease severity.

These studies provide the first demonstration of a serum factor in myasthenia gravis that blocks αBT binding to acetylcholine receptor at the normal human neuromuscular junction. It is presumed that this is the same factor that blocks the more sensitive extrajunctional, diffuse sarcolemmal acetylcholine receptor of denervated fibers. The factor may cause functional and structural damage to the postsynaptic membrane of the neuromuscular junction, and possibly the presynaptic membrane as well.

► [In myasthenia gravis a circulating factor that binds α-bungarotoxin to the acetylcholine receptor of either normal neuromuscular junctions or denervated sarcolemmal membranes is present in 68% of serums tested, whereas in both experimental denervation and human denervating illnesses the acetylcholine receptor becomes present diffusely along the muscle sarcolemmal membrane in denervated fibers. — Ed.] ◄

Radioimmunoassay of Myelin Basic Protein in Cerebrospinal Fluid: Index of Active Demyelination.

Elevated values of protein or IgG or both are found in the cerebrospinal fluid of patients with multiple sclerosis, and myelin fragments have also been found in the fluid. Steven R. Cohen, Robert M. Herndon and Guy M. McKhann[2] (Johns Hopkins Univ.) assayed cerebrospinal fluid from 303 patients for the presence of myelin basic protein. Forty-seven patients had multiple sclerosis, 4 had other forms of demyelination and 252 had a variety of other neurologic diseases. The samples were subjected in a "blind" manner to a radioimmu-

Fig 31. — Presence of myelin basic protein in cerebrospinal fluid. Hatched area represents number of samples in each group with myelin basic protein. Nondemyelinating neurologic diseases included neuroblastoma, arthrogryposis, temporal arteritis, collagen vascular disease, peripheral neuropathy, cerebellar degeneration, microcephaly, neurosyphilis, seizures, Guillain-Barré syndrome, unknown neuron disease, trigeminal neuralgia, spastic paraplegia, malignant lymphoma, alcohol withdrawal, dementia, stroke, meningitis, migraine, moya-moya syndrome, progressive supranuclear palsy, motor neuron disease, glue-sniffing neuropathy, aneurysm, hydrocephalus, vasculitis and labyrinthitis. Myelinopathies other than multiple sclerosis included transverse myelitis and systemic lupus erythematosus, hereditary leukodystrophy, metachromatic leukodystrophy and central pontine myelinolysis. (Courtesy of Cohen, S. R., et al.: N. Engl. J. Med. 295:1455–1457, Dec. 23, 1976.)

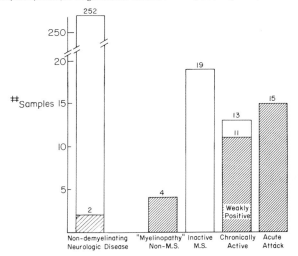

noassay for myelin basic protein that used ^{125}I-labeled basic protein.

The results are shown in Figure 31. In 19 patients with multiple sclerosis that was in remission and clinically active, no basic protein was demonstrable, whereas 11 of 13 with chronically active disease had low levels of myelin basic protein and all 15 with acute exacerbations had extremely high levels. Three patients showed a rapid fall in myelin basic protein after acute attacks, as they recovered rapidly from their neurologic symptoms. Two patients with nondemyelinative neurologic disease had myelin basic protein. They had extensive damage from strokes near the brain surface. Four other patients in whom the protein was demonstrated had myelinopathies, including transverse myelitis, central pontine myelinolysis and metachromatic leukodystrophy. One was a child who had symptoms identical with those of a sibling in whom autopsy showed a brain with little or no myelin.

Patients with active demyelinating diseases had high concentrations of cerebrospinal fluid myelin basic protein in this study, and those with multiple sclerosis in acute exacerbation had high values. The assay appears to be a useful index of active demyelination. Attempts are being made to increase its sensitivity to detect lower levels of basic protein in patients recovering from attacks. The basic protein may also be released into serum and urine. The properties of basic protein in cerebrospinal fluid are being studied to determine whether it is membrane bound and if the whole molecule or peptide fragments are present.

► [This radioimmunoassay of myelin basic protein in cerebrospinal fluid appears to be a useful index of active demyelination. J. W. Palfreyman et al. express the belief, however, that further data on the nature of the inhibiting factor in the cerebrospinal fluid are necessary before it can be identified absolutely as myelin basic protein (N. Engl. J. Med. 296:883, 1977). N. Baumann and F. Lhermitte report the finding of cerebrosides in the blood plasma during the evolutionary stages of multiple sclerosis (ibid., p. 884). – Ed.] ◄

Neurologic Complications of Systemic Disease

Eales's Disease with Neurologic Involvement. —*Part I. Clinical features in 9 patients.* —B. S. Singhal and Darab K. Dastur[3] (Bombay) have seen 9 patients with central nervous system involvement and the typical ocular changes of Eales's disease since 1966. The disease usually consists of periphlebitis, neovascular formation and recurrent retinal and vitreous hemorrhages. Neurologic involvement has not been described often.

All patients were male; the age at onset ranged from 11 to 40. The eye was involved first in nearly all patients. In 2 cases the ocular disease was active when the neurologic findings appeared. Five patients had bilateral ocular involvement. Perivenous sheathing was noted in all patients and recent or old hemorrhages in the retina in 5. Three patients showed neovascular formation and 6 had advanced changes of retinitis proliferans. Optic pallor was noted in only 2 patients. Four patients had old patches of chorioiditis or chorioretinitis.

The neurologic illness was acute or subacute in most patients. The spinal cord was mainly involved except in 1 patient who presented with seizures and hemiparesis. The mid or lower dorsal cord was predominantly affected. Moderate to severe loss of power, spinothalamic involvement, and a sensory loss were all noted in most patients. Bladder involvement was present in all 8 patients with myelopathy. Partial improvement was seen in 7 of these patients but 4 had a relapse after initially improving. Cerebrospinal fluid protein levels and number of cells were significantly elevated in the acute or subacute phase of illness. The Mantoux test result was positive in 7 of 8 patients but chest films showed old tuberculosis in only 1 patient. All patients but 1

(3)   J. Neurol. Sci. 27:313–321, March, 1976.

received antituberculosis therapy and 6 also received corticoids. Improvement was slight. Two bedridden patients died of chronic renal failure from pyelonephritis. Seven were left with mild to moderate disability.

The salient clinical picture in most of these patients was one of acute or subacute myelopathy after an ocular episode of Eales's disease. The picture did not indicate any known neurologic disorder occurring concurrently with the ocular disease. The association appears to be specific.

Part 2.—Pathology and pathogenesis.—Dastur and Singhal[4] report the neuropathologic findings in a patient with Eales's disease with neurologic involvement. The patient acquired a retinal vasculopathy, followed first by signs of brain stem and cerebellar disease and then by a myelopathy; he died 4 years later of renal infection.

Autopsy showed mild chronic inflammation in the retina and subtotal demyelination of one optic nerve. The brain stem and cerebellum showed extensive vasculopathy, with various stages of venous change from proliferation and dilatation to hemorrhage, and thickening with hyalinization. The perivenular brain tissue, especially of the cerebellum, often showed demyelination, with relative axonal preservation, but no inflammation. Similar but less marked venopathy was seen in the dorsal spinal cord, with ascending degeneration of Goll's columns and descending degeneration of the lateral columns (Fig 32). The lateral columns were maximally affected in the middorsal region of the cord, where near-total demyelination was observed. The kidneys showed severe chronic inflammatory and degenerative changes with extensive lymphocytic infiltration and fibrosis or frank hyalinization of most glomeruli.

The essential pathologic changes in this patient were mild chronic inflammation and gliosis in the retina, a vasculopathy of varying stages with patchy partial demyelination and degeneration of the sensory tracts and motor pathways in the spinal cord. Eales's disease with central nervous system involvement appears to constitute a separate syndrome of vasculopathy with episodic demyelinating retinoencephalomyelopathy. The syndrome may develop as a hypersensitivity mechanism similar to that seen in tuberculous

(4)   J. Neurol. Sci. 27:323–345, March, 1976.

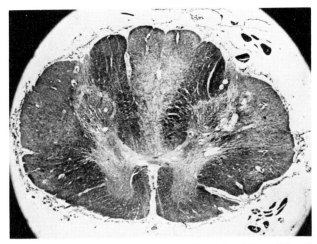

Fig 32. — Transverse section through D1 level of spinal cord shows diffuse demyelination in lateral column and medial part of posterior columns. Note dilated veins in right posterior horn. Klüver-Barrera; reduced from ×9. (Courtesy of Dastur, D. K., and Singhal, B. S.: J. Neurol. Sci. 27:323–345, March, 1976.)

encephalopathy. The vessels in the neuroglial tissue of the retina and optic nerve exhibit a predilective susceptibility to the noxious agent. Liberation of proteins from the breakdown of these tissues may render the vessels and parenchyma of the white matter of the spinal cord and brain susceptible, resulting in subsequent episodes of vasculopathy and demyelination.

► [In this article and the preceding one the clinical and pathologic features of Eales's disease are described. The characteristic picture is that of an acute or a subacute myelopathy, along with retinal changes that include periphlebitis, hemorrhages and neovascular formations. The etiology of the disease is uncertain, but hypersensitivity to a variety of allergens, notably to tuberculosis, needs to be considered. — Ed.] ◄

Inherited Metabolic Diseases of the Nervous System are summarized by Roscoe O. Brady[5] (Natl. Inst. of Health).

Reasonably good evidence exists that inborn enzymatic defects are the underlying cause of nearly 150 metabolic disorders; in many, central and peripheral nervous system damage occurs. A disorder of amino acid metabolism, phenylketonuria (PKU), is the most common heritable metabo-

(5) Science 193:733–739, Aug. 27, 1976.

lic disorder involving the central nervous system. Conceivably, a compound such as phenylpyruvic acid could interfere with pyruvate carboxylase or pyruvate decarboxylase, impairing carbohydrate metabolism and interfering with the large energy requirement of the brain. The altered behavior of PKU patients may result from abnormalities of catecholamine metabolism.

Nervous system malfunction occurs in several disorders in which carbohydrate metabolism is abnormal. Pompe's disease, with excessive glycogen in nerve cells in the central nervous system, is an example. Disorders of complex carbohydrates that may involve the nervous system include the mucopolysaccharidoses. Presumably, once the catabolism of surface glycoproteins is initiated, most of the reactions involved in their degradation occur after endocytosis of the partly modified components.

Abnormal enzymology has been well established for 10 heritable disorders of lipid metabolism. Lipid catabolic disorders include Gaucher's disease, Niemann-Pick disease and Tay-Sachs disease, in which excessive quantities of sphingolipids accumulate in various tissues. Enzyme replacement is potentially important in disorders such as Tay-Sachs disease, where the central nervous system is primarily involved. Deficiencies of synthetic enzymes are involved in a new type of hereditary abnormality of the nervous system, disorders of lipid anabolism. An example is the hereditary form of sudanophilic leukodystrophy (Schilder's disease), in which deficiency of a thiolase may be operative.

Some forms of epilepsy and perhaps certain psychiatric disturbances may be found to be inherited metabolic disorders. Eventually, this reasoning may be extended to biochemical explanations of variations in individual skills and talents.

▶ [This is a timely overview of hereditary metabolic disorders that result in nervous system dysfunction. Therapeutic approaches for the correction of such disorders are discussed where appropriate. — Ed.] ◀

Secondary Metabolic Encephalopathy: Diagnosis and Treatment are discussed by Joel R. Saper[6] (Univ. of Michigan).

Secondary metabolic encephalopathy (SME) is a diffuse

(6) Postgrad. Med. 59:122–128, May, 1976.

brain disturbance caused by an extracerebral process. Unlike the primary metabolic encephalopathies, the secondary forms often are reversible. Major underlying causes include oxygen deprivation, systemic metabolic disease and toxic drug effects. Mental changes often occur early in the course of SME. Occasionally, the neurologic findings are suggestive. Most metabolic causes of cerebral dysfunction tend to depress some functions while sparing others. The respiratory system is especially vulnerable to metabolic insult, and abnormal respiratory patterns may have prognostic and anatomic localizing value. Acute and chronic forms of lung disease are extremely important causes of SME; acute hypertension is a less common cause. Other causes include nonketotic hyperglycemic coma, uremia and drug intoxication. The drugs implicated include marijuana and lysergic acid diethylamide, glutethimide and anticholinergic agents.

Early diagnosis of SME is essential. A detailed medical history is necessary. Demonstration of diffuse or, less often, focal neurologic abnormalities along with metabolic derangement or signs of toxicity from an exogenous agent supports the diagnosis. The EEG is reliable in diagnosis and in following disordered cerebral function. Appropriate support of vital functions must not be delayed, even if the underlying cause of SME is undetermined. Neurologic and extracerebral functions must be monitored. Accurate diagnosis and treatment of cerebral edema are essential. Seizures are common in patients with SME and must be treated but excess anticonvulsant medication should be avoided if possible. Intravenous anticonvulsant therapy is indicated for status epilepticus. Clinical improvement of cerebral function may occur for weeks after effective treatment for the process underlying SME.

► [This article calls attention to the potential reversibility of metabolic encephalopathy secondary to an extracerebral process. Because of this reversibility, early recognition is imperative. – Ed.] ◄

Neuropathology of Experimental Vitamin B$_{12}$ Deficiency in Monkeys. It is generally considered difficult to induce vitamin B$_{12}$ deficiency in experimental animals. D. P. Agamanolis, E. M. Chester, M. Victor, J. A. Kark, J. D. Hines and J. W. Harris[7] (Cleveland) attempted to produce

(7) Neurology (Minneap.) 26:905–914, October, 1976.

prolonged pure vitamin B_{12} deficiency in rhesus monkeys by dietary manipulations under controlled conditions. Nine monkeys were fed a diet containing less than 500 pg vitamin B_{12} daily. Three received supplemental folic acid. Three control animals received the vitamin B_{12}-deficient diet plus 20 μg hydroxocobalamin every 2 weeks. Eight animals were started on the deficient diet in the fall of 1970 and 4 more were added 1 year later.

The deficient animals showed a progressive fall in serum vitamin B_{12} levels to 10 pg/ml by 13 months, in red blood cell vitamin B_{12} levels to 72 pg/ml by 20 months and in hepatic levels to 5% of basal levels at 21 months. After 6 months, all deficient animals excreted abnormal amounts of methylmalonic acid. Five monkeys had a gradual onset of visual impairment 33–45 months after starting on the deficient diet; 2 slowly became totally blind. Optic atrophy was seen in the animals given supplemental folic acid and more complete optic atrophy was seen in others not supplemented with folic acid. The animals also became thin and weak and had sparse body hair; paralysis developed in some in the hind limbs and tails.

Neuropathologic studies showed marked loss of myelin and axons in the optic nerves, lesions in the optic chiasm

Fig 33. – Degeneration of posterior and lateral columns of cervical cord in monkey on vitamin B_{12}-deficient diet plus supplemental folic acid. (Courtesy of Agamanolis, D. P., et al.: Neurology (Minneap.) 26:905–914, October, 1976.)

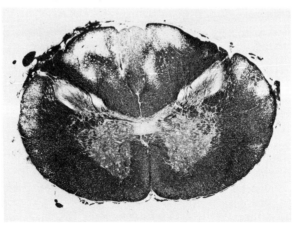

and tracts, and transsynaptic degeneration in the lateral geniculate bodies. The white matter of the spinal cord exhibited spongy change and dissolution, and infiltration of lesions by lipid-laden macrophages (Fig 33). Active lesions were seen in a number of cranial nerve roots in 5 of 6 deficient animals. Mild vacuolation of the central white matter was sometimes observed. The peripheral nerves and muscle were unaffected.

Vitamin B_{12} may be important in DNA synthesis, and impaired DNA synthesis may explain the hematologic abnormalities in vitamin B_{12} deficiency. Vitamin B_{12} is a coenzyme in the methylmalonyl COA mutase reaction, a key step in propionate metabolism, impairment of this step may lead to the production of abnormal fatty acids. This may be responsible in some way for central nervous system degeneration in vitamin B_{12} deficiency.

▶ [This is an interesting study. The lesions certainly closely resemble those found in vitamin B_{12} deficiency in man. One might wonder about blood studies in these animals and whether or not the animals developed anemia. In an article entitled "The Neurology of Vitamin B_{12} Deficiency: Metabolic Mechanisms," by E. H. Reynolds (Lancet 2:832, 1976), it is stated that both the neurologic and hematologic complications of vitamin B_{12} deficiency are the result of a secondary disorder of folate metabolism. — Ed.] ◀

CNS Manifestations of Diabetes Mellitus are discussed by Russell N. DeJong[8] (Univ. of Michigan). Involvement of peripheral nerves and nerve roots causes the most common neurologic manifestations of diabetes; whether there is specific involvement of the central nervous system (CNS) has not been well documented. The association of areflexia and marked proprioceptive disturbance with diabetes led to a concept of diabetic pseudotabes, in which there also may be bladder and bowel disturbances, impotence, trophic ulcers, neuropathic arthropathy and changes in pupillary response. Syndromes suggestive of tabes dorsalis and posterolateral sclerosis have been described in association with diabetes; however, most of the manifestations attributed to spinal cord involvement can be explained by involvement of other parts of the nervous system. Spinal tract degeneration has been demonstrated in diabetics (Fig 34), indicating that cord changes occur that may account for symptoms and signs of myelopathy.

(8) Postgrad. Med. 61:101–107, January, 1977.

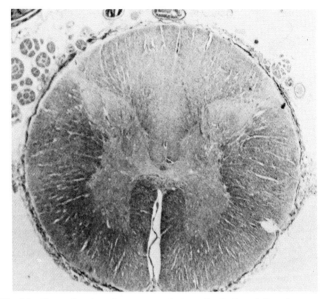

Fig 34.—Demyelination of posterior columns of spinal cord. Iron hematoxylin-van Gieson stain. (Courtesy of DeJong, R. N.: Postgrad. Med. 61:101–107, January, 1977.)

Few reports of parenchymal brain involvement in diabetes have appeared. Cranial nerve dysfunction probably is due to pathologic changes in the nerves themselves, not to changes in their brain stem nuclei. The EEG studies indicate a higher incidence of abnormalities in diabetics than in nondiabetics. Recent neuropathologic studies have shown diffuse degeneration of ganglion cells and nerve fibers in the cerebrum, brain stem and cerebellum of diabetics. Brain changes apparently do occur and may justify use of the term "diabetic encephalopathy."

Arteriosclerosis is common in diabetic patients and both focal and diffuse cerebral disease may occur on a vascular basis. Recent studies emphasize the importance of pathologic cerebrovascular changes as a basis for neurologic manifestations of diabetes. The cerebral changes may result either from a specific encephalopathy or from infarcts secondary to arteriosclerotic changes; statistically, the latter are much more important because of the prevalance of arteriosclerosis.

▶ [The editor might be criticized for having his own article in the YEAR BOOK. He does feel, however, that physicians are not as aware as they should be that the central nervous system, as well as the peripheral and autonomic nervous systems, may be affected in patients with diabetes mellitus. — Ed.] ◀

Neuro-ophthalmology

Movement Phosphenes in Optic Neuritis: New Clinical Sign. Floyd A. Davis, Donna Bergen, Charles Schauf, Ian McDonald and William Deutsch[9] recently saw 2 patients with multiple sclerosis and optic nerve involvement who reported fleeting, bright flashes of light when in the dark, which were phosphenes induced by eye movement. Seven other patients with retrobulbar neuritis or multiple sclerosis, or both, also had this phenomenon. Analysis revealed striking analogies with Lhermitte's sign.

Most patients had light flashes only with horizontal eye movement. In 2 cases, this occurred unilaterally and corresponded with the side of known optic nerve involvement. The flashes lasted 1–2 seconds and were not maintained even on persistent lateral gaze. The phenomenon could be fatigued by repeated eye movements but reappeared after several minutes of rest.

"Movement phosphenes" occur most often in older subjects and are especially frequent in myopes; vitreous "floaters" are almost always seen in these patients. The association of prominent movement phosphenes with optic nerve demyelination suggests that phosphene genesis in these patients may be in the optic nerve rather than in the retina. Movement phosphenes may be the visual equivalent of Lhermitte's sign, which consists of trunk and limb paresthesias precipitated by quick neck flexion in patients with diseases affecting the posterior columns of the spinal cord. In multiple sclerosis, this phenomenon probably is due to altered excitability of demyelinated posterior column fibers. The precise mechanism by which mechanical stimulation of nerve fibers occurs is unclear.

The acute development of movement phosphenes suggests optic nerve demyelination, provided that other causes are excluded. Confirmation of an optic nerve lesion in such cases

---

by evoked potential studies or red-free photography of the retinal nerve fiber layer may provide objective evidence for dissemination of lesions where multiple sclerosis is suspected.

► [This is an interesting and important contribution. The authors show that patients with multiple sclerosis may have eye movement-induced phosphenes. The authors believe that the mechanism of this phenomenon is similar to that which underlies the Lhermitte sign. – Ed.] ◄

Explanation of Eye Movements Seen in Internuclear Ophthalmoplegia is presented by Jordan Pola and David A. Robinson[1] (Johns Hopkins Univ.). The oculomotor deficits in internuclear ophthalmoplegia are thought to be due to a lesion of the medial longitudinal fasciculus (MLF). Loss of adduction of the ipsilateral eye is explained by excitatory fibers rising in the MLF to innervate medial rectus motoneurons on the same side, but other aspects of the eye movements have not been well explained. Results of recording from the fibers of the MLF in the behaving monkey have now been evaluated in light of the possibility of inhibitory as well as excitatory fibers running in the MLF.

A horizontal saccade is made by a pulse step of neural activity in the monkey, part of which rises to medial rectus motoneurons on MLF fibers. If inhibitory fibers run in the MLF, each MLF must carry both the excitatory and inhibitory activity required for contralateral, horizontal saccades. Interruption of these fibers removes not only excitation from the ipsilateral medial rectus, but inhibition from the contralateral medial rectus. Such a lesion also disturbs the correct relationship between the pulse and the step and creates abnormal saccades. Most fibers had firing rates associated with vertical eye movements, whereas a smaller population was associated with horizontal eye movements. High discharge rates were noted during contralateral saccades, with silence during ipsilateral saccades. Commands for saccades and position holding are not delivered to the oculomotor nucleus on separate sets of fibers, but rather the same fibers carry both signals.

These findings explain why, in internuclear ophthalmoplegia, the ipsilateral eye adducts slowly and inadequately, while the opposite eye has nystagmus in abduction. If this

(1) Arch. Neurol. 33:447–452, June, 1976.

model is correct, it implies that a lesion of the MLF is a sufficient diagnosis, because it does not require the assumption, for instance, that the nystagmus in abduction indicates more complicated or extensive pontine lesions.

► [These facts make it possible to explain why in internuclear ophthalmoplegia the eye on the side of the lesion adducts slowly and inadequately, while the opposite eye has nystagmus in abduction. – Ed.] ◄

Hemorrhages with Optic Nerve Drusen: Differentiation from Early Papilledema. Roger A. Hitchings, James J. Corbett, Jan Winkleman and Norman J. Schatz[2] report 5 cases of optic nerve drusen that emphasize the difference between papilledema and drusen with hemorrhages.

The optic discs were elevated and had blurred, irregular margins consistent in appearance with buried drusen. Central cupping was absent. Variable findings in the 5 patients, all of them aged 16 or younger, included subretinal, arcuate hemorrhage, absence of spontaneous venous pulsations, flame hemorrhages and areas of hyperpigmentation surrounding the optic disc. One patient had bilateral disc elevations with exposed drusen and a serous retinal detachment with subretinal hemorrhage of the macular region in one eye. Visual acuity was normal or near-normal in the other patients.

Papilledema can be distinguished easily from optic disc drusen in most patients. Some confusion may arise in the late stages of papilledema, where multiple refractile bodies may appear. These "pseudodrusen" are located superficially in the substance of the optic disc and usually are seen at the disc margins; they probably represent degenerated axons. Nerve fiber layer defects or "gutters" also may be observed. The flat, white disc of chronic atrophic papilledema bears no resemblance to the elevated discs of optic nerve drusen. Examination with a red-free ophthalmoscopic filter after pupillary dilatation will facilitate the distinction. Other family members should be examined when drusen are suspected. Fluorescein angiography often is helpful.

► [The differentiation between early papilledema and drusen of the optic nerve is often difficult. This is especially true if there are hemorrhages into optic nerve drusen. – Ed.] ◄

Ocular Myopathy (Progressive External Ophthalmoplegia) with Neuropathic Complications. P. B. Croft, J.

(2)   Arch. Neurol. 33:675–677, October, 1976.

C. Cutting, E. C. O. Jewesbury, W. Blackwood and W. G. P. Mair[3] (London) reviewed 335 reported and 13 personal cases of ocular myopathy, or progressive external ophthalmoplegia. The personal series included 8 male and 5 female patients, and there was no unusual sex distribution in the review series. A positive family history was reported in 37% of the reported cases. Symptoms generally tended to be first noted in the 3d decade.

Ophthalmoplegia or other abnormalities may lead to a search for help after many years of mild ptosis. Most patients exhibited both ptosis and external ophthalmoplegia but 18 patients had ptosis independent of ophthalmoplegia and 16 had ophthalmoplegia without ptosis. Bilateral facial weakness occurred in 15.5% of the reported patients. The neck muscles were affected in 9.5% of the patients and the limb muscles in 19%. Cerebellar involvement occurred in 9% of the reported patients and in 2 personal patients. Corticospinal tract involvement was noted in 4%, peripheral neuropathy in 2% and perceptive deafness in 4%. Organic mental disorder was reported in 2%.

A rise in cerebrospinal fluid protein was sometimes found without associated neurodegenerative disease. Electromyographic and nerve conduction studies tended to indicate a myopathic condition of affected facial, neck and limb-girdle muscles. The findings in 1 patient indicated a myopathic rather than a neurogenic cause of the progressive ptosis and ophthalmoplegia. Previous histologic studies of proximal limb muscles have also indicated a myopathic rather than a neurogenic change.

In addition to the simple myopathic manifestations of this disorder, a number of more complicated neurologic disturbances may develop. It seems likely that a general metabolic disturbance may be present in some patients. Whether the primary change is in the mitochondria of many different types of tissue has not been determined.

► [This study, like other recent ones, suggests that progressive external ophthalmoplegia is a part of a wide spectrum of syndromes. Possibly all of them are part of a general metabolic disorder. – Ed.] ◄

(3)   Acta Neurol. Scand. 55:169–197, March, 1977.

Neuropathies

Neuropathy in Upper Extremity after Open Heart Surgery. Joseph C. Honet, James A. Raikes, Adrian Kantrowitz, Stewart E. Pursel and Melvyn Rubenfire[4] (Detroit) reviewed data on 7 patients, who had neurologic abnormalities in the upper extremities after cardiac surgery by a sternum-splitting approach, and the results of electromyography in another 11 consecutive patients, who underwent similar surgery. Four of the latter patients had upper extremity neurologic abnormalities. Two of these 4 patients were asymptomatic.

All lesions could be postulated to occur within the brachial plexus, the most common area being the median cord, but lesions were also noted in the posterior and lateral cords and the upper trunk. Four of the 11 patients examined had abnormal electromyographic findings. One patient had an onset of unilateral symptoms after brachial artery catheterization and before surgery, although the symptoms worsened and became bilateral after surgery. Several other patients, who had intra-aortic balloon pumping for cardiac augmentation, had neurologic lesions in the leg in which the femoral artery was used for pump insertion. There were many similarities in the present patients, but no one totally common feature other than the site of surgical incision and retraction of the sternum was noted. Arterial procedures were not performed on the abnormal extremities.

This problem appears to be due to stretching injury of the brachial plexus from retraction of the sternum, which in turn causes retroclavicular displacement of the clavicle. It is possible, however, that an ischemic neuropathy could result from intra-arterial procedures in some cases. Physicians who may have an opportunity to evaluate patients having open heart surgery should realize that neurologic deficit

(4) Arch. Phys. Med. Rehabil. 57:264–267, June, 1976.

may occur in the upper extremity, and that stretching of the brachial plexus is a possible cause.

▶ [When open heart surgery is performed through a median sternotomy incision, retraction of the sternum may cause a stretching injury of the brachial plexus. – Ed.] ◄

Folate-Responsive Neuropathy: Report of 10 Cases. Folate deficiency is not universally accepted as a cause of neuropathy, despite observed improvements in neuropathy after folate administration. Mohammad Manzoor and John Runcie[5] (Glasgow) report data on 10 patients aged 52 – 93 years with a characteristic neuropathy and severe folate deficiency. The 8 men and 2 women had a loss of tendon reflexes at the knee and ankle, impaired or absent vibration sense and bilateral extensor plantar responses. Folic acid was given orally in a dose of 10 mg 3 times daily. Two patients initially received several doses of chlorpromazine. The patients' serum vitamin B_{12} levels were normal. Psychiatric intervention was not necessary.

All patients had grossly reduced serum folate levels but no relationship with macrocytic anemia was apparent. In 1 patient a low serum vitamin B_{12} level, thought to be due to ileal dysfunction, rose quickly and spontaneously to normal when folic acid was administered. The neuropathy was completely reversed in 3 cases and in 2 others, the only residual abnormality was incomplete recovery of vibration sense in the legs. Three other patients improved significantly, whereas 2 showed no reflex or sensory improvement, even after 15 months' treatment in 1 case. All patients noted an improvement in mood and psychosis resolved dramatically in 2 cases. Psychic improvement was apparent within 2 weeks of the start of treatment and preceded the improvement in reflex abnormalities by many weeks or even months.

Folate therapy led to significant reversal of a neuropathy clinically indistinguishable from subacute combined degeneration of the spinal cord in these folate-deficient patients. The hematologic and neurologic effects of chronic folate deficiency may be completely dissociated. The nervous system is more vulnerable to long-standing folate deficiency. A normal hemoglobin level does not exclude severe folate-depen-

(5) Br. Med. J. 1:1176 – 1178, May 15, 1976.

dent neuropathy, and macrocytosis is masked by concurrent iron deficiency. One of the present patients presented with iron deficiency anemia and exhibited macrocytosis when the anemia was corrected; spastic paraparesis progressed rapidly during the same period.

▶ [These findings indicate the need to review orthodox concepts of the role of folate acid in maintaining the integrity of the nervous system. — Ed.]

Prognostic Significance of Electrodiagnostic Studies in the Guillain-Barré Syndrome. Various clinical features are not useful prognostically in patients with the Landry-Guillain-Barré (LGB) syndrome. P. T. Raman and G. M. Taori[6] (Christian Med. College, Vellore, India) studied serial nerve conduction and needle electromyography in 50 cases of LGB syndrome. The patients, aged 3 – 70 years, were hospitalized during 1968 – 72. Motor conduction velocities were determined in the median and lateral popliteal nerves in all patients; in 39 patients, the ulnar nerve also was examined. Sensory potentials were evoked in the median nerve in 39 cases and conduction velocity was determined in the distal sensory division of the radial nerve in 28 cases by antidromic stimulation in the forearm.

Thirty-one patients had gross abnormalities of nerve conduction and no fibrillation potentials during the illness; 25 of these (80.6%) recovered rapidly and well. Nineteen patients had profuse fibrillations in the first 4 weeks of illness, with or without nerve conduction deficits. Only 31.5% of these patients recovered well and marked residual deficits were more common than in the other group; involvement of the lower limbs was often more severe in the patients in this series. Muscle wasting was correlated with profuse fibrillation potentials. Hospitalization was prolonged in the group with profuse fibrillations.

Two populations are found among patients with LGB syndrome. In one, demyelination seems to be the main pathologic change, with significant fibrillation potentials lacking. Axonal damage is minimal or absent and the prognosis is good. In the second group, profuse fibrillation potentials are present, often in the 1st month after onset, indicating significant axonal damage. Associated conduction abnormalities may or may not be present. The prognosis is

(6)   J. Neurol. Neurosurg. Psychiatry 39:163 – 170, February, 1976.

poor. Parameters such as sensory impairment, cerebro-spinal fluid pleocytosis or the degree of rise in cerebrospinal fluid protein are not helpful in differentiating these two types of LGB syndrome.

▶ [This study indicates that if profuse fibrillations are found in patients during the first 4 weeks of illness with Guillain-Barré syndrome with or without nerve conduction deficits, the prognosis is poorer for recovery without residuals than if no such fibrillations are found. The authors conclude that electrophysiologic studies are not only of value in the diagnosis, but also are a reliable prognostic index in this syndrome. — Ed.] ◀

Chronic Polyradiculoneuropathy of Infancy: Report of Three Cases with Familial Incidence. Michael Kasman, Lawrence Bernstein and Sidney Schulman[7] (Univ. of Chicago) describe 2 siblings and another child having a syndrome of progressive muscular weakness and wasting, closely resembling Werdnig-Hoffmann paralysis. The 2 siblings were the only offspring of their parents. Autopsy was done of 1 sibling and the third child.

The mother of the siblings had bilateral pes cavus and possibly blunted pinprick sensation in the hands, lower legs and feet. Motor nerve conduction velocities and sensory latencies were normal in both parents; electromyographic study of the mother gave negative results. The father of the third patient had had a neurologic disorder from early childhood or infancy, with an awkward gait and possibly recent weakness and incoordination; examination showed signs of a well-developed symmetric sensory-motor polyneuropathy.

Both autopsies showed a complete absence of myelin almost everywhere in the spinal cord and peripheral nerves (Fig 35). Only a few isolated, single nerve fibers in the cauda equina and cranial nerve roots were covered with thin myelin sheaths. The myelin loss did not extend into the glial portions of the roots. Nerve fibers seemed normal except for a greater irregularity of caliber in many individual fibers. No phagocytic or inflammatory cells were seen in the cranial or spinal roots or in the sciatic nerve. Sheath cells were moderately increased in number and collagen fibers were considerably increased. A reduction in myelin was seen in a sural nerve biopsy specimen from the affected father; a muscle specimen showed typical, severe denervation atrophy.

These children had unusual variations of inherited poly-

(7)   Neurology (Minneap.) 26:565–573, June, 1976.

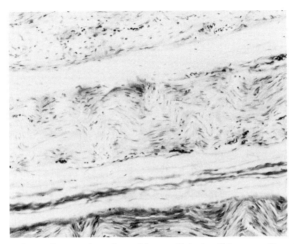

Fig 35.—Total absence of myelin and hypercellularity (Schwann cells and fibroblasts) in sciatic nerve. Klüver-Barrera; reduced from ×40. (Courtesy of Kasman, M., et al.: Neurology (Minneap.) 26:565–573, June, 1976.)

radiculoneuropathy. Some of these cases clinically resemble infantile spinal muscular atrophy of Werdnig-Hoffmann paralysis. The protein content of cerebrospinal fluid is very likely to be elevated in children with polyradiculoneuropathy but not in those with Werdnig-Hoffmann paralysis.

► [Although the neurologic disorder in these children resembles, to a certain extent, that found in Charcot-Marie-Tooth disease and the hypertrophic neuropathy of Dejerine-Sottas disease, it is difficult to classify it as either of these diseases as they presently are defined. The elevation of the cerebrospinal fluid protein level distinguishes this disorder from Werdnig-Hoffmann paralysis. — Ed.] ◄

Pain in Peripheral Neuropathy Related to Rate and Kind of Fiber Degeneration. Peter James Dyck, Edward H. Lambert and Peter C. O'Brien[8] (Mayo Clinic and Found.) studied the association of foot pain with the rate and type of nerve fiber degeneration and with the ratio of large to small fibers in sural nerves in 72 patients with peripheral neuropathy.

A compound action potential recording was obtained on sural nerve biopsy specimens from all patients. Estimates of the rate and type of myelinated nerve fiber degeneration

(8) Neurology (Minneap.) 26:466–471, May, 1976.

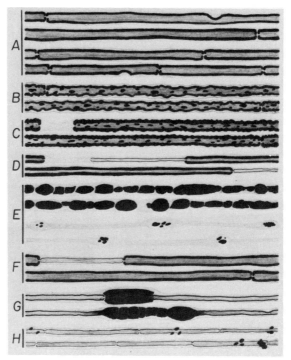

Fig 36. – Drawing of teased fiber descriptive conditions. **A,** fiber of normal appearance. **B,** fiber with excessive irregularity of myelin. **C,** fiber with segmental demyelination and variability of myelin thickness between internodes of less than 50% (demyelination without remyelination). **D,** fiber with segmental demyelination and variability of myelin thickness between internodes of more than 50% (demyelination and remyelination). **E,** fiber that has had myelin degeneration into linear ovoids and balls (wallerian and axonal degeneration). **F,** fibers with variability of myelin thickness between internodes of more than 50% (includes fibers with intercalated internodes). **G,** fibers with excessive variability of myelin thickness in internodes to form "globules" or "sausages." **H,** fiber with adjacent myelin ovoids or balls (probably regenerating fiber). (Courtesy of Dyck, P. J., et al.: Neurology (Minneap.) 26:466–471, May, 1976.)

were based on an evaluation of teased fibers (Fig 36). Pain was present in 76% of patients with acute fiber degeneration and in 15% of those with other types of fiber degeneration, a highly significant difference. The respective average ages were 55.1 and 29.9 years, but no meaningful age effect on painfulness was noted.

The frequency of condition E teased fibers, fibers degenerating into linear rows of myelin ovoids and balls, was increased with increasing grade of pain. No significant difference between median A and C potentials was found between the patients with acute fiber degeneration and the others. No significant differences between patients with and without pain were seen. A comparison of amplitudes of A and C potentials and their ratio in the nerves of patients with and without pain in the group with acute fiber degeneration also showed no significant difference.

Pain in peripheral neuropathy is associated with the rate and kind of nerve fiber degeneration. Patients with acute breakdown of myelinated fibers (wallerian or axonal degeneration) tend to have pain more often and to a greater degree than those with more chronic forms of nerve fiber degeneration. This difference is not due to a different proportion of large to small fibers remaining after nerve degeneration. The ratio of remaining large to small fibers does not seem to influence painfulness, an effect anticipated by the proponents of the gate theory of pain; these findings do not support this theory.

▶ [Patients with acute breakdown of myelinated fibers either by wallerian or axonal degeneration tend to have pain more often and to a greater degree than do patients with more chronic forms of nerve fiber degeneration. – Ed.] ◀

Giant Axonal Neuropathy Caused by Industrial Chemicals: Neurofilamentous Axonal Masses in Man. John G. Davenport, Donald F. Farrell and S. Mark Sumi[9] (Univ. of Washington, Seattle) describe 2 patients in whom a symmetric polyneuropathy developed after contact with acrylamide and methyl n-butyl ketone (MBK). One patient had worked with raw acrylamide for 6 months. The other had worked for up to 14 hours daily for 4 months with lacquer compounds as a furniture finisher; methyl n-butyl ketone had been substituted for methyl isobutyl ketone 2 months before the patient had begun the work.

In both cases, sural nerve biopsy specimens showed diffuse fibrosis, loss of nerve fibers and enlargement of several axons, both with and without myelin sheaths (Fig 37). Focal dilatation of the myelin sheath was a common finding in teased fibers. Neurofibrillary tangles were seen in en-

(9)   Neurology (Minneap.) 26:919–923, October, 1976.

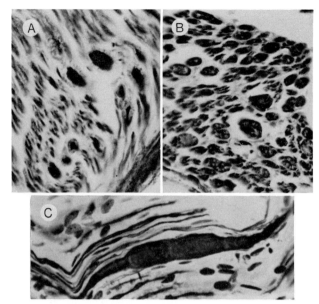

Fig 37. —Swollen axons in sural nerve biopsy specimens; luxol fast blue-Holmes stain. **A,** acrylamide neuropathy; original magnification ×420. **B,** MBK neuropathy. Large axons appear to contain neurofibrillary tangles; reduced from ×380. **C,** MBK neuropathy. Focally enlarged axon is seen on longitudinal section; original magnification ×250. (Courtesy of Davenport, J. G., et al.: Neurology (Minneap.) 26:919–923, October, 1976.)

larged axons in some fibers of the patient exposed to MBK. Electron microscopy showed bundles of fine filaments 10–15 nm thick, packed into numerous axons. Both normal-sized and enlarged axons were affected. Very few neurotubules were identified in affected regions.

These patients had clinical features typical of the neurotoxic syndromes caused by acrylamide and MBK. The most prominent findings from nerve biopsy specimens were accumulation of neurofilaments and an increase in mitochondria and dense bodies in affected axons. Similar changes can be produced by n-hexane, and a comparable picture has been found in the 3 reported cases of giant axonal neuropathy, all children with progressive polyneuropathy, who had had no apparent contact with any known toxins. Even without ultrastructural study, sural nerve biopsy specimens can give clinically important evidence of the focal axonal enlargements that appear to be the pathognomonic features of these toxic neuropathies. Both of the present patients recovered nearly completely in the year after their conditions were diagnosed; each currently has mild symmetric weakness of the ankle extensors and absent ankle jerks.

► [Sural nerve biopsy is an important diagnostic test in identifying cases of peripheral neuropathy caused by these chemicals. – Ed.] ◄

Mononeuritis Multiplex in Boeck's Sarcoidosis.

D. Kömpf, B. Neundörfer, C. Kayser-Gatchalian, L. Meyer-Wahl and K. Ranft[1] (Univ. of Heidelberg) present data on 2 patients with mononeuritis multiplex who were found to be in the early phases of Boeck's sarcoidosis. Neither had cranial nerve deficits. The clinical signs and electromyographic and neuropathologic results are compared with literature data.

Although etiologic clarification of polyneuritides and polyneuropathies with symmetric distribution of peripheral neurologic deficit presents few problems as a rule, a mononeuritis multiplex-like distribution pattern such as observed in the present 2 patients (Fig 38) may make initial etiologic classification difficult.

CASE 1. – Woman, 36, was admitted after a 3-week history of general dejection, fatigue and temperatures up to 101.5 F, accompanied by intermittent cramplike upper abdominal pain and vomiting. The physical status and blood picture were unremarkable; radiologic examination showed bilateral nodular hilus enlargements, which were egg-sized on serial films and suggested the diagnosis of Boeck's disease. A lymph node biopsy specimen from the scalenus region confirmed the diagnosis.

CASE 2. – Woman, 40, first reported bilateral swelling of the wrists with pain in the 1st to 3d digits 4 years earlier. This rapidly receded with cortisone medication but reappeared on conclusion of this regimen. Within 3 years, the pain extended to both arms, radiating from the wrist to the shoulder bilaterally, with nocturnal swelling of the hands. A 2-day treatment with cortisone relieved the pain. However, neurologic examination showed a mononeuritis multiplex-like deficit pattern and chest x-ray showed polycyclic lumping of hili bilaterally. Histologic investigation of a cherry-sized lymph node from the supraclavicular region showed marked epithelioid cellular granulomatosis and confirmed the diagnosis of Boeck's disease.

_____

(1) Nervenarzt 47:687–689, November, 1976.

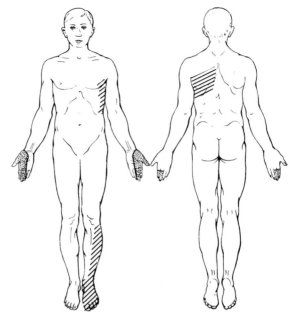

Fig 38. – Peripheral neurologic deficit in Case 1 *(hatched area)* and Case 2 *(stippled area)*. (Courtesy of Kömpf, D., et al.: Nervenarzt 47:687–689, November, 1976; Berlin-Heidelberg-New York: Springer.)

Such an involvement of peripheral nerves with a mononeuritis multiplex-like distribution pattern within the context of Boeck's sarcoidosis, particularly without accompanying cerebral nerve deficit, is rare. In Colover's compilation only 9 such patients were mentioned. There are two possible mechanisms for lesions of the nervous system (peripheral or central) in Boeck's sarcoidosis: a direct lesion of structures by epithelioid cellular granulomas or degenerative lesions with focal or ascending-descending demyelinization, in which, based on histologic investigations for this latter mechanism, the involvement of the small vessels could be under discussion.

► [Electromyographic and neuropathologic studies have shown that mononeuritis multiplex may be present in sarcoidosis. – Ed.] ◄

Guillain-Barré Syndrome and Hodgkin's Disease: Three Cases with Immunologic Studies. Guillain-Barré syndrome (GBS) is thought to be an immunologically mediated disease caused by delayed hypersensitivity to peripheral nervous system myelin or a component thereof. Much evidence suggests that some patients in certain stages of Hodgkin's disease are immunologically suppressed. Robert

Fig 39. — Perivascular lymphocyte infiltration in peripheral nerve trunk (brachial plexus) characteristic of Guillain-Barré syndrome (acute idiopathic polyneuritis). **A,** proliferation of Schwann cells has occurred. **B,** perivenular nature of the infiltrate is more evident. Hematoxylin-eosin; reduced from ×260. (Courtesy of Lisak, R. P., et al.: Ann. Neurol. 1:72–78, January, 1977.)

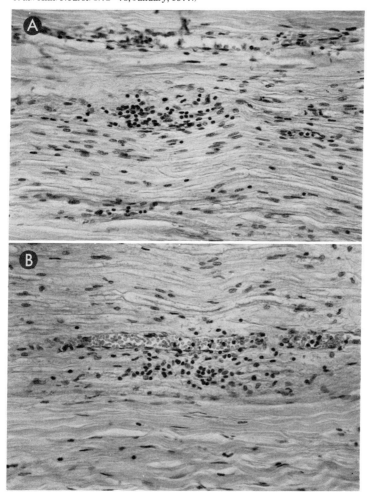

P. Lisak, Madeline Mitchell, Burton Zweiman, Edward Or-
rechio and Arthur K. Asbury[2] (Univ. of Pennsylvania) saw 3
patients who had GBS in association with Hodgkin's disease, all of whom were immunosuppressed.

Man, 52, with stage IVB Hodgkin's disease had paresthesias and
progressive weakness of several days' duration. He had last received vincristine 3 weeks before hospitalization. The cerebrospinal fluid protein level was 92 mg/dl. Mild to moderate weakness
and minimal sensory findings were noted. The patient failed to respond to skin test antigens or to show an in vitro lymphocyte proliferative response to standard antigens. In vitro response to phy-
tohemagglutinin (PHA) was low normal. The serum IgG level
increased; there were 60% E rosettes and 13% EAC rosettes. Reduced distal motor latency and minimally depressed motor conduction velocities were noted 5 days after the onset of symptoms; the
number of polyphasic potentials was increased and that of motor
units was reduced. The disease progressed rapidly, with facial
diplegia and depressed bulbar function and the patient died of
respiratory complications. Autopsy showed changes typical of
idiopathic polyneuritis (Fig 39).

Partial immunosuppression was demonstrated using in
vivo and in vitro methods in 3 patients with Hodgkin's disease and GBS. Guillain-Barré syndrome has been associated
with other conditions in which degrees of immunosuppression may occur. Under certain circumstances, partial and
perhaps transient immunosuppression could be a contributing factor in triggering an autoimmune disease of the peripheral nervous system. This postulate can be investigated
directly, both experimentally and in patients with GBS.

▶ [Under certain conditions, partial and perhaps transient immunosuppression can be a contributing factor in triggering an autoimmune disease of the peripheral nervous system. – Ed.] ◄

Mortality in Diabetic Autonomic Neuropathy. Certain complications of diabetes are associated with a high
mortality. D. J. Ewing, I. W. Campbell and B. F. Clarke[3]
(Royal Infirm., Edinburgh) followed 37 patients with clinical features of diabetic autonomic neuropathy for 33
months; several died during this time. The 31 men and 6
women had a mean age of 47 years and a mean duration of
diabetes of 18.5 years. Thirty patients were reexamined

(2) Ann. Neurol. 1:72–78, January, 1977.
(3) Lancet 1:601–603, Mar. 20, 1976.

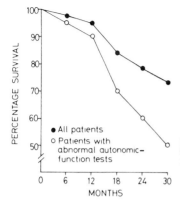

Fig 40. — Survival curves in 37 diabetic patients with autonomic neuropathy. (Courtesy of Ewing, D. J., et al.: Lancet 1:601 – 603, Mar. 20, 1976.)

18 – 24 months after initial assessment and their vascular reflexes were retested. Six other patients died before retesting and 1 had moved but was alive and well.

Ten patients (27%) died (Fig 40), 6 of renal failure, 2 of cerebrovascular accident, 1 of hypoglycemic coma and 1 in "sudden death." Six patients had autopsy. Age, duration of diabetes and duration of symptoms of autonomic neuropathy did not distinguish the survivors from those who died. No significant differences in presenting clinical features were noted. Ten of the 20 patients with initially abnormal Valsalva's or handgrip test results have died but none of the 17 with initially normal test results have died. Seven of 15 patients with an initial blood urea level of over 6.6 mM/L have died compared with 3 of 22 with normal levels. Symptoms of peripheral neuropathy did not distinguish the two groups of patients. Differences in resting blood pressure and retinopathy were not apparent.

One of the survivors with abnormal initial test results had normal test results on follow-up with no change in symptoms. Symptoms or other diabetic complications worsened in 5 other patients, all of whose tests remained abnormal. Four of 13 patients with initially normal test results who had impotence alone, had borderline abnormalities of autonomic function; 3 of these had other symptoms of autonomic neuropathy. Of 4 patients with other clinical features of autonomic neuropathy initially and normal autonomic function tests, 3 remained normal, 2 improved symptomatically and 1 deteriorated and had abnormal autonomic function test results.

This study delineated a group of end-stage diabetic patients whose major features were clinical autonomic neuropathy and abnormal autonomic function test results. Half of these patients were dead within 2½ years, although it is impossible to say that the deaths were caused by the autonomic neuropathy. Autonomic neuropathy can be added to those diabetic complications associated with an especially high mortality.

► [In diabetic patients with clinical features of autonomic neuropathy, simple tests of autonomic function are a good guide to prognosis. A high mortality rate is found in these patients whose tests gave abnormal results. — Ed.] ◄

Diabetic Polyneuropathy: Importance of Insulin Deficiency, Hyperglycemia and Alterations in Myoinositol Metabolism in Its Pathogenesis is discussed by Albert I. Winegrad and Douglas A. Greene[4] (Univ. of Pennsylvania). There is no effective prevention or treatment of diabetic polyneuropathy, and its pathogenesis is unknown. Neuropathologic studies have excluded occlusive arterial disease and diabetic "microangiopathy" as major factors, and most workers now believe the syndrome to be conditioned by some chronic metabolic disturbance. Overt polyneuropathy is associated with pathologic changes that are most prominent in the distal parts of the peripheral nerves, including loss of myelinated and unmyelinated nerve fibers, segmental demyelination, Schwann cell proliferation and an increase in connective tissue elements within the nerve. Insulin deficiency and hyperglycemia appear to have primary roles in the pathogenesis of impaired nerve conduction velocity in animals with acute diabetes. Some have suggested a so-called dying-back neuropathy in diabetic polyneuropathy, involving impaired axonal transport of proteins synthesized in the neuron.

The development of impaired motor nerve conduction velocity in acute induced diabetes is related to a secondary derangement in regulation of free myoinositol in nerves. Dietary myoinositol over a wide range has a major role in determination of plasma and nerve concentrations in nor-

(4) N. Engl. J. Med. 295:1416–1421, Dec. 16, 1976.

mal rats. The effects of insulin deficiency and hyperglycemia on peripheral nerve conduction velocity appear to be mediated by a defect in myoinositol metabolism, reflected by decreased nerve myoinositol concentrations. The importance of high concentrations of free myoinositol in mammalian tissues is unknown, and it is difficult to predict how the peripheral nerve may be affected by defective regulation of its myoinositol concentration. Many data have been obtained from in vitro studies of whole nerve segments, and these findings are difficult to interpret.

The effects of insulin deficiency and hyperglycemia on diabetic patients merit serious consideration. These factors are probably not controlled by present treatments. The marked variability in development of overt diabetic polyneuropathy suggests that genetic and environmental factors may influence its pathogenesis.

▶ [Hyperglycemia, insulin insufficiency and altered myoinositol metabolism all seem to be implicated in the pathogenesis of diabetic neuropathy. Disturbances in the sorbitol pathway also seem to play a part. Genetic factors doubtlessly influence the pathogenesis of the syndrome, but whether or not environmental factors also are significant is still to be proved. – Ed.]

Facial Diplegia. Sudden facial diplegia or recurrent facial palsy is rare but may be seen initially as the only symptom of a systemic illness. Michael I. Weintraub[5] (New York Med. College) reports 2 cases showing how bilateral facial palsy in the absence of the Guillain-Barré-Strohl syndrome can be the only initial manifestation of infectious mononucleosis.

CASE 1. – Girl, 15, had sore throat, adenopathy and swallowing difficulty and, 10 days later, facial discomfort and difficulty speaking. A bilateral peripheral facial palsy was documented. A slide test for mononucleosis gave positive results and Epstein-Barr virus titers were strongly positive. Both facial nerves could be stimulated easily 1 week after the onset of facial diplegia. A short course of prednisone was given and notable clinical improvement occurred over the next few months.

CASE 2. – Girl, 15, had a peripheral right-sided facial palsy without preceding infection, followed in 2 months by a severe sore throat and left-sided peripheral facial palsy. A short course of prednisone was given and almost complete reversal of symptoms occurred over the next 2 months. The Monospot test for mononucleosis gave positive results.

(5)   Arch. Otolaryngol. 102:311–312, May, 1976.

Facial diplegia can occur at all ages; it may be seen in association with traumatic delivery, the so-called Möbius syndrome, myotonic dystrophy, myasthenia gravis, pontine gliomas, viral infections and sarcoidosis. Postimmunization reactions also can produce facial nerve dysfunction. Melkersson's syndrome is a rare entity that includes recurrent facial palsy. The slide test for infectious mononucleosis is extremely important. Infectious mononucleosis should always be included in the differential diagnosis of sudden facial diplegia.

► [Although sudden facial diplegia is rare, when it does occur it is generally believed to be a part of the Guillain-Barré syndrome. This author describes 2 patients who have this condition in the absence of the Guillan-Barré syndrome. Whenever sudden facial diplegia occurs, a differential diagnosis should include infectious mononucleosis and the patient should be carefully evaluated for the presence of underlying systemic disease. – Ed.] ◄

Amyloidosis with Plasma Cell Dyscrasia: Overlooked Cause of Adult-Onset Sensorimotor Neuropathy. John L. Trotter (Washington Univ.), W. King Engel (Natl. Inst. of Health) and Thomas F. Ignaczak[6] (Univ. of Michigan) discovered erstwhile "primary" nonhereditary amyloidosis to be the overlooked cause of a predominantly sensory, painful, hyperesthetic distal neuropathy in 10 patients with previously undiagnosed disease.

The patients, with nonhereditary disease, were seen during 1965–74. All had abnormalities of the peripheral or autonomic nervous system; 2 had carpal tunnel syndrome. The mean age at the time symptoms began was 54 and the duration of illness at last examination was 2–10 years. Eight patients were men. None had a family history of neurologic disease.

Nine patients had pain in the distal lower limbs and 1 had hand pain. The pain was usually aching or burning. Distal numbness was an early complaint of all patients. Five noted significant distal hyperesthesia. Sensory symptoms were typically symmetric and progressed a variable distance proximally in the lower limbs before affecting the upper limbs and ventral trunk. Symptoms of autonomic dysfunction were prominent; these included impotence, orthostatic hypotension, constipation and diarrhea and hypohidrosis.

(6) Arch. Neurol. 34:209–214, April, 1977.

Seven patients had had fasciculations at some time. Three patients were totally areflexic when first seen.

Typical denervation changes were evident on electromyography. Motor nerve maximum conduction velocities were mildly slowed to unobtainable. All sural nerve and muscle biopsy specimens showed loss of unmyelinated and myelinated fibers and fibrosis and amyloid deposits in and around blood vessel walls. All patients eventually had evidence of more generalized amyloid deposition. Cardiac involvement was prominent. Seven of 8 patients had a monoclonal "spike" on serum electrophoresis. Seven had over 4% plasma cells in marrow specimens and 2 of them had "overt multiple myeloma." Four patients exhibited no response to treatment with melphalan and prednisone. Three patients have died of cardiac amyloidosis with heart failure and 1 survivor is on long-term hemodialysis for renal insufficiency.

The neuropathy in this form of amyloidosis appears to be secondary to a plasma cell-originating dysproteinemia. The mechanism of diffuse nerve damage in amyloidosis is not known but a toxic-metabolic process is favored.

► [Patients with the hereditary (Portugese) variety of amyloidosis have, in addition to severe polyneuropathy, orthostatic hypotension, constipation or diarrhea, and male impotence. These patients with a predominantly sensory, painful and hyperesthetic distal neuropathy, associated also with the above-listed symptoms, were found to have "primary" nonhereditary amyloidosis that was diagnosed by the finding of crystal-violet metachromasia of amyloid in fresh-frozen sections of nerve and muscle biopsy specimens. It was concluded that the neuropathy in this form of amyloidosis is secondary to a plasma cell-originating dysproteinemia. — Ed.] ◄

Spinal Cord Disease

Cervical Spondylotic Radiculopathy and Myelopathy: Long-Term Follow-up Study. F. Karl Gregorius, Thelma Estrin and Paul H. Crandall[7] (Univ. of California, Los Angeles) followed 96 patients operated on for severe cervical spondylotic myelopathy and radiculopathy for a mean time of over 7 years. The average age of the 63 men and 33 women was 51 years at the onset of symptoms and 53 years on admission. Myelopathy was present in 55 patients and radiculopathy in 41. All had had 1 operation after progressive deterioration despite conservative management. Anterior interbody fusion was done by the Cloward technique in 62 cases and laminectomy in 30. Four patients underwent posterior lateral laminectomy with foraminotomy.

Patients with radiculopathy were generally operated on for chronic unremitting pain and numbness. Results after a mean follow-up of 7.3 years were excellent in 13 cases, improved in 18, unchanged in 5 and worse in 5. Twenty-four of 38 patients evaluated had no disability, 10 had moderate disability and 4 were bedridden. Patients with myelopathy were most commonly operated on for progressively declining spinal cord function. On follow-up, 21 patients were excellent or improved, 10 were unchanged and 24 were worse. Nine patients were unimpaired and working full-time, 20 were moderately disabled and 24 were severely disabled. The only preoperative feature related to the outcome was sphincter disturbance. Disability tended to decrease after anterior interbody fusion and to increase after laminectomy.

A trend toward improvement in disability was seen after anterior interbody fusion in patients with myelopathy in this series. Myelographic evidence of block to contrast flow was not necessarily associated with a poor result. Atrophy of the cervical cord, seen on air myelography or at operation,

(7) Arch. Neurol. 33:618–625, September, 1976.

also did not necessarily imply a poor result. Age at admission did not influence the outcome in this series. The results were not related to the number of radiographic levels of disease.

▶ [A worsening disability in patients operated on for the treatment of cervical spondylotic myelopathy was associated with preoperative symptoms of sphincter disturbance and lower extremity weakness. In other patients, improvement was maintained for an average of 85 months. Postoperative changes in hand movement and distance walking were not correlated with numerous preoperative factors. Results of operations for relief of radiculopathy were consistently good. – Ed.] ◀

Narrow Lumbar Spinal Canal with "Vascular" Syndromes. Panayotis E. Karayannacos, David Yashon and John S. Vasko[8] (Ohio State Univ.) operated on 14 patients with a verified narrow lumbar spinal canal syndrome (lumbar spondylosis) during 1969 – 72; they had been admitted first to a vascular service because of symptoms and signs of vascular disease.

Three patients had typical intermittent claudication; 10 had atypical symptoms mimicking arterial or venous disease. In all cases, vascular disease was excluded before neurosurgical evaluation. The patients had cauda equina compromise from herniated disk, osteoarthritis and hypertrophic ligaments. Complete follow-up data were available for 3 patients with typical claudication and 4 with atypical features. Operation showed herniated intervertebral disks, osteophytic bone or hypertrophied ligamenta flava, or a combination of these. All patients benefited from lumbar laminectomy.

When patients with vascular-like symptoms are without arterial or venous disease, lumbar spondylosis should be considered: chronic incapacitating pain without vascular disease and electromyography provide clues. Myelography should be done even in the absence of neurologic signs, since plain spinal x-rays do not show the abnormality. The symptoms of a narrow spinal canal are not always typical of neurologic disease. The cause of intermittent claudication with narrow spinal canal has not been well defined. The vascular factor seems more important than the mechanical factor. The operation of choice generally is a wide laminectomy sufficient to decompress the involved cauda equina seg-

(8)   Arch. Surg. 111:803 – 806, July, 1976.

ments. The removal of herniated or extruded disks also may be necessary and foraminotomies of compressed nerve roots should be done. The operation is suited to the needs of each patient.

▶ [When patients with vascular-like symptoms are found to be free of arterial or venous disease, lumbar spondylosis should be considered. Plain x-rays of the lumbar spine may not show the abnormality. Myelography thus should be carried out even in the absence of neurologic signs. — Ed.] ◀

Diagnosis and Natural History of Spinal Cord Arteriovenous Malformations. W. Dennis Tobin and Donald D. Layton, Jr.[9] (Mayo Clinic) reviewed the records of 47 male and 24 female patients with established spinal cord arteriovenous malformations seen in 1940–75. Patients were aged $2\frac{1}{2}$–72 years but most were aged 30–70. Most of the lesions were in the middle and lower thoracic or thoracolumbar cord. Four lesions were extremely extensive. Only 2 of 8 patients under age 20 had cervical involvement. Arteriovenous malformation was suspected in only 10% of the 64 patients who presented without subarachnoid hemorrhage.

A slowly progressive course characterized 73% of the cases; 10% had an abrupt onset with subarachnoid hemorrhage. Most patients were diagnosed within 2 years after the onset of symptoms. Leg weakness with sensory loss, pain and early sphincter involvement was a common presentation. The location of pain was not a reliable indicator of the level of involvement.

Thirteen patients had severe deficits at diagnosis and 4 patients presented with essentially end-stage paraplegia and neurogenic bowel or bladder. Plain spinal films were not diagnostically helpful. Myelography did not permit a consistently correct prediction of the extent of the lesion or the degree of an anterior or intramedullary component. Eight of 38 patients who had angiography were shown to have a significant anterior component to their lesions and 4 had a significant intramedullary component.

Most spinal arteriovenous malformations are in the thoracic cord. The use of subtraction techniques, stereoscopy and transaxial tomography may allow better evaluation of the extent of intramedullary lesions. Di Chiro et al. (1967) and Baker et al. (1967) distinguished three angiographic

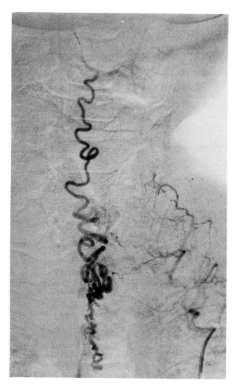

Fig 41. — Type III arteriovenous malformation at C7 – T2. Multiple arterial feeders were identified arising from thyrocervical and costocervical trunks. Lesion was located on dorsal surface of cord and was composed mainly of venous channels. (Courtesy of Tobin, W. D., and Layton, D. D., Jr.: Mayo Clin. Proc. 51:637–646, October, 1976.)

classes of cord malformation; type I, the single coiled vessel; type II, the glomus anomaly; and type III, the juvenile malformation (Fig 41). A more surgically relevant classification would divide all malformations into two groups, one with one or two arterial inputs and an essentially dorsal location and the other with multiple feeding vessels and more structural pleomorphism. The prognosis of arteriovenous malformations of the spinal cord requires further study.

► [It is of interest that these malformations occur more often in men than in women and that disturbances of micturition appear much earlier with these lesions than they do with disk syndromes or neoplasms. – Ed.] ◄

Brain Stem Dysfunction Related to Cervical Manipulation: Report of Three Cases. Fewer than 20 cases have been reported concerning the association of cervical manipulation and vertebrobasilar artery ischemia resulting in central nervous system symptomatology. S. Mueller and A. L. Sahs[1] (Univ. of Iowa) report 3 cases of vertebrobasilar ischemic damage after cervical manipulation. The cases represent a spectrum of symptomatology from mildest to relatively severe, but none of the patients died. Patients were seen over a 15-month period.

Man, 38, with mild headaches for 3–4 years believed to be emotional in origin, had had cervical and occipital headache after the most recent of several mechanical spinal adjustments; he also had nausea and vomiting, dizziness and inability to walk unaided. His speech was slurred and the right side of the face drooped. Examination showed marked dysarthria, peripheral facial palsy on the

Fig 42. – Left vertebral angiogram. Lateral "step-off" at C2 level. (Courtesy of Mueller, S., and Sahs, A. L.: Neurology (Minneap.) 26:547–550, June, 1976.)

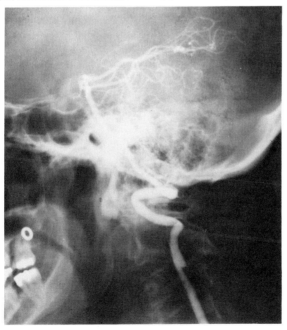

(1) Neurology (Minneap.) 26:547–550, June, 1976.

right, deviation of the tongue to the right and bilateral 6th nerve palsies. The right extremities were ataxic and pain sensation was reduced over the medial left calf. Arteriography showed an irregular right distal vertebral artery segment and a "step-off" at the C2 level in the left vertebral artery (Fig 42).

Ventriculography done 2 days later showed enlarged lateral ventricles; a contrast study showed a shift of the 4th ventricle to the left. A ventriculosubgaleal shunt was placed on the right. Craniectomy, done 8 days after admission, showed hemorrhagic infarction of the right cerebellar hemisphere. The patient improved slowly after operation. He returned to work 1 year after discharge, when speech and motor function had improved and the only symptom was occasional right-sided headache.

Angiography was not done on the other 2 patients, 1 of whom had an anterior dislocation at the C2 level after manipulation. Apparently, cervical manipulation precipitated compromise of posterior circulation in these cases, leading to brain stem or cerebellar ischemia. The trauma may be direct or indirect through alteration of a normal cervical bony alignment by the manipulation, compressing blood vessels and compromising blood flow. Neurologic dysfunction can range from minimal to severe in these patients.

► [It is reasonable to assume that cervical manipulation may cause a compromise in blood flow through the vertebrobasilar system, leading to brain stem or cerebellar ischemia. The possible dangers of such manipulation should always be borne in mind. — Ed.] ◄

Vascular Disease

Platelet Aggregation, Stroke and Transient Ischemic Attack in Middle-Aged and Elderly Patients. Platelet aggregation at areas of endothelial damage has been postulated as the initiating event in the formation of the atheromatous plaque; platelet aggregates in the bloodstream could act as microemboli. James R. Couch and Ruth S. Hassanein[2] (Univ. of Kansas) evaluated platelet aggregability in patients with history of recent transient ischemic attacks (TIAs) or who were at least 7 days post thrombotic stroke, and in age-, sex- and race-matched controls. No patient had used drugs that might alter platelet aggregation. Platelet aggregation was examined by the optical density method. The 39 study patients, aged 38–89 years, included 18 "young" and 21 "old" patients.

Platelet aggregability was increased significantly in young stroke patients compared with young controls at most adenosine diphosphate (ADP) concentrations. Older stroke patients and controls did not differ significantly. Percentage disaggregation was significantly less for young stroke patients than for young controls for aggregation tested at 1.7 μM ADP. Platelet aggregability was not influenced by time since stroke. Older control subjects showed a highly significant increase in platelet aggregability compared with younger ones but no such age effect was seen in stroke patients.

These data suggest that platelet aggregability is increased in young patients with stroke and increases with age. The degree of platelet aggregability is not a function of the interval between stroke and testing, excluding the acute poststroke phase. Platelet hyperaggregability is a significant risk factor for stroke in middle-aged and elderly patients but this risk factor may be relatively more important in middle-aged or younger subjects. Alternately, stroke pa-

(2) Neurology (Minneap.) 26:888–895, September, 1976.

tients aged 35–60 years may represent a unique subgroup with platelet characteristics different from those in older stroke patients. More data are needed to determine which of these hypotheses is more tenable.

▶ [This study suggests that platelet aggregability is a significant risk factor for stroke that is relatively more important in the younger than in the older patient. — Ed.] ◀

Prevalence of Cerebral Hemorrhage and Thrombosis in Japan: Study of Major Causes of Death. Vascular lesions of the central nervous system, especially cerebral hemorrhage, generally are accepted as the most common cause of death in Japan, a country that is unique in the world in this respect. About one fourth of all deaths in Japan are caused by vascular central nervous system lesions, and the ratio of hemorrhage to thrombosis is high. Martin G. Netsky (Vanderbilt Univ.) and Toru Miyaji[3] (Osaka Univ.) found that these beliefs are artifacts of diagnosis and recording and that malignant neoplasms are the major cause of death in Japan. Review was made of causes of death from 1920 to 1965 from death certificates.

A large diagnostic error in certification of cerebrovascular diseases, especially cerebral hemorrhage, was found. Comparison of death certificate data with data from autopsies done throughout Japan showed major discrepancies. Malignant neoplasms were the major killer, vascular lesions of the central nervous system constituting 4.5% of deaths. Cerebral thrombosis exceeded cerebral hemorrhage, and a predilection for the North was not evident.

The autopsy data, however, had many deficits, notably selection factors, age and sex distribution, and quality of reports, and a small number in relation to total deaths. Autopsies performed by the Atomic Bomb Casualty Commission (ABCC) have greater validity. The group studied had age and sex characteristics of the mortality group in Japan, and the quality of data was relatively high. The ABCC findings also revealed that malignancy was the major cause of death (30.4%). Vascular lesions of the central nervous system were the fifth most frequent cause of death. Cerebral thrombosis slightly exceeded hemorrhage in the ABCC series.

(3) J. Chronic Dis. 29:711–721, November, 1976.

Clinical data further substantiate the concept that the rate of fatal cerebrovascular disease in Japan is similar to that in the United States. It is suggested that the high rate of cerebrovascular disease, and especially of cerebral hemorrhage, in Japan is an artifact of diagnosis and recording methods.

► [It appears that in Japan, as in the United States and probably as in most other countries, data from death certificates cannot be relied on to give valid information. – Ed.] ◄

Positional Cerebral Ischemia. L. R. Caplan and S. Sergay[4] (Harvard Med. School) describe 4 patients with occlusive cerebrovascular disease in whom dramatic transient central nervous system deficits developed when the patients were raised from the supine position. Postural sensitivity was present early in the stroke syndrome but remitted after several weeks.

Woman, 56, with classic migraine for many years, noted transient numbness of the right hand 2 days before hospitalization and right limb weakness on admission. The husband witnessed a gradual increase in right-sided weakness and a slow disorganization of speech, followed by gradual improvement. Examination showed severe right hemiplegia, paraphasic verbal errors, poor localization of tactile stimuli on the right and visual inattention. The blood pressure was 170/100 mm Hg.

The patient was placed in the supine position and improved markedly. Carotid angiography showed complete occlusion of the left internal carotid artery at the carotid bifurcation in the neck, with collateral circulation from the external carotid artery filling the middle cerebral artery via the left ophthalmic artery. The right internal carotid artery was moderately stenosed at the bifurcation. The patient sat up the next morning and developed severe aphasia and right hemiplegia. She improved when placed in Trendelenburg's position. Hemiparesis and poor speech returned when the patient sat up over the next 6 days, without postural blood pressure change. After day 11, the patient sat and gradually walked without difficulty and by day 21 no deficit remained. The patient was well 3 years later.

All patients had documented occlusive cerebrovascular disease; 2 had basilar artery occlusion. All had had transient ischemic attacks and a fluctuating clinical course. Striking deficits occurred with the patients erect. Patients with posterior circulatory disease had respiratory arrest,

(4) J. Neurol. Neurosurg. Psychiatry 39:385–391, April, 1976.

stupor and bilateral brain stem signs. The patients were kept supine for 3 weeks and then were mobilized slowly and carefully. One patient had cerebral infarction but the others had no significant deficits.

Position in bed may be critical in some patients with occlusive cerebrovascular disease, especially those with fluctuating signs. These patients should be kept either supine or in Trendelenburg's position and should be mobilized gradually, with caution, on a trial-and-error basis.

▶ [In 4 patients with occlusive cerebrovascular disease documented angiographically, there were recurrent episodes of dramatic transient clinical worsening when the patients were raised from the supine to the sitting position even though postural hypotension was not present. Such patients should be maintained either supine or in Trendelenburg's position and, after a period best determined by trial and error, they should be mobilized gradually with caution and supervision.—Ed.] ◀

Comparison of Computerized Tomography and Radionuclide Imaging in "Stroke." Mokhtar H. Gado, R. Edward Coleman, Anthony L. Merlis, Philip O. Alderson and Kil Soo Lee[5] (Washington Univ.) compared computerized tomography (CT) and nuclide brain scanning in 40 patients with a final diagnosis of cerebrovascular accident. There were 28 patients with recent hemispheric infarction, 1 with recent cerebellar infarction, 7 with intracerebral hemorrhage and 1 with subarachnoid hemorrhage. The mean interval between CT and nuclide brain imaging was 1.8 days; it was less than a week in all patients. The CT scans were made with an EMI scanner and nuclide brain scans with a scintillation camera and $15-20$ mCi ^{99m}Tc-pertechnetate. Both rapid-sequence and static-image studies were carried out.

Among the 29 patients with recent infarction, 55% had abnormal CT scans and 69% had abnormal nuclide brain images. The CT abnormality consisted of decreased density of the brain tissue. Rapid-sequence scintigraphy was normal in 10 of the 20 patients with abnormal nuclide images. There was no increased uptake in 8 patients with recent infarction. Both studies were negative in 3 patients. None of 3 patients studied a year after stroke showed increased nuclide uptake, but both rapid-sequence studies showed a flip-flop phenomenon. The CT scan was positive in all 3 of these

(5)   Stroke 7:109–113, Mar.–Apr., 1976.

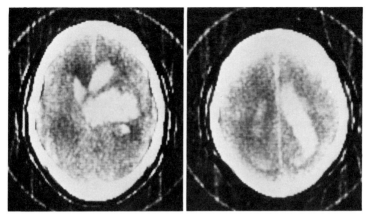

Fig 43. – Right intracerebral hematoma. Computerized tomography scan shows increased density caused by high x-ray absorbency of clotted blood in deep portion of right cerebral hemisphere. Blood clot extended into lateral ventricle. (Courtesy of Gado, M. H., et al.: Stroke 7:109–113, Mar.–Apr., 1976; by permission of the American Heart Association, Inc.)

patients. Nuclide imaging was more often positive a week or longer after the incident but this was not true of CT studies. Intracerebral hematoma was detected by CT in all 7 patients (Fig 43) and in all patients the nature of the lesion was determined, as distinct from infarction, by its high density. The nuclide studies showed increased uptake indistinct from infarction in 2 patients; the other 5 had normal nuclide studies.

The incidence of abnormalities on CT scanning in patients with cerebral infarction is comparable to that with nuclide imaging, but CT is far superior in cases of intracerebral hematoma. Only CT will distinguish intracerebral hematoma from cerebral infarction. The two study methods are complementary in evaluating patients with stroke.

► [This study indicates that computerized tomography was far superior to radionuclide scanning in detecting intracerebral hematomas and distinguishing them from cerebral infarction, but each technique has its value in the study of patients with cerebrovascular disease. – Ed.] ◄

Bulbar Infarctions. – *Systematic study of lesional topography in 49 cases.* – J.-J. Hauw, P. Der Agopian, L. Trelles and R. Escourolle[6] (Hôp. de la Salpetriere, Paris) made a

(6) J. Neurol. Sci. 28:83–102, May, 1976.

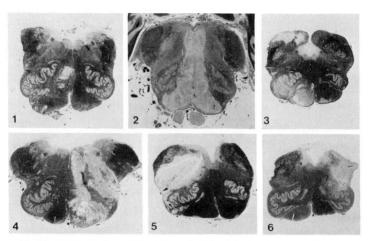

Fig 44. – Isolated infarct of the right medial area. Note involvement of the anterior part of the medial lemniscus and that, more discrete, of the pyramidal fascicles. Embedded in celloidin; Loyez stain. (Courtesy of Hauw, J.-J., et al.: J. Neurol. Sci. 28 83–102, May, 1976.)

pathologic study of 33 patients with 49 medullary infarcts. After removal of the arterial supply the brain stem was sectioned perpendicular to its longitudinal axis. The medulla oblongata was then examined microscopically, at various levels.

Twelve medial infarcts were seen in 10 patients. Ischemic lesions were found in only 2 cases (Fig 44), and in 1 of them the lesions were bilateral. Three cases had no other medullary lesion. In 6 cases there was, in addition, a lateral medullary infarct, which was homolateral 4 times, contralateral once and associated with a bilateral infarct once. The dorsal region was affected by an infarct in 3 cases (homolateral in 2 cases and contralateral in 1 case).

Thirty lateral infarcts were seen in 29 patients. The inferior salivatory nucleus (or its area) seemed injured in 5 cases, but because of its small size and difficulty in precise identification, it was excluded from the study. The external part of the ventral lamina of the olive was slightly affected in 1 case. The ependyma was always spared, except when there was concomitant involvement of the dorsal region.

Seven dorsal infarcts were seen in 7 patients. When a dorsal infarct was associated with a lateral infarct on the same side, it seemed difficult to differentiate the two lesions. In 1 case the presence of lesions of different ages helped to make this distinction. None of the lesions was isolated. Three were associated with a lateral infarct on the same side and 2 with a homolateral medial infarct; 1 was associated with a lateral infarct on the opposite side and 1 with a lateral infarct on the same side and a contralateral medial infarct.

No infarcts involving the olivary region were observed. This appeared to be due to the possibilities of supply by both lateral and medial vessels. Moreover, it is probable that there are rich craniocaudal anastomoses in this region.

Study of vascular lesions in 26 patients. — Escourolle, Hauw, Der Agopian and Trelles,[7] as the second part of a study of bulbar infarcts, investigated the arrangement of arterial lesions in 26 patients with 38 bulbar infarcts. In 10 patients, only the intracranial vessels (Fig 45) were examined. In the other 16, the entire arterial system which supplies the brain was removed and dissected.

Three medial infarcts were located on the right, 3 on the left and 2 bilaterally. Occlusion of the termination of the vertebral artery homolateral to the infarct opposite the ostium of its anterior spinal branch and the arterioles of the foramen caecum was the cause of 7 cases in 5 patients. Study of 6 cases in 4 patients revealed a thrombosis on an

Fig 45. — Arrangement and vascular lesions in 10 cases of bulbar infarcts in patients in whom only intracranial vessels were examined. Black areas indicate atheroma (indented: ulceration); hatched areas indicated occlusion. (Courtesy of Escourolle, R., et al.: J. Neurol. Sci. 28:103 – 113, May, 1976.)

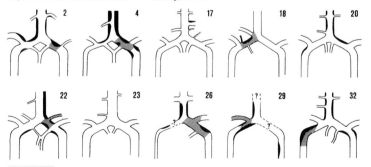

(7)   J. Neurol. Sci. 28:103 – 113, May, 1976.

atheromatous plaque in 4 cases, a probable embolus of cardiac origin in 1 case and occlusion of a vertebral artery at its origin in the other.

There were 9 lateral infarcts on the right side, 12 on the left and 1 bilaterally. Among 14 occlusions of the homolateral vertebral artery (of 23 lateral infarcts), 13 were due to a thrombosis of atheromatous origin. The other case was secondary to a blood clot originating from the ostium of the vertebral artery, the site of a severe atheromatous stenosis (90%).

Three dorsal infarcts were located on the right and 2 on the left. Etiology of the dorsal infarct is caused by occlusion of the trunk of the posterior inferior cerebellar artery. Of the 5 cases, 4 involved isolated occlusion of the trunk of the homolateral posterior inferior cerebellar artery. In 3 of these cases, it was due to a thrombosis which developed on an atheromatous plaque; in the other case, it was secondary to an embolus of cardiac origin. In the 5th case, the thrombotic occlusion of the vertebral artery involved the ostium of the inferior cerebellar artery.

► [This article and the preceding one give the results of an extensive study of medullary infarction that demonstrates that medullary infarcts are seldom single. Medial infarcts are related most often to occlusion of the vertebral artery, whereas lateral infarcts may also follow occlusion of the vertebral artery, especially near the origin of the posterior inferior cerebellar artery, but may also result from isolated occlusions of the latter artery. – Ed.] ◄

Pathologic Basilar Artery is described by J. Danziger, S. Bloch and H. Podlas[8] (Johannesburg). Malformations and variations in position of the basilar artery occur and an adequate evaluation of this artery is essential when pathology related to the posterior fossa is suspected. Aneurysms usually occur at the origin or bifurcation of the basilar artery. They may be small or large; when small, the clinical manifestations are due to subarachnoid hemorrhage. Giant aneurysms encroach on neighboring structures and present as mass lesions. Curvilinear calcification may be seen behind the clivus in these cases. Air studies will show posterior displacement of the brain stem. Vertebral angiography will define the vascular etiology but may not show the full extent of the aneurysm.

(8) Clin. Radiol. 27:309–316, July, 1976.

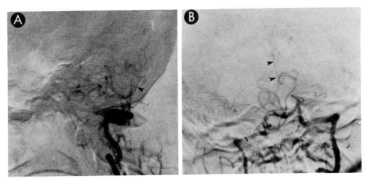

Fig 46. – Left vertebral angiogram. Lateral (**A**) and anteroposterior (**B**) projections with subtraction, demonstrating nonvisualization of basilar artery. Contrast material has refluxed down contralateral vertebral artery. Vermal branch of posterior inferior cerebellar is seen *(arrowheads)*. (Courtesy of Danziger, J., et al.: Clin. Radiol. 27:309–316, July, 1976.)

Tortuosity may be seen in arteriosclerotic patients. Air study may show features of a normal-pressure hydrocephalus. With extreme tortuosity of the artery the brain stem is displaced backward. When arteriovenous malformations receive an arterial supply from the basilar artery or its branches, the vessel becomes enlarged and elongated. Some patients with basilar artery occlusion have an adequate collateral circulation and survive. Occlusion usually occurs distal to the origin of the posterior inferior cerebellar arteries (Fig 46) but it may extend more proximally to involve a vertebral artery and the posterior inferior cerebellar artery arising from it. The distal extension of the occlusion is usually just proximal to the origin of the superior cerebellar arteries. Vertebral angiography may show partial or no filling of the basilar artery. Most basilar artery occlusions are due to arteriosclerosis.

The basilar artery may be displaced anteriorly by intra-axial tumors or tumors lying posterior to the brain stem or posteriorly away from the clivus by extra-axial posterior fossa tumors. However, posterior displacement of the brain stem may also be produced by pathology of the posterior 3d ventricle, pontine tumors or aqueductal stenosis in infants.

▶ [Vascular anomalies of the basilar artery can mimic many intracranial diseases. In this article, various abnormalities of the artery are discussed, as well as the displacements of the artery secondary to mass lesions in the posterior fossa. — Ed.] ◄

Use of Holter Electrocardiographic Monitor in Diagnosis of Transient Ischemic Attacks. Transient ischemic attacks are episodes of reversible central nervous system insufficiency, occurring as part of the complex of cerebrovascular atherosclerosis. Eugene B. Levin[9] (Univ. of Califor-

Fig 47. — Continuous Holter monitor strip, as patient fainted. Note asystole. (Courtesy of Levin, E. B.: J. Am. Geriatr. Soc. 24:516–521, November, 1976.)

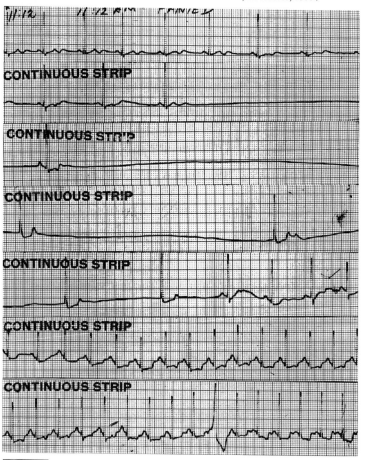

(9) J. Am. Geriatr. Soc. 24:516–521, November, 1976.

nia, Irvine) reviewed the results of Holter continuous ECG monitoring in 204 patients during the past 2½ years at a small community hospital.

The findings in a man aged 70, who had blackouts and whose only physical abnormality was faintness on slight pressure on the right carotid artery, are shown in Figure 47. The sick sinus syndrome was present in about 16% of patients. Pacemakers were inserted in 54 patients, in 24 because of the sick sinus syndrome, in 16 for sinus bradycardia and in 14 for heart block. Nine of the bradycardic patients, all those with heart block and 17 of those with sinus syndrome had significant cerebral symptoms. There was little morbidity and no mortality after pacemaker implantation.

Cardiac events can produce transient ischemic attacks and strokes in the elderly and in patients with a compromised cerebral circulation. A patient with central nervous system insufficiency of any degree should receive a complete medical workup, including continuous ECG monitoring by the Holter technique. This monitoring may reveal previously undetected cardiac abnormalities that can be alleviated by suitable drugs or by a pacemaker. In many cases the cerebral symptoms disappear after cardiac therapy. The Holter monitor is a valuable tool in evaluating patients with cerebrovascular insufficiency.

Long-Term ECG Monitoring in Patients with Cerebrovascular Insufficiency. Use of the Holter monitor permits monitoring of patients to detect transient dysrhythmias that may be associated with generalized or focal neurologic symptoms. Lawrence C. McHenry, Jr., James F. Toole and Henry S. Miller[1] (Bowman Gray School of Medicine) describe 10 patients with cerebrovascular insufficiency who had long-term Holter ECG monitoring to detect dysrhythmias associated with cerebrovascular symptoms. Nine patients were admitted with neurologic symptoms suggestive of cerebrovascular insufficiency and 1, because of two episodes of syncope. The patients were monitored for up to 24 hours with the Holter monitor. Eight patients had transient ischemic attacks or reversible ischemic deficits, and 2 had mild residual deficits from a completed stroke. Four of the former patients had symptoms in the internal carotid distri-

(1) Stroke 7:264–269, May–June, 1976.

bution and the rest, in the basilar-vertebral system. Four patients were hypertensive.

Four patients had no abnormalities on Holter ECG monitoring. The other 6 had a variety of cardiac dysrhythmias. They included frequent premature atrial or ventricular contractions, intraventricular conduction abnormality, suggestive Wolff-Parkinson-White syndrome, and questionable junctional rhythm. There were no persistent dysrhythmias, but frequent conduction defects of bradycardia occurred in 6 patients, and 1 had a changing pacemaker. The most common abnormal angiographic finding was carotid stenosis. Only 1 patient required a cardiac pacemaker. Three patients had carotid endarterectomies.

Over half of these patients had disturbances in cardiac rhythm or conduction that could have been directly associated with, or suggested an etiology for, the patient's neurologic event. Conflicting reports on the cardiac findings in patients with cerebrovascular insufficiency emphasize the need for further studies using prolonged cardiac monitoring in such patients.

► [Disturbances of cardiac rhythm and conduction may be responsible for cerebrovascular insufficiency in some patients. This can be demonstrated by the use of long-term ECG monitoring. — Ed.] ◄

Cerebral Ischemic Events Associated with Prolapsing Mitral Valve. Neurologic disturbances in patients with prolapsing mitral valve (PMV) have been noted in passing. Henry J. M. Barnett, Michael W. Jones, Derek R. Boughner and William J. Kostuk[2] (Univ. Hosp., London, Ont.) report transient and persistent cerebral ischemic events in 12 patients with PMV. The patients were encountered during a prospective trial of platelet-inhibiting drugs in cases of transient ischemic attacks and partial nonprogressing stroke. Cardiac monitoring was carried out for 24 – 72 hours. No study patient had significant extracranial or intracranial atherosclerotic disease on cerebral angiography. There were 215 cases of proved PMV and 154 patients with transient ischemia and nonprogressing stroke during the 4-year study period.

Seven men and 5 women aged 18 – 67 years had PMV and cerebral ischemic events. One of the women was taking an

(2) Arch. Neurol. 33:777–782, November, 1976.

oral contraceptive. No patient was hypertensive. Four patients had periodic bouts of chest pain, 5 had palpitations and 2 had light-headedness and faintness. The echogram showed PMV in 8 cases. Cardiac monitoring showed ventricular tachycardia in 1 patient, who died suddenly 2 years later. All patients had typical angiographic features of PMV. Eight patients had multiple neurologic attacks, and 4 had single attacks. The more frequent episodes were typical of transient ischemic attacks. Nine patients had transient hemiparesis or major stroke. Four of the 6 patients who had repeat angiography a year or more later when recurrent events developed had an occluded intracranial artery. One patient had an occluded posterior cerebral artery appropriate to symptoms of visual disturbances.

The ischemic events in these cases appear to be related to emboli emanating from the abnormal mitral valve, with or without an associated paroxysmal cardiac arrhythmia. Treatment for these PMV patients will include antiarrhythmic agents, possibly anticoagulants, and possibly drugs that interfere with platelet function. Cardiac monitoring is important in patients with transient ischemic attacks or partial nonprogressive stroke, especially in younger patients with normal cerebral angiographic findings.

► [Cerebral ischemic events may be related to emboli emanating from an abnormal mitral valve with or without associated paroxysmal cardiac arrhythmia. These may occur in patients younger than those who commonly have transient ischemic attacks and may occur in the absence of hypertension, coagulation defects or arteriosclerotic cerebrovascular disease, or in those receiving contraceptive therapy. – Ed.] ◄

Limitations of Doppler Cerebrovascular Examination in Hemispheric Cerebral Ischemia. The Doppler cerebrovascular examination has appeared to be a potentially valuable means of noninvasive assessment of carotid artery dynamics. George E. Bone and Robert W. Barnes[3] (Iowa City) attempted to characterize more clearly the role of this examination in the clinical evaluation of patients with carotid territory ischemic syndromes.

Doppler findings and arteriograms of 56 consecutive patients with resolved hemispheric stroke or hemispheric transient ischemic attacks were reviewed. None had severe, fixed neurologic deficits. Eighteen patients had a history of

(3)   Surgery 79:577–580, May, 1976.

previous focal hemispheric stroke, whereas 38 had had recurring transient hemispheric cerebral ischemic attacks. All patients were men; their average age was 60 years. Reduced frontal artery flow was demonstrated during arterial compression by the Doppler ultrasonic technique. Directional flow was assessed in the frontal artery with compression of the infraorbital and facial arteries, as well as the superficial temporal artery. Transient compression of each common carotid artery was also carried out. This technique was 99% accurate in detecting 75% or greater stenosis or occlusion of the internal carotid artery in a series of 453 examinations.

Examination of the ipsilateral carotid system was abnormal in 8 of 18 patients with resolved hemispheric stroke. Angiograms showed complete internal carotid occlusion in 4 cases, and over 75% stenosis in the other 4. Eight of 10 patients with normal Doppler findings had less than 75% stenosis, and 2 had no extracranial carotid lesion. The Doppler findings were abnormal in 10 of 38 patients with transient ischemia. Angiograms showed 6 significantly stenotic lesions and 1 at 60% stenosis. Seventeen of the 28 patients with normal Doppler findings had internal carotid lesions of potential clinical significance that were amenable to carotid endarterectomy. The overall accuracy of the Doppler study in detecting hemodynamically significant stenosis or occlusion was 94% in this series, but the accuracy in terms of operable lesions was only 31%.

The Doppler technique provides a rapid means of noninvasively detecting hemodynamically significant carotid artery lesions. The examination may prove useful in evaluating carotid bruits, determining the operative priority of bilateral carotid lesions, detecting postendarterectomy thrombosis and assessing nonhemispheric cerebrovascular symptoms.

► [This article and a similar one by the same authors (Clinical implications of the Doppler cerebrovascular examination: A correlation with angiography, Stroke 7:271, 1976) indicate that the Doppler examination has only an adjunct role in the evaluation of patients with hemispheric symptoms of cerebrovascular occlusive disease. In such patients the Doppler examination is not an appropriate criterion in making the decision of whether or not to proceed with angiography. — Ed.] ◄

Subcortical Arteriosclerotic Encephalopathy (Binswanger's Disease): Vascular Etiology of Dementia. Vascular dementias are usually engendered by extensive cortical softenings, but occasionally they are derived from the diffuse white matter degeneration of subcortical arteriosclerotic encephalopathy (SAE) or Binswanger's disease. Peter C. Burger, J. Gordon Burch and Ulf Kunze[4] report a case of this unusual cerebrovascular disorder.

Man, 51, was hospitalized 6 times in 1 year for progressive dementia. Personality change, with impaired memory and easy fatigability, was initially accompanied by episodic ataxia, intermittent dysarthria and deterioration of handwriting. Left frontal slow wave EEG changes and elevated cerebrospinal fluid protein were found. Examination showed psychomotor retardation and positive snout and suck reflexes. Sequential EEGs showed diffuse deterioration of the background activity. Cisternography showed ventricular reflux, delayed clearance and absent sagittal activity after 24 and 48 hours. An air study showed marked ventricular dilatation and minimal free-convexity air. The patient became incontinent and completely disoriented, with frontal release signs, ataxia and mild left hemiparesis. Shunt malfunction was ruled out but angiography gave evidence of a subdural hemorrhage, and the patient's condition improved after evacuation of a hematoma. Subsequently a subdural empyema at the craniotomy site was drained successfully. Myoclonic jerks, mutism and lethargy preceded the

Fig 48.—Arteriole in centrum semiovale is markedly thickened. White matter is pale and contains small cystic spaces and reactive astrocytes. Hematoxylin-eosin–Luxol fast blue; original magnification ×225. (Courtesy of Burger, P. C., et al.: Stroke 7:626–631, Nov.–Dec., 1976; by permission of the American Heart Association, Inc.)

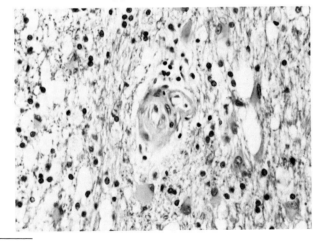

patient's death in marked obtundation and with bronchopneumonia.

The brain at autopsy showed moderate to severe atherosclerosis of the large vessels at the base and of the more peripheral middle cerebral artery branches. A cystic infarct was present in the right frontal lobe and another in the left parietal lobe. An organized subdural empyema was present over the right frontal lobe. Most of the lacunar infarcts were old, but a few were recent. Vascular changes were marked throughout the brain. Large confluent areas of white matter pallor were seen in the centrum semiovale (Fig 48) and cerebellar white matter and brain stem, representing decreased axon density and degenerating myelin.

This case is a dramatic example of progressive dementia in SAE. The white matter lesions clearly exceeded the watershed regions, but could have begun there. Binswanger's disease must be considered in cases of dementia, even in the presence of normal angiographic findings and in the absence of sustained hypertension and significant localizing neurologic signs.

► [This case demonstrates the need to consider vascular disesae as an etiology of dementia, even in the absence of localizing neurologic signs. — Ed.] ◄

Superior Sagittal Sinus Thrombosis. Dennis M. Gettelfinger and Emre Kokmen[5] (Univ. of Michigan) report 7 cases of superior sagittal sinus (SSS) thrombosis in adults unrelated to intracranial infection or neoplasm. The diagnosis was made antemortem in these cases.

Woman, 27, was admitted with left calf pain 5 days before she delivered a normal infant. Heparin therapy was given, with improvement, but severe bifrontal and left temporal headache occurred 2 days post partum, and worsening headache, vomiting and unsteadiness of gait were observed 5 days later. Platelets numbered 41,000/cu mm. Heparin was discontinued and the platelet count was 115,000/cu mm 4 days later. A brain scan was normal but an EEG was moderately abnormal and the patient was intermittently confused. The opening lumbar pressure was 270 mm cerebrospinal fluid and the protein content was 43 mg/100 ml. Dexamethasone was begun. Cerebral angiography showed extensive thrombosis of deep and superficial veins bilaterally, with occlusion of almost the entire SSS. Phenytoin treatment was instituted, but early papilledema and bilateral extensor plantar reflexes were observed. Heparin was given by continuous infusion and urokinase

(5) Arch. Neurol. 34:2–6, January, 1977.

was given intravenously. A hematoma developed at a puncture site when the platelets numbered 69,000/cu mm and the fibrinogen concentration was less than 45 mg/100 ml. Incoherent speech and right hemiparesis developed, and another angiogram showed a large avascular left cerebral mass. The patient died 6 days later.

Autopsy showed extensive thrombosis in the SSS and both transverse sinuses as well as in meningeal and cerebral veins. A large infarction was present in the right parietal area and a swollen infarction in the right occipital lobe. The left hemisphere contained a massive recent hemorrhage in the internal capsule. The ventricles contained bloody fluid.

The clinical features of SSS thrombosis vary with the setting in which it occurs and the extent of associated occlusions of other cerebral vasculature. The pathogenesis also varies, depending on the clinical setting. A coagulopathy seems to be contributory to most cases. The definitive diagnosis of SSS thrombosis is made by angiography. The natural history and prognosis are highly variable; the clinical course can be benign. Two of 3 of the authors' patients who received anticoagulants died of hemorrhagic intracranial complications. Four patients who previously took anticoagulants recovered completely on other forms of therapy. More conservative therapy with antiedema agents and anticonvulsants seems to be indicated.

► [The risk of untoward complications when anticoagulants are used in treating superior sagittal sinus thrombosis is sufficiently great for the authors to recommend more conservative therapy with antiedema agents and anticonvulsants. – Ed.] ◄

Pure Motor Hemiplegia due to Cerebral Cortical Infarction. Pure motor hemiplegia may result from lesions at sites other than the internal capsule or basis pontis. Theoretically, an appropriately placed infarction in the cerebral cortex may lead to pure motor hemiplegia. Sudhansu Chokroverty, Frank A. Rubino and Carol Haller[6] report 3 cases; in 1, autopsy confirmed the lesion site.

Man, 83, had transient weakness of the right side of the body, followed in 1 hour by complete paralysis. The blood pressure was 210/100 mm Hg. A mild central facial paresis on the right was noted, with complete paralysis of the right upper limb and severe diffuse weakness of the right leg. The hemiplegic limbs were flaccid but muscle stretch reflexes were greater on the affected side. An extensor plantar response was elicited on the right. Sensory find-

(6)   Arch. Neurol. 34:93–95, February, 1977.

ings were normal. The strength of the right leg improved considerably but the right arm remained functionless after rehabilitation. The patient died 5 months later from cardiopulmonary arrest.

Autopsy showed severe generalized and moderate coronary atherosclerosis, obstructive emphysema, occlusion of the left renal artery and atrophy of the left kidney. The major cerebral arteries showed atheromatous plaques. Old cystic infarctions were present in the cerebral cortex and thalamus. A thalamic lacuna on the left involved the medial edge of the anterior part of the posterior limb of the left internal capsule. The capsular lesion measured 5 × 1 mm.

The cerebral cortical infarction in this patient involved the face, arm and leg areas of the precentral cortex but spared the inferior portion of the posterior frontal cortex and most of the parietal cortex. The EEG findings indicated that pure motor hemiplegia was due to a cerebral cortical lesion in another patient. In the third patient, computerized axial tomography suggested a cortical lesion in the appropriate site for pure motor hemiplegia, although it did not show involvement of the motor cortex. Infarction of the cerebral cortex may cause pure motor hemiplegia.

▶ [It is probable that most discerning neurologists have long been aware of the fact that cerebral cortical infarction may cause a pure motor hemiplegia. Among 850 unselected stroke patients, R. W. Richter et al. found only 25 (3%) whose disorder fit a clinical definition of pure motor hemiparesis. Brain scans suggested that this picture may be associated with larger brain lesions than had been suspected before, as well as with lacunar infarctions (Stroke 8:58, 1977). – Ed.] ◀

Joint Study of Extracranial Arterial Occlusion: IX. Transient Ischemic Attacks in the Carotid Territory. William S. Fields and Noreen A. Lemak[7] (Univ. of Texas) present a prospective analysis of 79 patients hospitalized with transient ischemic attacks (TIAs) in the carotid territory who were followed for 1 – 9 years. All patients recovered fully within 24 hours. None had had a previous stroke or operation on the neck vessels. Twelve patients had attacks of amaurosis fugax, 38 had hemispheric episodes, 13 had both types of carotid events and 16 had a mixture of carotid and vertebrobasilar features. The average follow-up was 49 months. There were 54 men and 25 women in the series; the average age on admission was 60 years.

(7) J.A.M.A. 235:2608–2610, June 14, 1976.

Fifty patients (63%) had no other transient carotid episodes or strokes during follow-up. Eleven patients had documented occlusion of the appropriate carotid artery, as did 2 patients with recurrent TIAs and 1 who had a fatal stroke. Nineteen patients (24%) died, 6 of strokes and 11 of myocardial infarction or congestive heart failure. New cerebrovascular events occurred in 37% of patients. Fourteen patients (18%) had strokes during follow-up; only 1 was taking an anticoagulant at the time of stroke. Eleven of the 14 had other high-risk factors. Fifteen patients, including 5 on anticoagulant therapy, had recurrent transient carotid attacks during follow-up. Older patients and those who had had multiple transient attacks had more new vascular events during follow-up. Hypertension was diagnosed in 48% of all patients and in 64% of those having strokes.

Anticoagulant therapy, usually with dicumarol, was given to 30 patients. Sixteen patients took a coumarin drug consistently for 2–6 years with no untoward reactions. Only 14% of patients were severely disabled on follow-up. About 6% of patients at risk in the 1st 3 years had a stroke in this series. Only 15% of patients had strokes causing serious disability or death during follow-up.

► [It is probably impossible today to collect data on the natural history of transient ischemic attacks, inasmuch as virtually all patients who have more than one or two such attacks are receiving either medical or surgical treatment. – Ed.] ◄

Double-Blind Trial of Glycerol Therapy in Early Stroke. A double-blind trial by Mathew et al. in 1972 supported the use of intravenous glycerol therapy for early stroke; this view was strengthened by studies by Gilsanz et al. in 1975. Olle Larsson, Norm Marinovich and Kenneth Barber[8] (Fremantle, Australia) assessed the usefulness of this treatment using stricter criteria to select patients.

Twenty-seven patients hospitalized within 6 hours of the sudden onset of focal neurologic deficit were included in the trial. None had transient ischemic episodes or neurologic signs that cleared within 24 hours. Patients were randomly allocated to intravenous therapy with 10% dextrose or 10% glycerol in 5% dextrose solution, given for 6 hours on consecutive days for up to 6 days. Twelve patients received glycerol and 15 had placebo solution.

(8)   Lancet 1:832–834, Apr. 17, 1976.

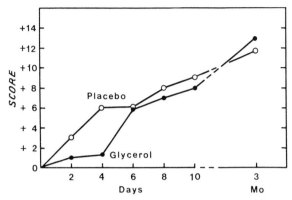

Fig 49. — Progressive change in mean scores of glycerol- *(black dot)* and dextrose-treated *(white dot)* groups in first 10 days and at 3 months. (Courtesy of Larsson, O., et al.: Lancet 1:832–834, Apr. 17, 1976.)

Four patients given glycerol and 5 given dextrose died in the 1st week of hospitalization; at autopsy, 5 were shown to have had massive cerebral hemorrhage and 2 to have had confirmed acute myocardial infarction. Ten placebo and 8 study patients lived longer than 10 days. Deficit scores in both groups are shown in Figure 49. Cerebrospinal fluid pressure changes were similar in both groups. Treatment of 2 healthy subjects with 500 ml 10% glycerol solution over 6 hours produced no significant change in serum osmolality or electrolyte levels.

Glycerol infusion produced no clinical improvement or change in serum osmolality in patients with early stroke in this study. This form of treatment has no place in the management of early stroke.

▶ [There has been considerable interest in attempts to reduce cerebral edema in patients with acute cerebrovascular incidents, especially cerebral infarction. According to this study, such procedures influence neither mortality nor improvement in neurologic status. — Ed.] ◀

Prognosis of Ischemic Stroke in Young Adults. Although ischemic stroke in young adults is rare, it is an important cause of persistent medical and social disability in this age group. The patient and family should be informed about the outlook as soon as possible after the stroke in order to plan appropriate future arrangements. Bengt Hindfelt and Olle Nilsson[9] (Univ. of Lund) report results of a long-term study of young patients with ischemic stroke, treated during 1965–75.

The 41 men and 23 women had a mean age of 30.8 when admitted with acute ischemic stroke. Most diagnoses were confirmed by selective angiography. All patients but 4 have been followed, the average follow-up being 51 months. Twelve patients were treated in the acute stage, most with anticoagulant therapy.

Two patients died of the stroke; both had middle cerebral infarcts. Five other patients died of other causes; none had recurrent ischemic stroke. Recovery was rapid in the first 2 months after the stroke. The prognosis of occlusions of the major vessels was unfavorable. In severely disabled patients, the lack of a predisposing condition appeared to be associated with a more favorable outcome. Fourteen patients had recurrent neurologic symptoms; 5 had postapoplectic epilepsy. Reinfarctions occurred in 4 patients. Three had brief episodes of transient neurologic dysfunction after the stroke. Five patients had relatively serious psychiatric manifestations, interpreted as reactive depression. Somatic disorders were few and usually irrelevant to the neurologic condition. All patients with a condition predisposing to stroke received prophylactic treatment if possible. Most patients have been able to resume work on a full- or part-time basis. Seven of 8 disabled patients had infarctions in the left internal carotid artery territory. The social prognosis has been excellent. All patients have obtained adequate home care after variable periods of rehabilitation.

The main impression from this study is that the prognosis of stroke in young adults is favorable. Mortality from stroke is low and the long-term mortality is due to causes other than cerebrovascular disease. The prognosis for neurologic recovery is favorable. Recurrences are rare.

Brain Infarction in Young Adults: With Particular Reference to Pathogenesis. Despite earlier studies, stroke in young adults remains an enigma. Bengt Hindfelt and Olle Nilsson[1] (Univ. of Lund) reviewed data on 64 adults, aged 16–40, who had acute ischemic stroke. Their

---

(9) Acta Neurol. Scand. 55:123–130, February, 1977.
(1) Ibid., pp. 145–157.

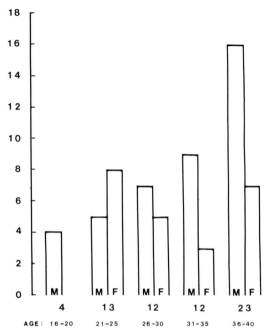

Fig 50. – Number of patients in various age categories (*M*, male; *F*, female). (Courtesy of Hindfelt, B., and Nilsson, O.: Acta Neurol. Scand. 55:145–157, February, 1977.)

mean age was 30.8 (Fig 50). There were 41 men and 23 women in the series, admitted during 1965–75. Angiography was done within 48 hours of the stroke in 58 patients.

In 2 patients, definite localization of the infarct was not possible. Two thirds of the infarcts were within the carotid territory and one-third were in the vertebrobasilar territory. The onset was typically acute. Nine of 16 patients with previous transient ischemic attacks had infarcts within the carotid territory. Only 4 patients had clinically evident cardiac disease but a considerable number had evidence of vascular disorders. Arterial hypertension was found in 12 patients. Four patients had diabetes and 3 were hypertensive as well and had evidence of advanced vascular disease. Four patients had had significant head trauma within a few days before the stroke. Eight women were taking oral contraceptives at the time of the stroke but other contributing factors were recognized in most of these patients. Three patients were chronic alcoholics and 1 was a narcotic addict. No contributory cause was identified in 19 patients, 15 of whom had stroke within the 6-month period of October to March. The variation in stroke incidence over the year was highly significant; strokes were minimal from April to September. Six of the 19 patients without obvious predisposing factors had overt symptoms of infection at the time of the stroke and 3 others had laboratory findings compatible with acute infection.

The pathogenesis of stroke in young adults differs from that of older age groups. Many patients in the present series had no predisposing factors, despite meticulous search and a broad concept of "predisposing cause." A prospective study is warranted to evaluate the importance of infection in the pathogenesis of stroke.

► [In this article and the preceding one, both on patients aged 16 – 40 years, it is brought out that cerebral infarction in young persons differs in many aspects from that in older people, especially in etiology and prognosis. Such predisposing factors as hypertension and hyperlipemia are rare, and one has to consider causes such as cardiac disease, arteritis, blood abnormalities, drug usage, pregnancy and the use of oral contraceptives. Recurrence is rare and late neurologic complications do not affect long-term prognosis, which is good in a large percentage of cases. – Ed.] ◄

Clinical and Angiographic Features of Carotid Transient Ischemic Attacks. Early recognition of symptomatic carotid artery stenosis offers the possibility of preventing stroke. Michael S. Pessin, Gary W. Duncan, Jay P. Mohr and David C. Poskanzer[2] (Harvard Med. School) analyzed data on 95 consecutive hospitalized patients with symptoms of transient cerebral ischemia who underwent angiography during a 2-year period. Transient ischemic attack was defined as a focal neurologic deficit lasting less than 24 hours, probably attributable to ischemia, and leaving no residua.

A bimodal distribution of angiographic findings was apparent (Fig 51). Intracranial branch occlusion was found in 4 patients with tight and 9 with open carotid arteries. Seven patients had further neurologic symptoms during or shortly after angiography, 6 in the same carotid territory. Fifty-two patients had transient hemispheral attacks, 33 had tran-

(2) N. Engl. J. Med. 296:358–362, Feb. 17, 1977.

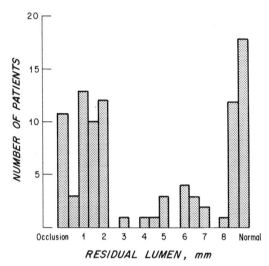

Fig 51. – Degree of carotid artery stenosis in 95 patients studied. (Courtesy of Pessin, M. S., et al.: N. Engl. J. Med. 296:358–362, Feb. 17, 1977.)

sient monocular blindness and 10 had both types of attacks. Recurrent attacks were notably of the same general type in the 67 patients affected. In no patient did transient hemispheral attacks and transient monocular blindness occur simultaneously.

Long-duration transient hemispheral attacks, lasting an hour or more, were significantly correlated with an "open" carotid artery in 17 of 22 patients. Eight of 10 patients having nonsimultaneous episodes of transient hemispheral attacks and transient monocular blindness had associated "tight" carotid artery stenosis. No reliable correlation was found between the angiographic findings and the type of attack or the number, spacing or detailed clinical features of individual transient ischemic attacks.

Distinct mechanisms that may produce transient ischemic attacks include cerebral embolism, lacunar disease and transient carotid occlusion. At least some transient ischemic attacks should be considered warnings of disaster. Transient attacks require consideration as symptoms, not as pathologic states. Their prognostic implications do not depend on their occurrence alone; the prognosis is more likely to depend on the underlying mechanism. Currently angiography is recommended in patients in whom an occult carotid stenosis or plaque may be present.

▶ [On the basis of the angiographic findings in these cases, one would assume that there are several distinct groups of patients who suffer from transient ischemic attacks in the distribution of the carotid arteries. Future studies based on grouping patients with transient ischemic attacks according to either the degree of carotid stenosis or the presence of carotid-branch ischemic disease (or both) may fruitfully elucidate not only basic mechanisms underlying transient ischemic attacks but also the prognostic factors that in turn may lead to more rational therapeutic approaches. — Ed.] ◀

Cerebral Ischemia: Role of Thrombosis and of Antithrombotic Therapy is discussed by Edward Genton, H. J. M. Barnett, William S. Fields, Michael Gent and John C. Hoak[3] (Study Group on Antithrombotic Therapy, Joint Committee for Stroke Resources). The socioeconomic importance of stroke is well-documented. Stroke is the third most common cause of death in the United States, accounting for about 200,000 deaths annually. Thrombosis-related ischemic strokes are the most common type.

As a first essential diagnostic step, cerebral hemorrhage should be identified, and cerebral embolism and thrombosis should then be distinguished. Progress has been slow in developing procedures for detecting impending or incipient thrombosis which are both accurate and practical for large numbers of patients. Procedures that are useful in diagnosing peripheral venous thrombosis may have little application to patients with impending stroke or transient ischemic attacks.

Present information indicates that anticoagulant therapy should be considered individually for the patient with ischemic cerebrovascular disease, depending on the pathogenesis of the cerebral lesion, the type of disorder and concurrent systemic disorders. Anticoagulant therapy carries a risk of hemorrhage. Indications for the use of anticoagulants in transient ischemia remain controversial; the evidence that anticoagulants reduce the incidence of recurrences is equivocal. In ischemic progressing stroke (stroke-in-evolution), anticoagulant therapy may have value in retarding the progress of the infarction. Anticoagulants have not

---

(3)   Stroke 8:150–175, Jan.–Feb., 1977.

proved useful in patients with completed stroke. Embolism of cardiac origin can be prevented with anticoagulants.

No clinical trial has established the efficacy of platelet function-suppressant drugs with respect to the end points of stroke and death. Although theoretically attractive, the use of thrombolytic therapy in acute cerebral ischemia appears to lack benefit and may be hazardous.

▶ [This study group has critically reviewed the extensive earlier reports of clinical trials of anticoagulants, platelet function suppressants and thrombolytic agents and reassessed according to present-day statistical standards the significance of the results. The information contained in this report should familiarize the reader with sufficient data to permit him to utilize antithrombotic agents under a variety of circumstances and to appreciate the contraindications and potential dangers in their use. — Ed.]

Diagnostic Procedures

Computed Tomography of Spinal Cord after Lumbar Intrathecal Introduction of Metrizamide (Computer-Assisted Myelography). Computer-assisted cisternography, which takes advantage of the "third circulation" rather than a gravitational-positional shift for the intracranial transport of contrast medium, is usually performed using metrizamide. Giovanni Di Chiro and Dieter Schellinger[4] (Georgetown Univ.) evaluated by computed tomography the ascent of metrizamide injected via the lumbar route through the entire spinal subarachnoid space up to the basal cisterns of the brain. The technique is termed "computer-assisted myelography."

Ten patients were studied. Six received metrizamide for evaluation of disk disease, 3 for neoblastic lesions and 1 for normotensive hydrocephalus. Contrast was given in a dose of 6 – 12 ml containing 180 – 270 mg iodine per ml. The lumbar injection was made over about a minute, with the patient kept prone for 15 – 20 minutes. Scans of the upper spine were generally obtained at 30 minutes and 1, 2, 3 and 6 hours, and scans of the head were obtained at 6 and, occasionally, 24 hours.

Clear visualization of all thoracic and cervical segments was obtained in all patients but 1. Thoracic distribution was evident by 30 – 60 minutes, and the cervical subarachnoid "ring" was well demonstrated at 1 – 2 hours. Conventional radiography of the spine failed to show metrizamide at the same levels. In 1 case no evidence of residual metrizamide was obtained. No metrizamide ring was recognized in 1 case of thoracolumbar cord ependymoma. An intradural meningioma acting as an anterolateral mass at C1 – C2 was framed by metrizamide in the computed tomography scan (Fig 52). No significant untoward effects were noted.

Computer-assisted myelography has demonstrated the

(4) Radiology 120:101 – 104, July, 1976.

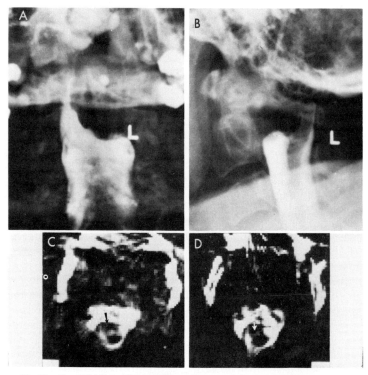

Fig 52. – Frontal (**A**) and lateral (**B**) myelograms, taken while patient was prone, in case of left anterolateral meningioma below foramen magnum at C1 – C2. Computed tomogram at level of lower half of C2 (**C**) and between C1 and C2 (**D**) show meningioma impinging on metrizamide-surrounded cord from in front (**C,** *arrow*) and left (**D,** *arrow*). (Courtesy of Di Chiro, G., and Schellinger, D.: Radiology 120:101 – 104, July, 1976.)

spinal ascent of metrizamide injected via the lumbar route. This method will provide information on the outline of the thoracic and cervical cord more accurately than will plain computer tomography. Computer-assisted myelography may also be performed after intraventricular injection of water-soluble contrast medium, taking advantage of the spinal descent of the cerebrospinal fluid. This should prove particularly interesting in the evaluation of central canal pathology.

► [This technique permits the demonstration of the metrizamide-containing subarachnoid spaces surrounding the thoracic and cervical spinal cord. — Ed.] ◄

Changes in Size of Normal Lateral Ventricles during Aging Determined by Computerized Tomography. Establishment of quantitative normative data on ventricular size is necessary for studying ventricular abnormalities in disease states, and computerized tomography (CT) is an ideal technique for such analysis. Stephen A. Barron, Lawrence Jacobs and William R. Kinkel[5] (Buffalo, N.Y.) performed CT in 135 normal subjects and measured ventricular

Fig 53. — Examples of normal computed tomography scans: **A,** 3d decade; **B,** 5th decade; **C,** 8th decade; and **D,** ventricles of man aged 101, who had mild dementia and is not included in statistical analysis. (Courtesy of Barron, S. A., et al.: Neurology (Minneap.) 26:1011–1013, November, 1976.)

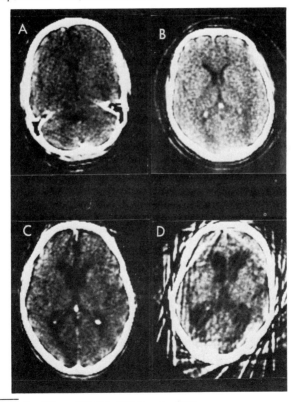

size by planimetry. The subjects' age range was 9 months to 90 years; none had evidence of neurologic disorder. In each age group by decade there were 7 female and 8 male subjects. Measurements were made from photographs of either the mid (level of foramina of Monro) or dorsal (level of bodies of lateral ventricles) portion of the lateral ventricles, whichever was larger.

Mean ventricular size increased gradually from 1.8% in the 1st decade to 6.4% in the 7th. Ventricular size then increased dramatically to 11.5% in the 8th decade and to 14.1% in the 9th decade. All increments in size except those between the 2d and 3d and between the 4th and 5th decades were significant. Widening of the cerebral sulci was noted in the 6th through 9th decades and became more prominent with increasing age, though it was never considered excessive for the subject's age. The pattern of enlarging ventricular size was not correlated with the degree of cortical atrophy. Representative CT scan appearances of ventricles during aging are shown in Figure 53.

Pneumoencephalography has not been practical for evaluating the ventricles of normal subjects, and alterations in ventricular size occur during and after the procedure. Postmortem studies have now resolved the question of variations in normal ventricular size during life. The CT scanning resolves these problems and has shown a gradual increase in ventricular size with aging, the greatest increase occurring in the 8th and 9th decades of life. The range of ventricular size was greatest in the 7th through 9th decades. Abnormalities of ventricular size may be more easily identified in younger than in older subjects.

▶ [These data are more valuable than those from pneumoencephalography or autopsy studies because computerized tomography is not subject to the artifact inherent in those procedures. — Ed.] ◀

Clinical vs. Quantitative Evaluation of Cutaneous Sensation. There is a need to test cutaneous sensation with graded, reproducible, quantifiable stimuli. Serial evaluations of cutaneous sensation might be used to follow diseases more accurately and to test the effects of various treatments on nerve function. Peter James Dyck, Peter C. O'Brien, Wilfred Bushek, Karen F. Oviatt, Kathleen Schilling and J. Clarke Stevens[6] (Mayo Clinic and Found.) evaluated cuta-

(6)   Arch. Neurol. 33:651–655, September, 1976.

neous sensation by both neurologic examination and quantitative assessment in 107 patients with various neuromuscular diseases. The Mayo touch-pressure system II involves supplying an electric pulse to a galvanometer motor attached to a stylus that produces a small skin depression, with 31 levels of stimulation resulting. Minnesota thermal disks were used to determine thermal discrimination on the dorsal surface of the hand and foot and a dolorimeter was used to estimate pricking-pain sensation.

Abnormal touch-pressure sensation was found in 66.7% of patients' feet and 55.4% of the hands. Thermal discrimination was abnormal in 28% of feet and 15% of hands and pricking-pain sensation in 18% of feet and 25% of hands. In a comparison of the clinical with the quantitative, the two methods produced the same conclusion for touch-pressure sensation in 66% of hands; in all cases of disagreement the quantitative measurement was abnormal and the clinical judgment normal. Comparative tests for thermal discrimination agreed in 78% of hands and 72% of feet. Agreement on pain sensation was obtained in about two thirds of patients at both test sites. In sural nerve biopsy specimens from 27 patients, the standard deviation of density of myelinated fibers in those considered normal by quantitative measurement of touch-pressure was markedly less than that arising from clinical evaluation.

There is reasonably good correlation between the recognition of abnormal cutaneous sensation by clinical methods and by quantitative methods and between decreased touch-pressure sensation and a decrease in large myelinated fibers in cutaneous nerves. Clinical neurologists tend to underestimate abnormalities of touch-pressure sensation.

▶ [A comparison of the evaluation of cutaneous sensation by neurologic examination and by quantitative assessment in patients with neuromuscular disease shows that there is a reasonably good correlation between the recognition of abnormalities of cutaneous sensation by clinical and quantitative methods. — Ed.] ◀

Computed Tomography in Diagnosis of Pseudotumor Cerebri. Michael S. Huckman, Jacob S. Fox, Ruth G. Ramsey and Richard D. Penn[7] (Rush-Presbyterian-St. Luke's Med. Center) examined the accuracy of computed tomography (CT), in 17 female patients with a clinical diagnosis

(7) Radiology 119:593 – 597, June, 1976.

of benign intracranial hypertension, because of the morbidity attending pneumoencephalography and angiography. The patients exhibited true papilledema, had normal neurologic findings and had normal cerebrospinal fluid findings apart from pressure, had a normal EEG and brain scan and had normal angiographic findings. No mass was found at CT and ventricular size was normal. Either improvement or no worsening was observed in the patients followed.

The ventricles were initially thought to be smaller than those in normal subjects. Ventricular sizes in the 17 female patients, whose mean age was 26.5 years, were compared with those of 27 normal females in the same age range. The difference in mean ventricular sizes between these groups was not significant.

Patients with papilledema, headache, normal mentation, a normal EEG and nuclide image and no lateralizing neurologic signs should be examined by CT, with and without contrast infusion. If the ventricles are normal and no mass is detected, further radiodiagnostic tests need not be done unless the patient's neurologic condition deteriorates. It is premature to say that all these patients will ultimately have only benign intracranial hypertension.

▶ [On the basis of this study and others cited, there would appear to be almost no instances in which invasive neuroradiologic procedures would be required to confirm the diagnosis of pseudotumor cerebri. Other studies have showed this to be the case also in the diagnosis of so-called normotensive hydrocephalus. — Ed.] ◀

Orbicularis Oculi Reflex in Brain Death. The evoked response in the orbicularis oculi muscle produced by stimulation of the supraorbital nerve has an early unilateral (R1) and a late bilateral (R2) component. The afferent path of this reflex is the trigeminal nerve, and the efferent is the facial nerve. The central paths are not well understood, but these must involve connections between the trigeminal and facial nuclei.

A. J. Mehta and S. S. Seshia[8] (Univ. of Manitoba) studied the orbicularis oculi (blink) reflex in 3 children who fulfilled accepted criteria of brain death. A portable electromyographic device was utilized; the supraorbital nerve was stimulated percutaneously with the cathode over the supraorbital foramen. The facial nerve was stimulated with

---

(8) J. Neurol. Neurosurg. Psychiatry 39:784–787, August, 1976.

the cathode placed anterior to the mastoid process. The early and late components of the orbicularis oculi reflex were absent bilaterally in all 3 patients. A response to peripheral facial nerve stimulation was obtained in all.

The R1 response is affected by intrinsic and extrinsic pontine lesions, whereas the R2 component is involved by lateral medullary lesions, and its absence in coma may suggest diffuse suppression of the reticular system. Both components of the orbicularis oculi reflex can be lost with combined hemispheric and brain stem dysfunction, and coma due to depressant drugs may be associated with a reversible loss of both components of the reflex. The reflex may be difficult to obtain during stages 2 – 4 of sleep.

Where criteria of brain death exist, in the absence of hypothermia and coma due to depressant drugs or metabolic disturbance, a bilateral absence of the early and late components of the orbicularis oculi reflex suggests that the brain stem is irreversibly involved.

► [These preliminary observations suggest that the study of the orbicularis oculi reflex is a simple, objective bedside neurophysiologic test of brain stem function, complementing the EEG in the diagnosis of brain death. – Ed.] ◄

Therapy

Reversal of Tricyclic Overdosage-Induced Central Anticholinergic Syndrome by Physostigmine. Tricyclic antidepressant poisoning has received little attention until recently. Paul C. Holinger and Harold L. Klawans[9] (Michael Reese Hosp. and Med. Center, Chicago) report a case of prolonged coma caused by tricyclic antidepressant overdosage and reversed with physostigmine. The duration of coma before reversal by physostigmine is the longest known in the literature.

Woman, 55, with many previous hospitalizations for depression, was discharged from a psychiatric hospital 4 days before being admitted after taking an overdose of amitriptyline. Unknown but small amounts of chlorpromazine and benztropine had also been ingested. The patient was comatose and responded only to deep pain. Examination 4 hours after lavage and the extraction of many pills showed 1 + tendon reflexes, flaccid muscles and responsiveness only to deep pain. Myoclonic jerks and choreoathetoid movements of the limbs were observed, and 60 mg phenobarbital was given every 4 hours. Intubation was necessary because of worsening hypoventilation. Fever developed, and antibiotics were administered. Bilateral lung infiltrates subsequently appeared.

Physostigmine was begun after 64 hours of known coma, and the patient quickly began moving her arms and opened her eyes. Physostigmine was given for 3½ days, finally in a dose of 4 mg every 2 hours, along with 1 mg methylscopolamine every 4 hours. Phenobarbital was discontinued. The myoclonus ceased after physostigmine administration. Consciousness fluctuated but gradually improved, and the patient was extubated 8 days after physostigmine therapy. The lungs cleared gradually.

This patient, after ingesting a tricyclic drug along with a phenothiazine and an antiparkinson drug, had prolonged coma complicated by the iatrogenic use of phenobarbital to control seizure-like activity. Phenobarbital may have contributed to the depression of consciousness and respiration. This case supports the anticholinergic basis of the clinical

(9) Am. J. Psychiatry 133:1018–1023, September, 1976.

manifestations of overdosages and also the hypothesis of a decrease in acetylcholine relative to dopamine in the basal ganglia in choreiform states. The myoclonus seen in this patient and in others may be a result of decreased serotonin uptake into serotoninergic neurons and a subsequent increase in serotonin at the synapse, caused by tricyclic antidepressants.

► [This report supports the anticholinergic basis of the clinical manifestations of tricyclic overdosage and provides information on the role of acetylcholine and dopamine in psychiatric and movement disorders. It also dramatically illustrates the need for accurate diagnosis and treatment. — Ed.] ◄

Evaluation of Baclofen Treatment for Certain Symptoms in Patients with Spinal Cord Lesions: Double-Blind, Crossover Study. Clinical manifestations of spinal cord lesions include, in the chronic stage, flexor and extensor spasms, other released cutaneous reflexes and loss of precise autonomic control. The involuntary spasms are often accompanied by severe pain and emptying of the bowels and bladder. Gary W. Duncan, Bhagwan T. Shahani and Robert R. Young[1] (Harvard Med. School) conducted a double-blind study of baclofen in patients with "spasticity" secondary to spinal cord disease.

All patients had had stable spasticity for at least 3 months and had no fixed contractures. Muscle relaxants were withheld for at least a week before the study. Baclofen and placebo were given for 4-week periods at a 1-week interval. The dose of baclofen was 5 mg 3 times daily and increased no more often than every 3 days up to a maximum of 100 mg daily or until maximal improvement occurred.

Twenty-two patients completed the trial. Eleven had a clear diagnosis of multiple sclerosis, of an average duration of 12.3 years. The other patients had been ill for 5.1 years. There were 11 patients of each sex. Disability varied considerably; 8 patients were able to walk. Spasms were significantly reduced in number during baclofen therapy (Fig 54) and those that did occur were less intense and of shorter duration. Both flexor and extensor spasms were affected. Nocturnal spasms improved in all but 1 of 12 patients who were affected. Eleven of 20 patients with significantly increased resistance to passive leg movements were improved

(1) Neurology (Minneap.) 26:441–446, May, 1976.

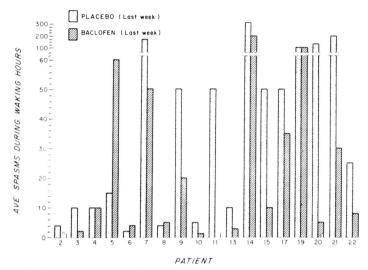

Fig 54. — Average daily number of spasms during last week of baclofen and placebo treatment periods in 18 patients with spontaneous daytime spasms. (Courtesy of Duncan, G. W., et al.: Neurology (Minneap.) 26:441 – 446, May, 1976.)

by baclofen and only 1 on placebo. The "spastic" gait was improved in 5 of 7 ambulatory patients. Clonus was dramatically reduced in 1 patient. Strength did not improve during the trial. One patient had severe spasms while on baclofen and was withdrawn from the study. Mild side effects were more frequent on baclofen, but side effects were insignificant.

Baclofen is useful in the symptomatic treatment of patients with spinal cord lesions who are troubled by certain components of "spasticity." "Positive" components are benefited by the drug but "negative" symptoms such as weakness are not.

▶ [In evaluating a new mode of therapy for relief of spasticity, one must consider selectively the response of individual components of such a global syndrome. In this study, baclofen was found to be useful in the treatment of flexor and extensor spasms and increased resistance to passive movement of the legs but did not alter strength, gait, stretch reflexes or clonus. – Ed.] ◀

Neurologic Disorders Responsive to Folic Acid Therapy. Deficiency of folic acid in adults is not believed to produce symptoms of neurologic disorders, even though folate is present in the central nervous system and its cerebrospinal fluid concentration is considerably higher than its concentration in serum. M. I. Botez, M. Cadotte, R. Beaulieu, L. P. Pichette and C. Pison[2] (Montreal) describe 6 women aged 31–70 years who had folate deficiency and neuropsychiatric disorders.

Three women with acquired folate deficiency were depressed and had permanent muscular and intellectual fatigue, mild symptoms of restless legs, depressed ankle jerks, reduced vibratory sensation in the legs, stocking-type hypesthesia and long-lasting constipation. Xylose absorption was abnormal. The marrow was megaloblastic in only 1 patient, and she and another had jejunal mucosal atrophy. All 3 patients recovered on folic acid therapy.

The 3 other women were members of a family with the restless legs syndrome, fatigability and diffuse muscle pain. One also had subacute combined degeneration of the spinal cord and renal disease, but not megaloblastosis; she improved dramatically on large-dose folic acid therapy. The other 2 women had minor neurologic signs and were controlled with 5–10 mg folic acid daily. The Achilles tendon reflex time was prolonged in some of these patients. Three further families with the restless legs syndrome and mild neurologic disturbances are presently under study; all have folate deficiency. Dominant transmission has been reported in this syndrome.

Unrecognized, treatable folate deficiency may be the basis of a well-defined syndrome of neurologic, psychiatric and gastroenterologic disorders. The restless legs syndrome may represent the main clinical expression of acquired and familial folate deficiency in adults. About 4–13% of the Canadian population are at high risk, and about 32–59% are at moderate risk for folate deficiency. Patients with both acquired and inherited folate deficiency may remain moderately deficient for years. Folate deficiency in erythrocytes occurs only in the later stages of folic acid deficiency.

▶ [Although neurologic and psychiatric manifestations may develop in folate deficiency states and are responsive to folate therapy, the administration of folic acid to patients with pernicious anemia or other vitamin B_{12} deficiency states results in hematologic changes that lead to precipitation or aggravation of neurologic complications. – Ed.] ◀

(2)   Can. Med. Assoc. J. 115:217–222, Aug. 7, 1976.

**Long-Term Therapy of Myoclonus and Other Neuro-
logic Disorders with L-5-Hydroxytryptophan and Carbidopa.** Several clinical studies have shown the efficacy of
L-5-hydroxytryptophan (L-5HTP), the precursor of serotonin, in combination with carbidopa in the treatment of postanoxic intention myoclonus. Anoxic brain damage may
cause preferential degeneration of serotonergic neurons,
reducing brain serotonin formation, and this treatment may
reduce myoclonic movements by restoring brain serotonin
formation. Melvin H. Van Woert, David Rosenbaum, John
Howieson and Malcolm B. Bowers, Jr.[3] treated 14 females
and 9 males aged 16 – 74 years who had myoclonus. Thirteen
patients had postanoxic intention myoclonus and 5 had intention myoclonus from other causes. Two patients each had
essential myoclonus and myoclonus associated with idiopathic epilepsy and 1 patient had progressive myoclonus
epilepsy. Sixteen patients with other neurologic disorders
were also treated. The L-5HTP was given orally in a starting dosage of 100 mg daily, which was increased by 100 mg
every 2 or 3 days. Carbidopa was given orally in daily doses
of 100 – 300 mg. Placebos were substituted when definite
clinical changes occurred.

Cerebrospinal fluid 5-hydroxyindoles increased markedly
during treatment in 2 patients with familial essential myoclonus. Over 50% overall improvement in postanoxic intention myoclonus occurred in 61% of cases, and 3 patients had
over 90% improvement, Improvement has been sustained;
some patients have been treated for over 3 years. Maximum
daily doses of L-5HTP ranged from 400 mg to 2 gm. The
treatment had no marked effect in the other study patients
or in patients with other neurologic disorders. Most patients
had anorexia, nausea and diarrhea at the outset, which responded to prochlorperazine or trimethobenzamide. Three
patients had dyspnea and hyperventilation early in the
course of therapy. Mental stimulation was observed in several patients. Cerebrospinal fluid 5-hydroxyindoleacetic
acid was 35% lower in study patients than in controls and
was increased by treatment with L-5HTP and carbidopa.

This treatment appears to be safe for long-term manage-

(3) N. Engl. J. Med. 296:70– 75, Jan. 13, 1977.

ment of patients with myoclonus. The dose of carbidopa used to inhibit the decarboxylation of levodopa in patients with Parkinson's disease is insufficient to inhibit L-5HTP decarboxylation completely.

▶ [It appears that a deficiency of brain serotonin is causally related to intention myoclonus and that the therapeutic action of L-5-hydroxytryptophan and carbidopa may be due to repletion of serotonin in regions of the brain where serotonergic neurons have degenerated. – Ed.] ◀

Physostigmine in Familial Ataxias. R. A. Pieter Kark, John P. Blass and M. Anne Spence[4] (Univ. of California, Los Angeles) conducted a randomized, double-blind trial of the effects of physostigmine on 12 patients with spinocerebellar degenerations. Five patients had Friedreich's ataxia, 4 had olivopontocerebellar atrophy and 1 each had cerebellar cortical atrophy, combined cerebral and cerebellar cortical atrophy and the Ramsay Hunt syndrome. A 1-mg dose of physostigmine salicylate was dissolved in 10 ml normal saline for intravenous use. Three patients had short-term studies for 2 consecutive days. Methylscopolamine was given intravenously before the infusion of 1 mg physostigmine or saline alone. Eight patients were included in long-term, double-blind trials of 4 periods, each of 3 months' duration (Fig 55).

In short-term studies, subtest scores improved after physostigmine injections, indicating less ataxia. Physostigmine sometimes caused bradycardia, fainting and abdominal discomfort, despite administration of methylscopolamine. Because methylscopolamine prevented double-blind comparisons of physostigmine and saline, subsequent patients were given physostigmine orally. All scores after oral administration were better than before. By either route, maximal effects were seen within 15–40 minutes; speech usually was affected before the upper limbs. No effects were seen after 2 hours; there were no side effects from the oral dose.

In the long-term studies, ataxia scores were better on physostigmine than on placebo despite disease progression. Only 1 patient had side effects, which resolved when the dosage was reduced to 0.5 mg every 2 hours. Three patients were unable to distinguish between the effects of physostigmine and placebo during the trial.

---

(4) Neurology (Minneap.) 27:70–72, January, 1977.

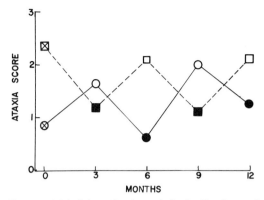

Fig 55. – Crossover trial of physostigmine and placebo. Results are shown for the 2 patients, a girl aged 9 *(circles)* and woman aged 22 *(squares),* both with Friedreich's ataxia, who had two trial periods on each tablet. Before treatment, *crossed circle* or *square;* and on physostigmine, *black circle* or *square;* and on placebo, *clear circle* or *square.* (Courtesy of Kark, R. A. P., et al.: Neurology (Minneap.) 27:70– 72, January, 1977.)

The improvement in ataxia seen with physostigmine administration in this study raises the possibility that deficient activity of some cholinergic mechanism may be involved in the pathophysiology of Friedreich's ataxia, cortical cerebellar atrophy and cerebral and cerebellar cortical atrophy. In the doses used, physostigmine is not a treatment for ataxias. Further trials of physostigmine and other cholinergic agents are needed to determine the nature of the pharmacologic effect, the possible correlation with specific diseases and possible efficacy.

► [This study is an interesting and possibly a significant one. Further therapeutic studies, however, are certainly indicated to determine whether physostigmine is, in fact, of therapeutic value in the familial ataxias and related disorders. – Ed.] ◄

NEUROSURGERY

OSCAR SUGAR, M.D.

Introduction

Neurosurgeons may have felt themselves on the outside of the current arguments about legislative control of abortions if they were not directly involved for religious or ideological reasons. Few have considered the more basic question: "Shall the government (be it state or federal) have the power to regulate the specific type of medical and surgical treatment that may be given to a patient?" The courts have long been involved in deciding whether certain persons shall have specific operations (or administration of blood) with or without the consent of the person or his guardian, and now the issues have included neurosurgeons and psychiatric physicians who are involved in (or might become involved in) psychosurgery. On Monday, May 23, 1977, the *Federal Register* (Vol. 42, pp. 26317–26332) included the Report and Recommendations of the National Commission for the Protection of Human Subjects of Biomedical and Behavioral Research entitled "Use of Psychosurgery in Practice and Research." The Department of Health, Education and Welfare completed its own review of the report and evaluated it during the comment period that ended in July. Comments were made particularly in reference to the use of recommendations in medical practice and medical research. The Commission was to study the use of psychosurgery in the United States during the 5-year period ending December 31, 1972. Psychosurgery was defined to mean brain surgery on "normal brain tissue of an individual who does not suffer from any physical disease, for the purpose of changing or controlling the behavior or emotions," or on "diseased brain tissue . . . if the sole object is to control, change or affect any behavioral or emotional disturbance." Surgery for relief of epilepsy and movement disorders was excluded from this definition, as was electroconvulsive therapy. The Commission also decided to exclude brain operations that interrupt sensory pathways for relief of pain from the definition of psychosurgery, but to include procedures to relieve the emotional response to persistent pain.

The first three chapters of the report provide a short history of the use of psychosurgery, the focus of public concern, a description of the issues raised and a discussion of various legal approaches. The studies performed under the contract of the Commission form Chapter 4 – and these are the subject of the last article, by Barbara J. Culliton, in this YEAR BOOK. It is of interest that in Teuber's study group, the relief experienced by 9 of the 11 patients whose presenting symptom was persistent pain was complete or nearly complete. All but 2 would recommend surgery to others and preferred operation to electroconvulsive therapy, yet such pain-relieving operations are considered psychosurgery and electroconvulsive therapy is not! Chapter 5 of the report deals with a conference held to explore the possible implications for minority groups, because fears had been expressed that psychosurgery would be used primarily against these groups – fears that have not been based on statistics or historical facts.

The American Psychiatric Association's spokesman supported a national registry of psychosurgical patients, without obvious evidence of a consideration of the dangers of publicity and violations of privacy that could occur. Other proposals to have the Commission scrutinize any medical procedure or research proposal that threatens people's lives or dignity are clearly fanciful, because on the surface this would involve virtually any operation, and especially any operation on the brain for any purpose, including the removal of benign and malignant brain tumors or aneurysms. Congressman Stokes proposed legislation based on a premise that psychosurgery has no therapeutic value because the indications for it do not depend on identifiable brain pathology and while no psychosurgical operations have been successful, many have been failures (and he cited three poor results). His other premises for prohibiting psychosurgery (in federally supported health care facilities – a term that might be construed, with the Hill-Burton act, to mean virtually every hospital of sufficient size to consider neurosurgical alleviation of disease) include the invention that psychosurgery deprives the patient from obtaining proper redress of grievances and has potential use as a tool for repression of minorities, dissenters and the poor. The assumption of lack of therapeutic value in psychosurgery is not only contradicted by the Commission's investigations, but by every reputable neurosurgeon and psychiatrist who has had patients operated on for relief of mental distress.

Doctor Heilman, of the International Neuropsychological Society, Inc., said that ablative neurosurgery always produces a defect in behavior. Experience with hemispherectomies certainly shows the ablative procedures may indeed improve behavior and can make life more fruitful and enjoyable for the brain-damaged epileptic patient. Dr. Charles Fager of the Congress of Neurological Surgeons put forth the guidelines endorsed by the International Society of Psychiatric Surgery, which seem to me to be rational and protective of the rights of the individual. A number of other groups were represented in person or by written statements; the suggestions of the National Association for Mental Health, Inc., are strange in that the proposed procedure was to be reviewed and approved by at least two other neurosurgeons; I do not believe neurosurgeons are qualified to select patients for such procedures, nor do I think legal counsel should be present for any final decision in a given case.

Review of recommendations by the Commission affirms the decision not to ban psychosurgery, but it is still the opinion of the Commission that the safety and efficacy of the surgical procedures have not been demonstrated to the point of permitting them to be considered "accepted practice." Safeguards should include review by an independent review board of the decision to operate, review of consent provisions, performance of preoperative and postoperative evaluations and additional safeguards for patients involuntarily confined or incapable of giving consent. Children are not to be automatically excluded from psychosurgery, but operations on them are to have additional approval from a national psychosurgery advisory board and a court of competent jurisdiction. The Commission did not believe the literature was sufficient to establish the safety and efficacy of particular procedures in response to particular symptoms or disorders. The Secretary of the Department of Health, Education and Welfare is encouraged to support studies to evaluate the safety and efficacy of psychosurgical procedures. He is instructed to impose strict sanctions up to and including withholding of federal funds to insure compliance with the recommendations. When the Department publishes regulations, the Congress should pass necessary legislation to assure adherence to them.

The foundation for disparagement of the early operations (generally termed "frontal lobotomy") based on the side effects (often important and discouraging) and occasional failure to cause improvement is emotional. I recently received word from a patient's sister who was trying to arrange the request of the patient for postmortem brain donation; the patient had returned to work after "frontal lobotomy" in 1944, with useful and enjoyable life until retirement in 1969 but now with nursing home existence — due to problems with the vascular supply to the legs! Surely such anecdotal reports are not to be ignored for lack of that fetish, "controlled series." Disparagement of psychosurgery because of its lack of refinement in the 1940s and 1950s is, I believe, similar to disparagement of aneurysm surgery in the same years as compared to the 1970s. Progress does occur. The argument that some brilliant researcher may come up with a new chemical treatment for mental disorder and hence no irreversible surgery should be done is insufficient in view of the present suffering of patients. Operative treatment of parkinsonism declined abruptly after the coming of L-dopa and its combinations, but occasional patients still fail to respond or have too many side effects from the medication. Why should we not give patients who have mental illness just as real as those with basal ganglion disease the same opportunity to improve while research on better techniques continues? Sympathectomy for arterial hypertension was not the definitive answer for that problem, but managed to help many patients until proper medications were developed. No operation is devoid of dangers and side effects, yet psychosurgical ones are singled out for damnation. Not all epileptic brains have recognizable gross or microscopic lesions, yet when medical control fails, operation is accepted and is understood not to be infallible. If we were to find a focus of electric abnormality (for instance, in the septal nuclei) in patients with obsessive disease, would that then make operations for relief more palatable?

I, too, would like to see better records kept and better conclusions drawn from records of those undergoing psychosurgery, but implicitly to find fault with psychosurgeons because not all of their cases are reported (the "literature" already is burdened with too many case reports) is ascribing mischief where none is intended.

Implicit in many of the criticisms and fears voiced to the Commission is the concept that psychosurgery implies subsequent lack of control to the point of permitting others to dictate behavior. To the best of my knowledge, automatons in this sense have not been created by any neurosurgical procedure. Indeed, the earlier operations were followed by the opposite — that is, by activities that are best considered as lack of control by outsiders, by willfullness or by uninhibited behavior, if you will, but not by mind control.

As in other segments of our civilization, so in this one the direction from the Federal Government (though directed primarily to enterprises funded by it) will surely be taken to create guidelines for all such psychosurgical procedures. This indeed is the threat to the doctor-patient relationship implicit in the psychosurgery affair; if the Federal Government can intervene in abortions, why not in cingulumotomies; and if in psychosurgery, why not in radical breast surgery or in cosmetic surgery — or even in the use of Laetrile?

It will be interesting to see what comments come in to the Department of Health, Education and Welfare and what regulations come out.

OSCAR SUGAR, M.D.

Brief Interesting Notes

The volume of the skull can be directly measured in cadavers by sealing the foramina with latex and pouring in water or by filling them with peas. According to Muke et al. (Fortschr. Geb. Roentgenstr. Nuklearmed. 125:219, 1976), who have used radiographs and planimetry in setting up calculations to estimate skull volumes in vivo, the water technique is probably slightly more accurate. They believe the volume is most accurately and simply determined from the product of greatest width (transverse diameter) and area of the median plane.

In Rhodesia, the skulls are thicker in women than in men! Ross et al. (S. Afr. Med. J. 50:635, Apr. 10, 1976) measured skull caps at autopsy, using similar loci in 218 skulls from black and white adults (50–59 in each category). The skulls of white women were thickest; the skulls of white men were thinnest. The thin skull of the white man is related to a large brain pan area.

In a study of formalin-fixed pineal glands from Ugandans, Mugondi and Poltera (Br. J. Radiol. 49:594, 1976) found 125 that were calcified on x-ray. The incidence increased with age; none was calcified in the 1st decade. Glands from females were more often calcified than those from males. After age 10, calcification occurs in 68% of Ugandans, and 43% should be detected by radiography of the skull. It appears not to interfere with pineal gland function (whatever that may be!). The weights of the glands were less overall than in other reported series. The authors suggest that this may be due to more exposure to light in the equatorial region from which these autopsies came.

The anterior choroidal artery can be related to a line passing from tuberculum sellae to internal occipital protuberance, making an angle of 20–35 degrees with Twining's line, and frequently one of 25–30 degrees. Theron (Ann. Radiol. (Paris) 19:223, 1976) also uses both an anterior choroidal point that corresponds to the entry of the artery into the temporal horn and a plexal point that corresponds to the retrothalamic segment of the artery. The choroidal point usually is indicated after a small undulation, with a decrease in caliber, disappearance of the artery or division into several thin branches. Theron points out how these arteriographic references can be used to detect space-occupying masses.

A girl aged 3 years had a midline vertex swelling that appeared chiefly with her lying down or straining. It was shown well by technetium scan in the recumbent position according to Rodermond (Radiol. Clin. (Basel) 45:272, 1976). The varix communicated with the superior sagittal sinus via 2 minute canaliculi. These were plugged and the varix removed successfully.

The source of bleeding in the spinal canal in newborn infants may be difficult to determine. It may even be from the trauma of the spinal puncture. Chaplin et al. (Pediatrics 58: 751, 1976) determined the percentage of fetal hemoglobin in bloody cerebrospinal fluid and compared this with the percentage in the vascular bed. In children who have had transfusion of adult blood after subarachnoid hemorrhage is suspected, there will be a significantly increased proportion of fetal hemoglobin in the bloody cerebrospinal fluid if this is due to subarachnoid hemorrhage, but no difference if the bloody fluid is due to trauma. Of course, this method cannot be used if there has been no transfusion.

A nicely illustrated article by Shapiro and Robinson on embryogenesis of the occipital bone (Am. J. Roentgenol. 126: 1063, 1976) points out the origin of this bone from cartilage except for the membranous origin of the interparietal portion. This is separated from the supraoccipital portion by the mendosal sutures. There is no normal midline suture or synchondrosis, so a radiolucency in the midline of the supraoccipital segment is considered to be a fracture.

At times, hemicraniectomy may be followed by progressive weakness. Tabaddor and La Margese (J. Neurosurg. 44: 506, 1976) report such a case with rapid reversal of cranioplasty. I have encountered a similar case with bone removal for osteomyelitis after craniotomy for subdural hematoma. Repair may be delayed with infection, but probably should not be postponed long when hemicraniectomy is done for decompressive purposes.

Hemangioblastomas above the tentorium are rare and are distinguished with difficulty and uncertainty from angioblastic meningiomas. The diagnosis in the case of Perks et al. (J. Neurol. Neurosurg. Psychiatry 39:218, 1976) is reinforced by the coincident polycythemia (hematocrit, 59%, hemoglobin, 19.3 gm/dl; and red blood cell mass, 65.5 ml/kg (normal 28 ± 8 ml/kg).

Aloia et al. (Am. J. Med. 61:59, 1976) have studied body composition and skeletal metabolism after pituitary irradiation in 9 acromegalic patients. Total body levels of calcium, phosphorus, sodium, potassium and chloride were studied by neutron activation analysis by the Brookhaven 54 detector. Phosphorus, sodium and potassium were reduced toward normal ratios, whereas total body calcium was reduced to levels observed in osteoporosis, associated with vertebral compression fractures in 2 patients. The authors believe risk of fracture can be reduced by giving adequate calcium and sex hormone replacement therapy to hypogonadal acromegalic patients.

Batnitzky et al. (J.A.M.A. 237:148, 1977) reemphasize the risks of implanting epidermal fragments into the spinal canal when lumbar punctures are done with needles lacking stylets or with ill-fitting stylets. They give case histories of 3 children encountered in an 18-month period, all of whom had one or more lumbar punctures 3.5 – 6 years earlier and all of whom had intraspinal epidermoid tumors.

The liver responds in various ways to neoplasia elsewhere in the body. In a woman aged 57, whose case is reported by Henderson and Grace (J. Clin. Pathol. 29:237, 1976), the serum alkaline phosphatase level was elevated as the major laboratory abnormality with malignant schwannoma of the sciatic nerve. The isoenzyme pattern showed an increased fast liver band and appearance of slow liver and biliary bands. Liver scan, liver inspection and biopsy and inguinal nodes were normal. Recovery from hip disarticulation has been uneventful (2-year follow-up). The alkaline phosphatase pattern reverted to normal.

Arrangement and relative concentration of motor and sensory fibers at various points in the course of the ulnar nerve are reflected in the correlation of clinical and electrodiagnostic features in the study of ulnar nerve lesions at the elbow. Among the crucial findings listed by Bhala (Arch.

Phys. Med. Rehabil. 57:206, 1976) are absence or abnormality of evoked sensory action potentials in the 5th finger and motor conduction velocity less than 45 m per second across the flexed elbow. Abnormal electromyographic findings include increased insertional activity or signs of denervation in the 1st dorsal interosseus, abductor digiti minimi and flexor carpi ulnaris muscles.

The Martin-Gruber anastomosis refers to a communication in the forearm between the ulnar and median nerves. It is believed to occur in about 15% of the population. This anastomosis is considered by Iyer and Fenichel (J. Neurol. Neurosurg. Psychiatry 39:449, 1976) to be responsible for their 5 cases of carpal tunnel syndrome in which proximal stimulation of the median nerve yielded near-normal latency whereas distal stimulation produced prolonged stimulation. This phenomenon also explains partial or total sparing of thenar muscles from denervation when the median nerve is compressed at the wrist.

Facial nerve paralysis may recede spontaneously even when the nerve is excised during operation on parotid gland tumor. After describing such a case, Hakami and Masavy (Am. J. Surg. 132:394, 1976) review the English literature on such return of function. It seems probable that reeducation permits pathways to function between the cortex and the 5th cranial nerve, which has a number of preexisting anastomoses with the facial nerve. Others have reported retention of recovered movement after a second resection of the parotid gland, indicating the absence of ordinary facial nerve regeneration.

The otorhinolaryngologic literature is full of reports of etiology, diagnosis and treatment of so-called idiopathic peripheral facial paralysis (Bell's palsy). Ischemia is a commonly proposed etiology, usually ascribed to compression in the fallopian canal. Primary ischemia of the petrosal artery (a branch of the middle meningeal artery) deserves attention, according to Calcaterra et al. (Laryngoscope 86:92, 1976). They report 3 cases of facial paralysis after selective intra-arterial ferrosilicone embolization for extensive vascular meningiomas of the middle cranial fossa. Partial recovery of facial function has occurred. The angiographically vascular tumors were found to be avascular at operation.

When there is doubt as to the ability of a neurosurgical

patient to swallow without harming his respiratory tract, a simple test devised by Rossato and Wrightson (Surg. Neurol. 7:24, 1977) can be used. The patient swallows 10 ml Dionosil bronchographic contrast material (sterile oily propyliodone suspension) while seated. X-rays of the chest and upper abdomen taken within 30 minutes should show the contrast material only in the stomach. The bronchial tree will be partly outlined if pharyngeal protection is inadequate; the material disappears within an hour.

In order to establish how much of the sympathetic nervous system needs to be removed for Raynaud's disease in the upper limbs, G. Arnulf (J. Cardiovasc. Surg. (Torino) 17: 354, 1976) studied humeral blood flow in dogs by stimulating and resecting parts of the cervicodorsal sympathetic system, as well as by injecting epinephrine. Stellectomy is not necessary. Blood flow is increased by section between the 4th and 5th ganglia. Increase in flow is about the same for removal of T2–T4 ganglia as for removal of T3 alone; the larger resection gives more assurance. Decreasing effects come from removal of ganglia T6 and T7, and T8 has no vascular effect on the upper limb. Bilateral removal is needed for bilateral effects. Arnulf routinely uses a posterior approach via part of the 2d or 3d rib; he reserves the transaxillary approach (T4–T5) for obese patients without pulmonary or plural lesions, with removal of the ganglia of T2–T4.

Gildenberg (Rev. Inst. Nacl. Neurol. (Mex.) 10:11, 1976) has used the concept that spasmodic torticollis may be an aberration or imbalance of tonic neck reflexes. They may be altered by anterior root section (which is not really satisfactory), posterior root section (no longer performed because of large areas of anesthesia) or by adding input to the afferent limb of the reflex arc. He has inserted electrodes posterior to the cervical spinal cord via a lateral cervical approach for electric stimulation at about 1,000–1,200 Hz (more conventional analgesic stimulation of 250 Hz does not help torticollis). This was tried if transcutaneous stimulation helps. Of 18 patients, 2 were content with transcutaneous stimulators, 8 had no benefit from percutaneous techniques and 6 had dorsal column stimulators implanted after evaluation with transcutaneous and percutaneous stimulators. Results were excellent in 1 patient, good in 2, fair in 2 and poor in 1.

Anatomy and Physiology

Persistent Hypoglossal Artery, Diagnostic Criteria: Report of a Case. The persistent hypoglossal artery is not identical with its primitive precursor in the embryo; whereas the latter passes medially and anteriorly to the roots of the hypoglossal nerve, the former runs posteriorly and laterally to the nerve. The posteroinferior cerebellar artery may arise in the persistent hypoglossal artery, whereas in the embryo it originates in the lateral anastomotic channel. The cranial part of the persisting hypoglossal artery may be formed by the lateral anastomotic channel connected to the basal artery through a transverse anastomotic channel. Jan Brismar[1] (Univ. of Lund) reports the 26th case of persistent primitive hypoglossal artery.

Woman, 56, with history of migraine, had angiography after having a grand mal seizure followed by a transient right-sided hemiparesis. Common carotid angiography on the left showed a large frontal falx meningioma supplied by the anterior falx branch of the ophthalmic artery. Right-sided injection showed a wide artery branching off from the internal carotid 2 cm cephalad to the carotid bifurcation and running dorsal to the internal carotid in a cephalad direction, ending at the basilar artery. Selective angiography of the anomalous artery showed retrograde filling of hypoplastic vertebral arteries through a network probably involving the posteroinferior cerebellar arteries. Antegrade flow in the vertebral arteries was normal. The right internal carotid siphon was well filled through a wide posterior communicating artery on the right. On right-sided internal carotid injection, both pericallosal arteries and the posterior cerebral arteries filled via the wide posterior communicating artery.

The criteria suggested for persistent primitive hypoglossal artery include a persistent primitive hypoglossal artery leaving the internal carotid as an extracranial branch and passage of the vessel through the anterior condyloid foramen before joining the caudal part of the basilar artery. In

(1) Acta Radiol. [Diagn.] (Stockh.) 17:160–166, March, 1976.

the present case, hypoplasia of the left anterior cerebral artery, and probably also of the left posterior communicating artery, in early embryologic life may have placed too great a strain on the right internal carotid artery to allow it to assume the role of the primitive arteries in supplying the hindbrain. The role of these arteries also could not be assumed by the hypoplastic vertebral arteries.

Nonassociation of Adrenocorticosteroid Therapy and Peptic Ulcer. It is "known" that adrenocorticosteroid therapy often is complicated by the appearance or reactivation of peptic ulcers but the basis for this "knowledge" is difficult to define. Harold O. Conn and Bennett L. Blitzer[2] attempted to determine whether such an association really exists. Retrospective analysis was made of all prospective investigations of steroids or ACTH in the treatment of any disease in which adults were randomly selected to have either steroid or no therapy. There were 26 double-blind studies, including 3,558 cases, and also 16 prospective, controlled, non-double-blind studies that included 1,773 other cases.

Peptic ulcers occurred in 1% of control patients and 1.4% of steroid-treated patients in the double-blind studies, an insignificant difference. Rates of hemorrhage from and perforation of peptic ulcer were similar in both groups. In the non-double-blind studies, peptic ulcer occurred insignificantly more frequently in steroid-treated patients. Combining both groups of studies, the differences in frequency of peptic ulcer and in its complications were not significant. Hemorrhage of unknown origin occurred more frequently in placebo-control than in steroid-treated patients in both groups of studies. Combining the groups of studies, upper gastrointestinal hemorrhage of undetermined cause occurred significantly more often in control than in steroid-treated patients.

These data suggest that the frequency of peptic ulcer is not increased by steroid treatment. In the non-double-blind studies, analysis of duration of therapy revealed that treatment with steroids for more than 30 days was associated with significantly more cases of peptic ulcer than treatment for 1 month or less; however, long-term placebo therapy also

(2) N. Engl. J. Med. 294:473–479, Feb. 26, 1976.

was associated with a higher incidence of ulcer. Analysis of therapy dosage revealed no significant differences between high-dose and low-dose therapy. An association was found between peptic ulcers and the *total* dose of steroid administered. It is unlikely that the association of steroid therapy and peptic ulcer will ever be evaluated in a prospective, controlled manner. It should not be concluded that steroids are unassociated with the development of peptic ulcer. It is possible that high blood levels of unbound steroid are ulcerogenic.

► [Most of the neurologic disorders in patients in the control, double-blind and nonrandomized studies were "stroke." multiple sclerosis and Bell's palsy. What the outcome would be in patients with raised intracranial pressure associated with tumors and other disorders is unclear. However, if the incidence is truly small, then one might well consider returning to the use of aspirin instead of Tylenol as a pain reliever after craniotomy (and other neurosurgical procedures), in the hope that the salicylate therapy might inhibit the formation of venous thrombosis. My own totally uncontrolled series indicates a much lower incidence of venous thrombosis in the "old days" when aspirin was given for pain and (rectally) for control of elevated temperatures. – Ed.] ◄

Continuous Monitoring of Intracranial Pressure in Severe Closed Head Injury without Mass Lesions. Monitoring of intracranial pressure (ICP) is a familiar technique, but most previous reports on monitoring have involved heterogeneous patient populations. Alan S. Fleischer, Nettleton S. Payne and George T. Tindall[3] (Emory Univ.) present a report on a relatively homogeneous group of 40 patients with severe closed head injuries and no angiographic evidence of mass lesions, who underwent continuous monitoring. No surgical procedures were done. Only patients in grade III coma or worse were monitored. Patients were monitored continuously for 5 days to 2 weeks, usually with an intraventricular cannula attached to a subcutaneously implanted Rickham reservoir. The needle inserted percutaneously into the reservoir was changed every 12–24 hours. A subarachnoid screw was used in 8 cases. The ICP was considered significantly elevated if it exceeded 20 mm Hg in a sustained or repetitive fashion. Elevated pressure was managed by administering 20% mannitol and often by aspirating cerebrospinal fluid from the ventricle and by hyperventilation. All patients received 40 mg dexa-

(3) Surg. Neurol. 6:31–34, July, 1976.

methasone daily for 10 days. Elevated pressure was not refractory to treatment in any of the 40 patients.

Most patients had normal pressures; only 35% had elevated ICP. Patients with signs of brain stem dysfunction are as likely as those with less severe injury to have normal ICP. The ICP was not significantly related to prognosis in the entire group, but elevated pressures in grade III patients were associated with a worse prognosis. Functional survival was related to the absence of neurologic signs of brain stem dysfunction.

The value of continuous ICP monitoring in this type of injury is uncertain. Serious complications may occur with ICP monitoring, especially with intraventricular recording, and monitoring may not be indicated in severe head trauma when a mass lesion has been excluded by angiography or computerized axial tomography. Elevated pressure occurs in a minority of these patients, and, even when it is present and adequately treated, there is no apparent improvement in the overall results.

Analysis of Response to Therapeutic Measures to Reduce Intracranial Pressure in Head-Injured Patients. Hector E. James, Thomas W. Langfitt and Vijay S. Kumar[4] (Univ. of Pennsylvania) studied intracranial pressure (ICP) responses to various forms of treatment in 32 patients, aged 1 – 73, with suspected intracranial hypertension as a result of head trauma. Thirty-six recordings were made by the intraventricular cannula method. Closed head injuries, depressed fractures and subdural and epidural hematomas were present. All surgical lesions were treated promptly after diagnosis by cerebral angiography. An ICP recording was indicated for clinical evidence of brain swelling or anticipated brain swelling after surgery for intracranial hematoma. The ICP was recorded with a Scott cannula, inserted through a bur hole or twist drill hole 2 cm lateral to the midline at the level of the coronary suture into a lateral ventricle.

Thirty recordings showed an ICP over 20 torr and 6 were consistently below that level. The recordings of 2 – 301 hours in duration variously demonstrated a persistently elevated ICP, fluctuations in the forms of A or B waves of Lundberg

(4) J. Trauma 16:437 – 441, June, 1976.

and persistently low pressure. All patients received steroids in varying dosage. Cerebrospinal fluid drainage reduced the ICP immediately in all 11 instances. Hypertonic mannitol, hyperventilation and hypothermia were effective when they produced a fall in ICP of 10% or more of the control level. Hyperventilation reduced the ICP by 10–80% in 9 of 15 trials in 11 patients and caused no pressure reduction in 4 trials. Mild hypothermia of 32–36 C reduced the ICP in 4 of 11 trials but no reduction occurred in 4 instances. Moderate hypothermia of 27–31 C produced a response in 2 of 4 trials. Mannitol, given in a bolus of 0.18–2.5 gm/kg in 2–5 minutes, led to a reduction in ICP in 27 of 28 recordings in 17 patients, ranging from 10% to 98%. The only patient who failed to respond had a significantly increased regional cerebral blood flow at mannitol administration. Eleven of the 32 patients in the study died.

Withdrawal of cerebrospinal fluid was always effective but is not an effective permanent form of therapy for increased ICP in head-injured patients. Hypertonic mannitol administration was usually effective, whereas hyperventilation was least effective in the most severely ill patients. Hypothermia gave the poorest ICP responses.

▶ [Hyperventilation is more effective if the patient is paralyzed, and it is proper for therapy if there is some measure of effectiveness, such as intracranial pressure (via monitor). Deliberate paralysis removes criteria of the clinical state such as movement and state of consciousness. Persistently high intracranial pressure has such a poor prognosis that some clinicians discontinue treatment and give no supportive therapy in adults with persistently elevated pressure; if the patient is under age 18, however, supportive therapy is continued because of the exceptional young patient who may recover from persistently elevated pressure. — Ed.] ◀

Restricted Fluid Intake: Rational Management of the Neurosurgical Patient. It is possible that the water intake requirements for maintaining homeostasis are not as great in brain-injured patients as has been believed, since if the extracellular space is expanded with currently recommended amounts of fluid, brain edema will be adversely affected. Henry A. Shenkin, Honorio S. Bezier and William F. Bouzarth[5] (Philadelphia) maintained 10 patients having hemispheric brain tumors on an average of 1,055 ml 0.45% salt in 2.5% glucose solution every 24 hours. They were

(5) J. Neurosurg. 45:432–436, October, 1976.

compared with 10 patients previously maintained on an average daily intake of 1,995 ml 0.45% saline in 2.5% glucose solution and with a comparable series of patients given 24 mg dexamethasone and an average of 1,802 ml fluid daily.

Serum osmolarity remained within 1.5% of the average preoperative level in study patients, whereas an average decrease of 5% was seen with a greater fluid intake and an average decrease of 3.6% in steroid-treated patients. Serum sodium concentration did not change significantly in the study group, whereas it decreased an average of 2.2% in patients given large fluid loads and 3.8% in steroid-treated patients. Changes in body weight in the three groups generally reflected the changes in osmolarity and serum sodium. Hematocrit was reduced least in the steroid-treated patients. The blood urea nitrogen tended to decline in patients given large fluid volumes and to increase, though minimally, in the other groups.

Postoperative brain tumor patients given just over 1 L fluid daily are kept in homeostatic balance with respect to serum osmolarity and electrolytes. Fluid restriction should be used cautiously if hyperosmolar agents, diuretics or dexamethasone also are administered. A reduction in serum osmolarity and sodium may occur despite postoperative fluid restriction because of administration of excessive fluid during surgery or because of administration of humidified air.

► [The mechanism of coma in nonketotic hyperglycemic hyperosmolar coma is believed by Park et al. (J. Neurosurg. 44:409, 1976) to be related to shifts of free water from the cerebral extravascular space to the hypertonic intravascular space. This leads to intracellular dehydration, accumulation of metabolic products of glucose and brain shrinkage. Fatal complications include acute renal failure, terminal arrhythmia and vascular "accidents"; cerebral and systemic treatments are both disputed, particularly in reference to use of saline infusions, insulin resistance, monitoring of cerebrospinal fluid pressures and of serum and urine osmolarity. – Ed.] ◄

Variations in Local Cerebral Blood Volume as a Function of Mean Arterial Pressure in Man. B. Pertuiset, D. Ancri and G. Goutorbe[6] (Paris) describe a new method of measurement based on the use of radionuclides. A tracer that has a negligible rate of extravascular diffusion in

(6) Rev. Neurol. (Paris) 132:213–218, March, 1976.

a few hours is injected into the blood. In about 10 minutes the concentration is homogeneous in the blood compartment. In each region the radiotracer quantity is thus proportional to the blood volume. If the emitted x-ray energy is great enough, the measured activity will be proportional to the blood volume. Measurement of the activity in a cerebral region by use of an external probe indicates variations in blood volume. To have reliable counts, with stability of tagging and intravascular concentration, siderophilin tagged with [113m]In or the patient's erythrocytes tagged with ^{99m}Tc, at high specific activity, are used.

Under the effect of pressure variations, volume variations are registered continuously. Probes are placed opposite the different cerebral regions to be studied, but also opposite the face. Each yields information on the blood volume of a determined region. Correlations are established taking into account the recordings from opposite the face to evaluate and subtract the part that returns to the extracerebral circulation, when recording is with the cranium closed. In certain procedures, done after the flap is lifted during surgery, the recording gives a direct measurement of the variation in local cerebral blood volume.

Ten patients with meningeal hemorrhage related to rupture of an intracranial aneurysm were studied. Some were studied with the cranium closed and others, after the flap was lifted during operation.

The first recording was frontal, with the cranium closed. Mean pressure at the outset was slightly higher than 90 mm Hg. With perfusion of sodium nitroprussides, it decreased progressively to about 40 mm Hg. During this reduction, the blood volume increased regularly until it reached a maximum variation of 8.3% in relation to baseline volume, then diminished when the pressure rose due to cessation of perfusion with the hypotensive agent.

With the cranium open during operation, the recording was only that of the local blood volume. In 1 case in particular, rapid interruption of autoregulation was observed, from 80 mm Hg (mean arterial pressure at outset) to 50 mm Hg, causing a variation in volume on the order of 2.8%. Beyond 50 mm Hg, autoregulation was destroyed and volume varied in parallel with pressure, which caused a fall in the local blood flow elsewhere. When the pressure rises, it may be observed, due to loss of autoregulation, that volume and pressure vary in the same direction and that there is a volume which remains below the initial local blood volume for a given mean arterial pressure.

▶ [A fine review of physiology of cerebral blood flow by Lassen and Christensen appeared recently (Br. J. Anesth. 48:719, 1976). It emphasizes hazards of using painful stimuli to assess the level of coma in patients suffering from disorders such as tumor and trauma, lest there be an increase in blood flow and intracranial pressure. The authors calculate the lower limit of autoregulation to be 60 mm Hg mean arterial pressure (MAP); in normotensives the upper limit is at 130 mm MAP. Chronic hypertensives have their limits of autoregulation displaced to the right. The discussion of lactic acidosis, leading to vasomotor paralysis and loss of autoregulation, is very worthwhile. Segments of the article also deal with pharmacology of cerebral blood flow, including anesthetic gases. All gaseous anesthetic agents are vasodilators; the intravenous agents are vasoconstrictors — except for ketamine. The role of hyperventilation during recovery from anesthesia is discussed in the following article. — Ed.] ◀

Intracranial Pressure during Recovery from Nitrous Oxide and Halothane Anesthesia in Neurosurgical Patients. Intracranial pressure (ICP) is increased by all inhalational anesthetics through cerebral vasodilatation and the resultant increase in cerebral blood volume, particularly in patients with intracranial mass lesions. Hypercapnia adds to the vasodilating effect of anesthetics, whereas hypocapnia effectively counteracts it. P. B. Jørgensen and B. B. Misfeldt[7] (Univ. of Copenhagen) correlated the clinical state with arterial CO_2 tension and ICP in 7 patients recovering from anesthesia with nitrous oxide (N_2O) and halothane after surgery for intracranial disorders. Arterial, intracranial and central venous pressures and arterial CO_2 tension were measured. Five patients had operation for removal of tumors or hematomas and 2 had ventriculography. Patients were anesthetized with 50% N_2O in oxygen and 0.5 – 1% halothane and were hyperventilated with the same mixture for at least 10 minutes at the end of operation to maintain Pa_{CO_2}.

The mean Pa_{CO_2} value during hyperventilation was 24.1 mm Hg and the mean perfusion pressure value was 64.9 mm Hg. Only 1 patient had an elevated ICP during hypocapnia. After hyperventilation was stopped, the Pa_{CO_2} increased until spontaneous respiration began at a mean Pa_{CO_2} value

(7) Br. J. Anaesth. 47:977–982, September, 1975.

of 40.3 mm Hg; the mean ICP at this time was 17.9 mm Hg and the mean cerebral perfusion pressure (CPP) was 58.2 mm Hg. A mean of 19 minutes passed before spontaneous respiration began and another 6 minutes passed until respiration was adequate. With the patients awake, the mean Pa_{CO_2} value was 39 mm Hg and in all but 1 patient, the ICP was normal. The mean CPP at this time was 85 mm Hg. Central venous pressures were unchanged throughout the study.

Patients without evidence of marked brain swelling may be allowed to resume spontaneous respiration and may be awakened from N_2O-halothane anesthesia after intracranial surgery; however, some intracranial hypertension may occur even in these patients and a risk of hypercapnia exists. If severe brain swelling is evident at closure of a craniotomy, hyperventilation probably is indicated at least until N_2O and halothane have been eliminated, and probably for at least the next 24 hours, to minimize further brain swelling and to counteract development of secondary hypoxic and ischemic brain damage.

Origin of Intraventricular Hemorrhage in the Preterm Infant. G. Hambleton and J. S. Wigglesworth[8] (Hammersmith Hosp., London) examined the cerebral vessels in 19 preterm infants who came to autopsy in order to establish the basic anatomy of intraventricular hemorrhage and other cerebrovascular lesions. Vessels are inoculated with colored barium-gelatin solutions; usually a solution of red Colorpaque with 3% gelatin injected into the carotid arteries, is followed by an injection of blue Colorpaque with 5% gelatin through the same cannula to displace red solution into the capillaries and veins and leave the arteries colored blue. Study was made of 34 brains from infants of 24–40 weeks' gestational age who had died 8 minutes to 10 days postnatally. The specimens were examined by stereomicroscopy.

The immature brain exhibited a rich capillary bed in the terminal-layer region suplied mainly by Heubner's artery. Capillary channels drained directly into the terminal vein and its main branches. Study of 19 cases of spontaneous germinal layer hemorrhage, with or without intraventricular hemorrhage, failed to show rupture of the terminal vein

(8)   Arch. Dis. Child. 51:651–659, September, 1976.

or germinal layer infarction. In infants of up to 28 weeks' gestation, germinal layer hemorrhage was most frequent over the body of the caudate nucleus, whereas in older infants the hemorrhages were usually over the head of the caudate nucleus. Histologic study of 10 cases of germinal layer hemorrhage showed rupture at a capillary-vein junction in 1 case and fibrin masses adjacent to the vein wall in 2 others. Carotid artery injections caused prominent leaks within the germinal layer capillary bed, often adjacent to veins. Jugular vein injections in 2 subjects failed to rupture the terminal vein, but caused multiple vein ruptures at the junction of the deep and cortical venous systems; additional small ruptures in the germinal layer occurred in 1 of these 2 subjects.

Capillaries within the germinal layer may be ruptured by a rise in arterial pressure, especially under conditions of hypercapnia and hypoxia, resulting in germinal layer hemorrhage and subsequent intraventricular hemorrhage. High fibrinolytic activity in the germinal layer may allow propagation of the original hemorrhage. If this hypothesis is correct, meticulous care in monitoring Pa_{CO_2}, acid-base status and blood pressure is indicated in ill preterm infants, preferably with the use of continuous recording methods. At the same time it is essential to reduce handling of the infant to a minimum to avoid hypertensive episodes.

Diagnosis

Familial "Doughnut" Lesions of the Skull: Benign, Hereditary Dysplasia. The solitary calvarial "doughnut" lesion was first reported as an entity by Keats and Holt in 1969. All 21 cases have been found incidentally. Multiple rounded calvarial defects have been described in only 1 patient. John E. Bartlett and Pulla R. S. Kishore[9] (Univ. of Kansas) report data on 3 further cases of multiple calvarial doughnut lesions, with a familial relationship that follows an incompletely dominant sex-linked inheritance pattern.

The appearance in a man aged 18, the half-brother of 1 patient and the son of the other, is shown in Figure 1. The size of the multiple sclerotic calvarial lesions was variable, the central lucent zone becoming less apparent as the peripheral band of bony sclerosis increased. All 3 patients were males of the same kindred and all presented with a

Fig 1.—The doughnut appellation seems well suited to these sclerotic calvarial changes. (Courtesy of Bartlett, J. E., and Kishore, P. R. S.: Radiology 119:385–387, May, 1976.)

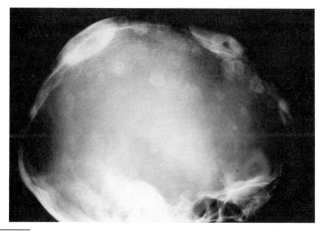

lumpy skull as the only clinical manifestation. A fourth family member was also reported to have a lumpy skull. No patient exhibited additional skeletal abnormalities. The histologic picture of one biopsy specimen was most consistent with hyperostosis.

These lesions are benign but their pathogenesis is obscure. The multiplicity of the lesions and their familial occurrence point toward a developmental abnormality. The father had had a lumpy skull since childhood, for over 40 years, and his lesions were smaller and much less well defined than those in the siblings. Multiple sclerotic doughnut lesions of the calvarium are characteristic enough to be distinguished easily from more significant pathology on clinical grounds.

Nitrous Oxide Encephalography: Five-Year Experience with 475 Pediatric Patients. Richard A. Elwyn, Wallace H. Ring, Edward Loeser and Garth G. Myers[1] (Univ. of Utah) used the characteristics of nitrous oxide in an attempt to provide patients undergoing gas pneumoencephalography (PEG) with a measure of operative safety, pain relief and postoperative comfort not previously afforded by other modalities. Studies were done on 538 pediatric patients having PEG, in 475 of whom N_2O was used; air was used in the 63 others. Infants up to age 1 year received 0.02 mg atropine per kg as premedication, whereas older children received hydroxyzine or diazepam orally, followed by pentobarbital or secobarbital and atropine. Anesthesia was induced with 70% N_2O in oxygen and 1 – 4% halothane and maintained by 0.25 – 1% halothane-N_2O-O_2 in N_2O-medium patients at the lightest level possible. Intrathecal gas instillation was carried out as anesthesia was continued with 65 – 75% N_2O and halothane.

No severe headache occurred in patients in whom N_2O was used as the contrast medium, but 44% of air-contrast patients had severe headache at 1 day. Only 3% of N_2O-contrast patients were vomiting at 24 hours, whereas 5% of air patients still vomited at 72 hours. All N_2O-contrast patients were discharged by 96 hours, whereas only 74% of air-contrast patients were discharged by this time and 5% remained in hospital at 144 hours. Radiologic results were sat-

(1) Anesth. Analg. (Cleve.) 55:402–408, May–June, 1976.

isfactory in 93% of N_2O patients and 81% of air-contrast patients. The N_2O injection ranged from 2 to 4 times the amount of cerebrospinal fluid removed. The usual duration of anesthesia was 1½ hours. Only minimal ventricular gas remained 15 minutes after cessation of the N_2O anesthetic. No neurologic complications or deaths occurred. Operative complications included 6 cases of marked bradycardia, 3 of severe hypotension in sitting patients and 2 cardiac arrests, 1 after inadvertent extubation.

This method of encephalography has resulted in a great reduction in postoperative discomfort and earlier discharge. The technique is both safe and effective. It is the first known application of gas physics used to provide patients with postoperative pain relief.

► [The assessment of headache was made only in children aged 6 and over (121 with N_2O and 18 with air injections). The authors consider headache related to the amount of gas injected, but it is more conventional to relate it to amount of cerebrospinal fluid removed, and statistics on this point are lacking. There might be some disadvantage in rapid removal of the ventricular gas in this technique should it be necessary to obtain additional films. However, the concepts offered concerning the same gas for injection and for anesthesia are interesting.

The criterion of cerebellar atrophy used by Kennedy et al. (Br. J. Radiol. 49:903, 1976) was width of two or more sulci in the vermis more than 2 mm. In 44 patients with cerebellar atrophy, there was a significant relationship between the severity of the atrophy and the severity of clinical cerebellar disease. Atrophy of cerebellar hemispheres was rarely found without vermis atrophy. Cerebral atrophy, found in 34 patients, was not correlated with cerebellar atrophy, but was most severe in patients with spinocerebellar degeneration, alcoholism, dementia and cerebrovascular disease. It is of interest that autopsies were available in 2 patients with moderate vermis atrophy on pneumography. Neither was thought to have atrophy by the pathologist; one brain of a patient with possible pseudotumor was normal macroscopically and microscopically. The other had changes consistent with those of cerebellar syndrome associated with carcinoma. – Ed.] ◄

► ↓ The advocates of decreasing medical costs particularly pick on the computerized tomography (CT) scanner as an expensive device that is being ordered too frequently by hospitals and private practitioners – without real regard for the amazing benefits this device has brought to diagnosis. We have been sharing access to a CT scanner for several years now, and sharing is *not* the answer for a hospital with a busy neurologic and neurosurgical service. The lack of access to such scanners for emergencies is a serious hindrance to the best care, and having to have the patient wait in the hospital for periods of days to a week or even 2 weeks is certainly not a cost-effective measure. – Ed. ◄

Computerized Tomography (The EMI Scanner): Comparison with Pneumoencephalography and Ventriculography. J. Gawler, G. H. DuBoulay, J. W. D. Bull and J. Marshall[2] (Natl. Hosp. for Nervous Diseases, London) compared EMI scans with conventional ventricular contrast procedures done in the same patients. Studies were done of 78 patients, aged 8 months to 73 years. Studies always were done within 3 weeks of each other. The initial EMI system, using the 80×80 matrix picture, was replaced by a high-resolution 160×160 matrix scan after the comparison study.

Identical conclusions were drawn from both study methods in 59 cases. Seven pneumoencephalograms were incomplete, 4 showing no ventricular filling. Five EMI scans in this group were normal and 2 showed cerebral atrophy. Two contrast studies showed distention of the anterior recesses of the 3d ventricle in patients with normal ventricular dimensions on both studies; 1 of these patients had cerebellar ectopia and the other had a small acoustic neuroma. Four pneumoencephalograms showed slight lateral ventricular enlargement or equivocal sulcal widening in patients with normal EMI scans. Six patients showed enlargement of the ventricular system on both studies but widened cortical sulci were seen only on scans in 3 cases and only on the pneumoencephalogram in 3. The temporal horns of the lateral ventricles were seen on EMI scans only when they were enlarged. Enlarged cerebellar sulci, present in 17 patients, were detected only by pneumoencephalography in 2 cases and only by EMI scanning in 2 others. Ventricular parameters measured directly on EMI scans were less than the equivalent dimensions on the contrast procedures. Computerized scans were valuable in monitoring the progress of several hydrocephalic patients having ventricular shunting operations.

The EMI scan is a safe method of diagnosing cerebral atrophy or hydrocephalus, precluding the need for conventional contrast procedures in many cases, and is ideal for monitoring disease progress or treatment effects. As computerized tomography becomes more sophisticated, the indications for conventional ventricular contrast procedures probably will decline.

(2) J. Neurol. Neurosurg. Psychiatry 39:203–211, March, 1976.

Some Limitations of Computed Tomography in Diagnosis of Neurologic Diseases are discussed by Kenneth R. Davis, Juan M. Taveras, Glenn H. Roberson and Robert H. Ackerman[3] (Harvard Med. School). Use of the EMI scanner has helped considerably in the diagnosis and management of many patients with neurologic disorders but the shortcomings of the technique have not received sufficient attention.

The computed tomography (CT) scan may fail to detect a small lesion or one with little difference in absorption coefficient from surrounding brain, before and after contrast enhancement. Extemely high or low absorption values of adjacent structures may interfere with detection of a lesion. Small vessels and details of larger ones are not observed on CT scans even after contrast injection. The fine detail of aneurysmal sacs and their relationships to parent vessels cannot be demonstrated. Many lesions appear similar on CT

Fig 2. – Four cases showing ringlike enhancement. Computed tomography scans after 300 ml meglumine diatrizoate *(top row)* and without contrast *(bottom row)*. **A,** proved infarction at surgery; preoperative diagnosis, abscess. **B,** surgically proved right frontal glioblastoma. **C,** surgically proved left frontal abscess. **D,** left frontal undifferentiated lung metastasis. (Courtesy of Davis, K. R., et al.: Am. J. Roentgenol. 127:111–123, July, 1976.)

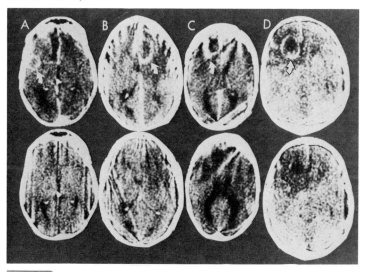

(3)   Am. J. Roentgenol. 127:111–123, July, 1976.

scans (Fig 2) and patients have been operated on because of a mistaken CT diagnosis of neoplasm. Errors commonly occur when plain studies are not obtained for comparison before contrast medium is used.

The overall accuracy of CT study in lesion detection has been high. Most often the problem is not whether a lesion has been detected but whether all the anatomical information necessary to institute treatment is available. Because many lesions are visualized so easily by CT, there is a temptation to cut short the diagnostic workup, sometimes to the detriment of optimal therapeutic results.

▶ [New uses for computerized tomography are being sought and found. Greitz (Am. J. Roentgenol. 127:125, 1976) reviews these, including detection of extremely small aneurysms using coned-down tomography and reconstruction in several planes. Dynamics of cerebrospinal flow, pharmacokinetics of contrast medium and blood volume alterations have been studied. Exact fixation of the head permits a diagnostic coordinate system that can be directly transferred to a therapeutic coordinate system such as used in stereotaxic treatments (Bergstrom and Greitz: ibid, p. 167).

Liliequist and Forssell (Acta Radiol. [Diagn.] (Stockh.) 17:399, 1976) point out that conventional use of the CT scanner makes the skull appear as a homogeneous structure. If a wide "window" is used, the range of EMI numbers may go up to 400, and new details appear. Of particular interest are: foramen magnum, hypoglossal canal, jugular foramen, internal auditory canal, occipital condyles, clivus and inion. Fractures through the skull base may be more easily evaluated with CT scanning than with conventional technique.

Different types of metastases may give variable CT pictures. Deck et al. (Radiology 119:115, 1976) found high-density lesions from melanoma, chorionic carcinoma, colonic carcinoma and osteogenic sarcoma. Low-density masses came from lymphoma and carcinoma of lung, breast and kidney. The last two may show increased density after intravenous injection of iodinated compounds. Comparisons of CT and radionuclide scans showed agreement in 61 patients. In 6 others, CT scan was correct; in 9, radionuclide scanning was more accurate. In 15, the disagreement could not be settled due to lack of inadequate investigation or follow-up. In general, CT scanning adds more information than radionuclide scans, especially concerning ventricular size and displacement. – Ed.] ◀

Computerized Tomography and Angiography in Subarachnoid Hemorrhage. B. E. Kendall, B. C. P. Lee and E. Claveria[4] (Nat'l Hosp. for Nervous Diseases, London) report the results of computer-assisted transverse axial tomography (CAT) in a small series of patients with subarachnoid hemorrhage with respect to its value in the preangiographic localization of bleeding sites. Review was

(4) Br. J. Radiol. 49:483-501, June, 1976.

made of data on 100 patients with multiple aneurysms and subarachnoid hemorrhage due to intracranial aneurysm. In 75 others with proved subarachnoid hemorrhage, CAT was performed from the day of bleeding to 90 days afterward. Three patients had two separate hemorrhages. Angiography was performed in all but 3 of these patients, usually within 2 weeks of the first CAT.

In 59 patients with multiple aneurysms, surgery was confined to the aneurysm that had bled and was by direct occlusion of its neck. The proportion of multiple aneurysms was nearly double when the posterior circulation was examined. Definite angiographic localizing features were absent in 43% of the patients. Thirty-four patients died within 2 months of initial bleeding, whereas the 66 survivors had a reasonably good prognosis; only 5 have died since the hemorrhage and only 1 death was due to intracranial hemorrhage.

Among 78 hemorrhages studied by CAT, 25 showed a local hematoma and 19 others a hematoma with surrounding infarction or edema (Fig 3). Infarction or edema alone was seen in 12 cases. Angiography showed causative aneurysms

Fig 3. – **A,** CAT, anterior communicating artery aneurysm. Note two areas of high density in frontal region bilaterally and another high density area midline anterior to 3d ventricle due to subfrontal and bifrontal hematoma. Two large low-density areas surround this lesion due to edema infarct in both frontal lobes. **B,** left carotid angiogram demonstrates anterior communicating artery aneurysm. There is separation of anterior cerebral arteries below the genu by hematoma. (Courtesy of Kendall, B. E., et al.: Br. J. Radiol. 49:483–501, June, 1976.)

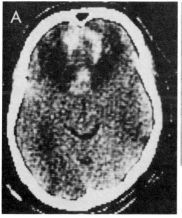
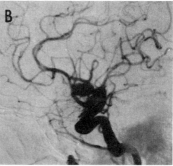

in 31 cases and angiomatous malformation in 11 of 57 hemorrhages in 54 patients. Two or more aneurysms were associated with 13 bleeds in 11 patients. Twenty-one hemorrhages had no focal signs on unenhanced CAT. In 56 of 75 patients, CAT alone localized or at least lateralized the site of hemorrhage.

Bleeding from incidental aneurysms is uncommon and it appears reasonable not to operate electively on most such aneurysms. If the site of bleeding can be approximately localized before angiography, the angiography should be directed primarily toward a detailed demonstration of the vessels adjacent to the CAT abnormality and extended to give any information relevant to surgical treatment. Further angiographic study to discover incidental aneurysms that have not bled is not necessary unless elective surgery on such lesions is contemplated.

▶ [The value of CAT scans in cerebrovascular disease is indicated by Kinkel and Jacobs (Neurology (Minneap.) 26:924, 1976). With one exception, each patient in this series who had a normal scan 48 hours after onset of symptoms ultimately was diagnosed to have had a transient ischemic attack. Abnormal scans were found in 98% of those with infarcts. Serial studies are needed to pick up initially normal scans that later change to abnormal or those with massive infarcts mimicking tumor. In general, infarcts have areas of decreased density whereas hemorrhages produce distinctly high-density scans. Many such hemorrhages appear clinically as thrombosis, and diagnosis of clot did not appear indicated by clinical study.

Postoperative neurosurgical care is made easier by CAT scanning according to Lin et al. (Neuroradiology 12:185, 1977). Differentiation of postoperative hematoma from edema, demonstration of adequacy of surgical resection and evaluation of the efficacy and complications of shunting hydrocephalic ventricles are demonstrated. The authors echo the request by others for plastic hemostatic clips to avoid the artefacts in CAT scans due to metal ones. — Ed.] ◀

Comparison of EMI and Radioisotope Imaging in Neurologic Disease. G. H. Du Boulay and John Marshall[5] (London) compared the information provided by isotope imaging before and after the introduction of computerized transverse axial tomography (EMI scanning) with that obtained from EMI scanning itself. Of 985 scintigrams made using ^{99m}Tc and the gamma camera in a 6-month period in 1973, 197 were reviewed. In a 6-month period in 1974, after introduction of the EMI scan, 897 scintigrams were ob-

(5) Lancet 2:1294–1297, Dec. 27, 1975.

tained, and in 290 of these an EMI scan was requested independent of the isotope study. Scintigrams were made with 10 mCi ^{99m}Tc intravenously after 400 mg potassium perchlorate orally. Where a vascular lesion was suspected, 15 mCi ^{99m}Tc was given.

The EMI scan was superior diagnostically to the isotope study in epilepsy of recent onset; it demonstrated atrophy as well as tumors. The EMI scan was clearly superior in cases of acute and progressive cerebral hemispheric lesions. In acute cases the EMI scan distinguished between infarction and hematoma. Both studies were less helpful in cases of acute and progressive posterior-fossa lesions. Both studies were rewarding in the investigation of headache of recent onset but the EMI scan showed more lesions than the scintigram. The EMI scan is useful in patients with dementia in excluding tumor and also by providing positive evidence of atrophy. Both studies were helpful in detecting structural lesions in cases of acute encephalopathy. Neither study was definitive in studying cases of visual failure. Both types of scan were extremely helpful in cases of tumor recurrence, but the EMI scan was superior to the isotope study, not only in detecting more tumor recurrences, but also in demonstrating associated atrophy, hydrocephalus and displacement of intracranial structures.

Computerized transverse axial tomography is superior to isotope scintigraphy in a wide range of neurological problems, in demonstrating lesions and showing the effects of lesions on the surrounding brain. Scintigraphy is not necessary as a screening test when EMI scanning is to be carried out. The cost of increased EMI scanning time will be largely offset by a reduction in the number of invasive studies required.

▶ [On the other hand, Kuhl et al. (Radiology 121:495, 1976) believe computerized axial tomography (CAT) information can be supplemented by results of radionuclide computerized tomography. Their Mark IV system used four detector assemblies, of eight separate detectors each, rotating around the head. Computerized data permit production of a scan that can show the results of local alteration of the blood-brain barrier to ingress of technetium or labeled red cells. Blood flow, blood volume and changes of small portions of the brain can be studied, in some ways, like autoradiography.

A comparison of radionuclide imaging and CAT scans also has been made by Alderson et al. (Neurology (Minneap.) 26:803, 1976). Both tests were done within 72 hours of one another (66% done within 24 hours). Disagreement was most common in the presence of acute cerebrovascular episodes; 3 patients had abnormal CAT scans and normal TC scans whereas 5 had abnormal TC scans and normal CAT scans. Tumors were picked up well by both techniques. Low-grade gliomas are less well detected with radionuclide scans, and hematomas are better seen with CAT scans. Of 67 patients with headache as the only complaint, 64 had normal scans with both techniques; 1 had a vascular malformation detected by both. Two had mild cortical atrophy detected only by the CAT scan.

The authors suggest that CAT scans will be better for focal presentations, seizures of recent onset and dementia. Patients thought to have cerebrovascular accidents will benefit from both. Patients with nonfocal presentations other than dementia and seizures can be screened adequately by nuclide imaging alone.

Many measurements can be made on CAT scans; among these are frontal ventricular dimensions, as calculated by Hahn and Rim (Am. J. Roentgenol. 126:593, 1976). Based on 200 normal subjects (age 10–81), they conclude that the cerebroventricular index is a reliable indicator of ventricular size. This is the ratio between the brain width and the distance between the outer borders of the lateral ventricles. The maximum bifrontal diameter of the frontal horns tends to increase slightly with age.

Computerized tomography differentiates well nonobstructive hydrocephalus, according to Wiggli et al. (Rev. Neurol. (Paris) 131:405, 1976). This test and radioisotope cisternography were done in 18 patients with progressive dementia. The CAT scans showed more dilated ventricles in patients with nonobstructive hydrocephalus than in those with cortical atrophy. Only with malresorptive hydrocephalus did the authors find "juxtaventricular edema," possibly due to transependymal absorption of cerebrospinal fluid.

In general, CAT scans give a more complete profile of malignant tumor characteristics than the EEG or ^{99m}Tc imaging in evaluation before and after chemotherapy and radiotherapy. Norman et al. (Radiology 121:85, 1976) found increased tumor size, central lucency and contrast enhancement in patients with clinical deterioration, with decrease in these characteristics in those who improved. In 9 of 33 patients who deteriorated, the CAT findings preceded clinical changes by an average of 2 months. Radionuclide imaging may fail to detect tumor or may pick up effects of surgery as well as tumor. Enlarged ventricles were often seen without obvious obstructive lesions and may be implicated in deterioration of some patients. – Ed.] ◄

Tumor Volume, Luxury Perfusion and Regional Blood Volume Changes in Man Visualized by Subtraction Computerized Tomography are discussed by Richard D. Penn, Randal Walser, Diane Kurtz and Laurens Ackerman[6] (Rush-Presbyterian-St. Luke's Med. Center). The most straightforward way to obtain a subtraction of a computerized axial tomographic (CAT) scan is by using negative transparencies of the pre- and postinfusion scans.

(6) J. Neurosurg. 44:449–457, April, 1976.

The only way to quantify the subtraction and to permit regional cerebral blood volume calculations is to use a computer subtraction technique. Subtracting scans require CAT density values that are linear with x-ray absorption over the range being subtracted.

Infusion scanning combined with subtraction allows the accurate delineation of tumor size and provides an estimate of increased blood volume within the mass plus breakdown of the blood-brain barrier. Subtraction CAT has been extremely useful in differentiating hemorrhagic from ischemic strokes. Variations in relative blood volume can be followed serially by subtraction CAT scanning. Once the normal blood distribution is known, the subtraction scan can provide a map of pressure variations in the intracranial vault. The large arteries at the base of the brain rarely are delineated on CAT infusion scans but the CAT scan can measure extremely small changes in overall tissue density.

The subtraction CAT scan is a picture of the blood distribution in the cerebral circulation. Subtracting scans should add to the diagnostic potential of CAT and provide a noninvasive way to study vascular changes in cerebral disease.

▶ [Regional blood flow has been calculated by Ladurner et al. (J. Neurol. Neurosurg. Psychiatry 39:152, 1976) by subtracting EMI numbers before and after injection of sodium iothalmate and adjusting for concentration of contrast material in the blood. A mean value of 5.7 ml blood per 100 gm brain was found for cortex and 5.1 ml blood per 100 gm brain for the thalamus. The authors consider their current efforts to need more work before this technique can be accurate enough for clinical use.

In 17 patients with a clinical diagnosis of pseudotumor cerebri (benign intracranial hypertension), Huckman et al. (Radiology 119:593, 1976) found normal ventricles by CAT scanning. They believe more invasive radiologic procedures are unnecessary in patients with pseudotumor if the scan shows normal ventricles without space-occupying lesion, infarct or arteriovenous malformation.

Movement of the patient threatens to invalidate CAT scanning. At the University of Pennsylvania Hospital, about 7% of patients need general anesthesia for this examination. Aidinis et al. (Anesthesiology 44:420, 1976) attribute this high percentage to a large pediatric case load and adults with head injury. They describe the mutual problems of radiologist and anesthesiologist regarding space, time for induction and scanning, equipment and other factors. Anesthesia is needed for uncooperative patients and for cooperative patients with movement disorders; sedation may not suffice when the head and neck must be flexed forward, possibly interfering with respiration. Oral intubation with thiopental-N_2O-O_2-relaxant technique is usually used, with a heating unit for small children. $-$Ed.] ◄

Subependymal and Intraventricular Hemorrhage in Neonates: Early Diagnosis by Computed Tomography. Cerebral intraventricular hemorrhage is one of the principal causes of death in premature infants. Most of these hemorrhages begin as small hematomas or hemorrhagic infarctions in the subependymal germinal matrix along the lateral cerebral ventricles. Paul H. Pevsner, Rafael Garcia-Bunuel (Johns Hopkins Univ.), Norman Leeds and Mitchell Finkelstein[7] (Albert Einstein College of Medicine) found that computed tomography (CT) may accurately detect subependymal and intraventricular hemorrhages during life. A survey was made of 709 neonatal and fetal autopsies performed in 1965 – 74, with anencephalic and macerated stillborn infants excluded. Eleven consecutive infant brains were evaluated with the EMI scanner, in 6 cases with the brain preserved within the calvaria.

There were 496 neonatal and 213 fetal autopsies in the survey, representing respective autopsy rates of 91% and 98%. Subependymal or intraventricular hemorrhage, or both, was evident in 154 (22%) of the 709 brains examined, of which 143 (29%) were newborns and 11 (about 5%) were stillborns. The rate in neonates weighing 1,000 – 1,500 gm was 52%. Five of 11 stillborn fetuses with hemorrhage showed subependymal bleeding only, as did 17 of the 143 neonates with hemorrhage. Eight of the latter group had intraventricular hemorrhage only. About two thirds of infants died within 2 days of birth; the longest survival was 3 months. Computed tomography scans showed a crescent-shaped parasagittal image of increased density in cases of intraventricular hemorrhage. The subependymal locus of hemorrhage was seen as a small protrusion or discontinuity along the lateral border of the ventricular hemorrhage. The scans could be nearly exactly superimposed on photographs of the corresponding brain slices.

This study showed an extremely close correlation between CT scan images of subependymal and intraventricular hemorrhage and the gross pathologic findings. Computed tomography scanning is an accurate means of diagnosing neonatal cerebral hemorrhage. It should now be possible to examine high-risk newborn infants to detect cerebral intraventricu-

(7) Radiology 119:111 – 114, April, 1976.

lar bleeding and its precursor, subependymal hemorrhage, at an early stage of evolution.

▶ [The special aspects of computerized scans in children are discussed by Harwood-Nash and Breckbill (J. Pediatr. 89:343, 1976). The physiologic status, airway patency, warmth and hydration must be considered. Paramount, however, is the problem of motion, requiring moderately heavy sedation and much patience. To be considered are presence of sutures, large subarachnoid cisterns and increased posterior fossa volume, among other factors. Many specific disorders, such as tuberous sclerosis, hydrocephalus and others, may be diagnosed by CT scan. — Ed.] ◀

CSF Enhancement for Computerized Tomography. Glenn H. Roberson, Jan Brismar, Alfred Weiss, Kenneth R. Davis, Juan M. Taveras, Paul F. J. New, Robert H. Ackerman and William V. Glenn[8] (Harvard Med. School) performed metrizamide cisternography, combined with hypocycloidal tomography, in 12 patients with possible posterior fossa or parasellar mass lesions. Computerized tomography (CT) was performed immediately after metrizamide cisternography. After premedication with phenobarbital and lumbar puncture under fluoroscopic control were carried out, 6.75 gm metrizamide in a concentration of 250–300 mg iodine per ml was instilled and transported to the basal cisternae by tilting. Hypocycloidal tomography and then CT scanning were done.

The CT scans showed enhancement of cerebrospinal fluid (CSF) attenuation values to 160–260 Hounsfield units (80–130 old EMI units) and produced sharp definition of the CSF-brain surface interface (Fig 4). In most patients the 4th ventricle was partially or wholly filled with metrizamide-enhanced CSF and the 3d ventricle usually remained free of metrizamide. The brain stem was outlined particularly sharply.

Metrizamide CSF enhancement appears to solve many interface difficulties by yielding clear definition of CSF-brain margins. Enhanced images of the cisternae are expected to permit earlier detection of small mass lesions that arise in or adjacent to the CSF pathways. Metrizamide cisternography by the combination of hypocycloidal and computerized tomography suggests the virtual replacement of air as a contrast agent for pneumoencephalography because patient tolerance of metrizamide appears to be better than

(8) Surg. Neurol. 6:235–238, October, 1976.

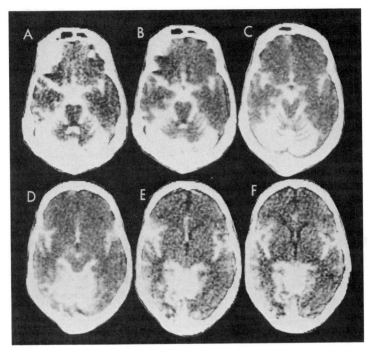

Fig 4.—Serial CT scans after cisternography, in ascending order from lowest level, *A*, to highest, *F*. In *A, B* and *C* progressively higher oblique sections of upper brain stem are visible, with sharply defined margins of brain stem. Posterolateral recesses of 4th ventricle are displayed in *A* and cerebellar folia are outlined in *B* and *C*. Supracellar cisternae are shown in *A, B* and *C*. The *D, E* and *F* levels include portions of superior vermis and show supratentorial regions as well, with 3d and lateral ventricles filled with cerebrospinal fluid. Sylvian fissures are distinctive and quadrigeminal cisterna is displayed. (Courtesy of Roberson, G. H., et al.: Surg. Neurol. 6:235–238, October, 1976.)

tolerance for air. An anticipated extension of this technique is the use of computerized body section scanning to image the spinal cord and lesions encroaching on the spinal subarachnoid space.

▶ [Drayer and Rosenbaum (Lancet 2:736, 1976) also have used metrizamide injected into the lumbar subarachnoid space for enhancement of CT scanning (over 60 cases). The normal interpeduncular and suprasellar cisterns were defined in detail. Five verified pituitary masses with suprasellar extension were mapped accurately prior to operation; in 2, the intravenously enhanced CT scan was normal. The authors believe this cisternographic technique further reduces the need for pneumoencephalography.—Ed.] ◀

Computed Coronal Tomography is described by Steven B. Hammerschlag, Samuel M. Wolpert and Barbara L. Carter[9] (Tufts-New England Med. Center Hosp., Boston). Computed tomography of the cranium with slices in the transverse axial (horizontal) plane is well established. Total body scanners, which eliminate the water-bath head-holder, allow more flexibility in positioning the patient's head and permit scans to be obtained in the coronal plane. With the Delta scanner, the gantry can be angled up to a maximum of 20 degrees to either side of the vertical plane. Coronal slices can be obtained with the patient prone with the head fully extended and the gantry angled 20 degrees forward, or with the patient supine with head fully extended and the gantry angled 20 degrees backward (Figs 5 and 6). A complete series of coronal tomograms from the supraorbital region to the occiput can be obtained with 6 scans (twelve 13-mm slices), and a full series is not always necessary. The ventricular system, including the foramen magnum region, can be covered by a series of 4 scans.

Coronal scans can be obtained directly with relative ease by this method. The segments of brain adjacent to the skull base are well demonstrated, especially the suprasellar re-

Fig 5 (left).—Patient position for coronal scanning. Patient is positioned prone with head fully extended and chin placed on head rest. *AC*, vertical position of the gantry; *BC*, position of the gantry after it has been angled forward 20 degrees. The angle of the scan is now 90 degrees to the orbitomeatal line, *OM*.

Fig 6 (right).—Patient is positioned supine with head extended fully. *AC*, vertical position of the gantry; *BC*, position of the gantry after it has been angled 20 degrees backward. The angle of the scan is now 90 degrees to the orbitomeatal line, *OM*.

(Courtesy of Hammerschlag, S. B., et al.: Radiology 120:219–220, July, 1976.)

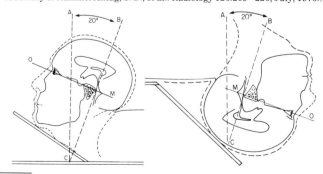

(9)   Radiology 120:219–220, July, 1976.

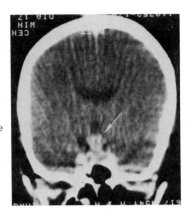

Fig 7. – Coronal scan at the level of the sella, with contrast enhancement. The floor of the sella and the sphenoid sinus are identified. A suprasellar tumor is present *(arrow)*. (Courtesy of Hammerschlag, S. B., et al.: Radiology 120:219–220, July, 1976.)

gion (Fig 7). The high convexity areas, obscured by the calvarium on transverse axial tomography, are also well seen. The falx and tentorium can be identified easily. Coronal tomography through the posterior fossa affords exceptional visualization of the foramen magnum region, including the cervicomedullary junction of the spinal cord. Computed coronal tomography may become another modality in the diagnosis of basilar invagination.

▶ [In the same journal (Radiology 120:217, 1976), Wolf et al. also show excellent computed tomography (CT) scans in conventional axial and coronal views. The relation to the ventricular and bony structures is well shown for acoustic tumor, tuberculum meningioma, vascular malformation of the corpus callosum, convexity meningioma and multiple metastases.

Even without coronal views, however, sellar and paraseller masses are well diagnosed. If the scans are negative (with contrast material), Nardich et al. (ibid., p. 91) believe angiography and pneumoencephalography are not helpful.

According to Jacobs and Kinkel (Neurology (Minneap.) 26:501, 1976), the CT scans in normal-pressure hydrocephalus may show significant cortical atrophy not revealed by pneumoencephalography. The air studies used only 50–70 ml air; however, autopsy confirmed the atrophy in some cases. There was no relationship between the presence or absence of cortical atrophy and clinical responses to ventricular shunting. Radionuclide cisternograms also were not correlated. Surprisingly, although most patients with improvement had small or normal-sized ventricles on followup, some patients with moderate improvement did not show smaller ventricles, although their shunts were working.

In a detailed article an evaluation of the posterior 3d ventricle by CT, Messina et al. (Radiology 119:581, 1976) also compare the findings with angiography, pneumography and radionuclide studies. In mass lesions, pneumography was most sensitive; for cerebral infarction, nuclide studies were most sensitive. Vascular lesions were best shown by angiography, but hematomas nearby, by CT scans. Pneumography is necessary when fine resolution is important. — Ed.] ◄

Noninvasive Angiography for Diagnosis of Carotid Artery Disease Using Doppler Ultrasound (Carotid Artery Doppler).

Screening methods to detect extracranial stenoses of cerebral vessels must fill the diagnostic gap between relatively fallible physical methods and invasive techniques. H. Keller, W. Meier, Y. Yonekawa and D. Kumpe[1] (Zurich) describe a procedure in which a bidirectional continuous-wave Doppler device gives information on disturbed carotid perfusion in the presence of moderate or greater stenosis. The device is placed manually over the supratrochlear, supraorbital and common carotid arteries of the prone patient, and the velocity signals are monitored by stereo earphones and on a three-channel recorder. Recordings are made from the supraorbital artery with and without compression of the superficial temporal artery, and supratrochlear artery recordings are made with compression of the common carotid arteries.

Of 800 patients having Doppler studies for symptoms of cerebrovascular failure, 186 underwent carotid angiography, 128 on the clinically relevant side and 58 on both sides. Five patients had repeat studies after the extracranial endarterectomy for suspected rethrombosis. Doppler studies detected 138 pathologic flow states in 123 patients. The corresponding angiograms showed 110 obstructions, 11 processes distal from the ophthalmic artery and 17 normal morphological situations. The most powerful criterion was reverse flow in the supratrochlear artery, followed by low diastolic common carotid flow, pathologic flow change in the supratrochlear arteries on common carotid compression, and a time delay in the rising phase of the systolic pulse wave of over 30 msec. Correspondence with angiography was noted in 82–87% of cases. Postoperative Doppler studies showed the short- and long-term hemodynamic effects of the surgery.

Carotid artery Doppler recording is a noninvasive, rapid examination method permitting the detection of hemody-

(1) Stroke 7:354–363, July–Aug., 1976.

namically significant obstructions in the carotid artery, with about 90% reliability. If used routinely, disorders in many potential stroke patients could be diagnosed before a stroke or even transient ischemic attacks occurred.

Anterior Inferior Cerebellar Artery in Mass Lesions: Preliminary Findings with Emphasis on Lateral Projection are presented by Thomas P. Naidich, Irvin I. Kricheff, Ajax E. George and Joseph P. Lin[2] (New York Univ.). The main trunk of the anterior inferior cerebellar artery (AICA) and the proximal parts of the rostrolateral, ascending, descending and caudomedial arteries define the brain stem and the petrosal aspect of the cerebellar hemispheres. The distal portions of these arteries define the occipital surface of the cerebellum. Abnormalities of the configuration of the AICA in the lateral projection may be identified on high-quality magnification-subtraction radiographs. They may be useful in the diagnosis of cerebellar hemispheric, intra-4th ventricular, and extra-axial posterior fossa masses.

Among extra-axial masses, a clival mass that displaces the pons posterosuperiorly results in traction on the fixed meatal loops and eventually in reversal of the curve of the main trunk of the AICA. Cerebellopontomedullary angle masses may cause striking arcuate displacements of the main AICA and its rostrolateral branch in the the lateral projection. Some angle masses reverse the normal posterosuperiorly convex curve of the ascending segment of the meatal loop. The infratentorial portion of a trigeminal neurinoma bows the AICA posteroinferiorly over a variable length of its course. Tentorial meningiomas produce a somewhat diffuse mass effect on the AICA, with generally inferior displacement.

Among the intra-axial masses, cerebellar peduncular and superior hemispheric masses cause anteroinferolateral displacement and elongation of the brachial segment. Inferior hemispheric and intra-4th ventricular masses may cause stretching and anteroinferior bowing of the biventral segments of the descending and caudomedial arteries. The lateral loop of the caudomedial artery is a useful indicator of mass effect at the anteroinferomedial aspect of the hemi-

(2) Radiology 119:375–383, April, 1976.

LATERAL
PROJECTION

STRAIGHT ANTEROPOSTERIOR
PROJECTION (RIGHT SIDE)

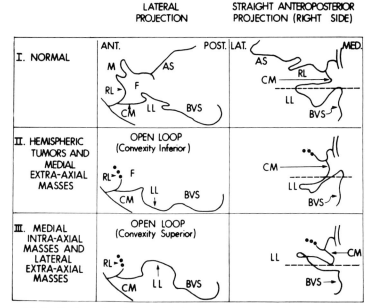

Fig 8. — Configuration of normal and abnormal lateral loops in lateral and straight anteroposterior projections. In Towne's projection this loop is normally partially closed. Note normal posteroinferior inclination of lateral loop in lateral projection. *BVS,* biventral segment; *CM,* caudomedial artery; *F,* floccular loop; *LL,* lateral loop; *M,* M segment; *RL,* rostrolateral loop. (Courtesy of Naidich, T. P., et al.: *Radiology* 119:375 – 383, April, 1976.)

sphere (Fig 8). In some cases a large medial extra-axial mass may also open the lateral loop with convexity downward by posteroinferior displacement of the caudal point and the entire proximal part of the loop.

▶ [The basis for the comparisons with normal findings appears in the same journal (*Radiology* 119:355, 1976). The authors dissected 32 inoculated human cerebella and integrated their findings with radiographs. The anterior inferior cerebellar artery bifurcates near the 6th nerve into the rostrolateral and caudomedial arteries. These define the position of the pontomedullary sulcus, supraolivary fossette, 5th to 11th cranial nerves, brachium pontis, flocculus, great horizontal fissure, posterolateral fissure, superior and inferior semilunar lobules, biventral lobule, foramen of Luschka and the choroid plexus of the lateral recess of the 4th ventricle. Magnification and high-quality subtraction are needed for identification of these landmarks.

Severe displacement of midline structures in angiograms may produce unusual thalamostriate and internal cerebral vein configurations, as shown by Winestock (J. Can. Assoc. Radiol. 26:235, 1975). When the vessels ipsilateral to a mass are seen in anteroposterior angiograms, the veins assume a configuration of infinity (ω) when the angiogram is done for masses contralateral to the side of the angiogram, the configuration is like "w." — Ed.] ◄

Arteriography of the Anterior Communicating Aneurysm. The anterior communicating aneurysm remains the most difficult intracranial aneurysm to delineate by routine angiography. It seldom is seen clearly in routine projections and only occasionally is well visualized on oblique or basal views. A. Kamisasa[3] (Saitama Med. School, Moro, Japan) proposes supplemental radiographic projections for evaluating this aneurysm. Studies were done with an adult skull and an iron ball simulating an anterior communicating saccular aneurysm. Good visualization of the iron ball was obtained in the anteroposterior (AP) oblique half-axial projection with a +30-degree central ray and a +20- to +30-degree skull rotation, the central point being 5 cm above the midsupraorbital ridge (Fig 9). A reverse oblique half-axial projection with a −20- to −30-degree rotation also proved effective. Good visualization was obtained in the orbital projection with a +30- to +40-degree rotation and with a −10-, 0- and +10-degree central ray. The reverse oblique orbital projection with −30- or −40-degree rotation and 0- or −10-degree central ray also proved effective. In the axial projection, visualization was better with an angulation of 90 degrees from the anthropologic baseline rather than from the orbitomeatal baseline.

These projections were used in 30 patients in whom the anterior communicating aneurysm was not well visualized on conventional AP and lateral views. Percutaneous carotid angiography was performed with 60% Conray or 65% Angiografin. The oblique half-axial and reverse oblique half-axial AP projections proved useful in patients with an aneurysm pointing either upward or downward. The oblique orbital and reverse oblique orbital AP projections proved valuable when the aneurysm pointed either upward or downward and the reverse projection was useful for an aneurysm projected to the side opposite the injection. They are especially valuable in showing the frequent anomaly of the circle of Willis.

---

(3) Neuroradiology 12:227–232, 1977.

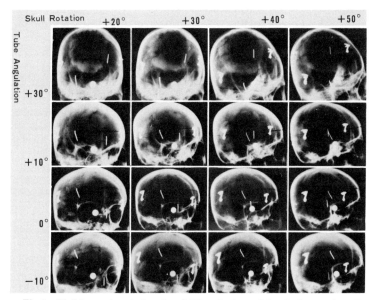

Fig 9.—Model experiment. A series of AP projections of the skull rotated at 10-degree intervals from +20 degrees to +50 degrees. The top line shows oblique half-axial projection with central ray angulation of +30 degrees. The second, third and fourth lines are oblique orbital projections. Note the better visualization of the iron ball in films with −10-degree, 0-degree angulation and +30-degree, +40-degree skull rotation. (Courtesy of Kamisasa, A.: Neuroradiology 12:227–232, 1977.)

The axial projection demonstrated the AP dimension and configuration of the aneurysm either arising at a right angle from the A1–A2 junction or the anterior communicating artery, with or without lateral deviation of the neck.

These projections are useful adjuncts to conventional projections in the study of anterior communicating artery aneurysms.

► [The angiograms were done by percutaneous carotid injection, a technique much decried by many neuroradiologists. Neurosurgeons may point out to their colleagues that Bergström and Jorulf (Acta Radiol. [Diagn.] (Stockh.) 17:577, 1976) contend that the femoral artery is much more susceptible to puncture spasm than the common carotid artery. For unilateral carotid angiography in infants, they prefer transcarotid catheterization to the transfemoral approach. — Ed.] ◄

Radioisotope Choroid Plexography: Preliminary Report is presented by R. Oberson and F. Azam[4] (Univ. of

Lausanne). Choroid plexus uptake of ^{99m}Tc has been considered a handicap in interpreting pertechnetate brain scans, but it may be of interest to enhance rather than to suppress the choroid plexus in vivo. It could become possible in this way to study physiologically and dynamically the structures commonly thought to be the main sources of ventricular fluid. A dose of unlabeled Solcocitran, containing 17 mg stannous citrate, is given 24 hours before the intravenous injection of 15 mCi ^{99m}Tc-pertechnetate; no perchlorate or sodium iodide solution is given. Plexography is done immediately and 1 and 3 hours after ^{99m}Tc-pertechnetate injection. Scintiphotographs are obtained in the frontal and lateral projections.

The choroid plexus of the lateral ventricles was demonstrated in 15 patients; in 10 others, the uptake was not as great because either iodine solution was given or the 24-hour interval between Solcocitran and ^{99m}Tc-pertechnetate administration was shortened. The interval may be shortened but should not be less than 3 hours. Subtraction technique may help eliminate the radioactivity of the sagittal sinus, which masks the choroid plexus of the 3d ventricle on the posterior frontal view. The plexus of the 4th ventricle is easily recognized deep in the posterior fossa.

Plexography may help detect an expanding lesion that deforms the homolateral ventricle and its plexus, especially in the region of the temporal horn and trigonum. It also may help show an active papilloma of the plexus and may differentiate tumors in the thalamic region. Blood pool activity can be responsible for visualization of the choroid plexus. Besides its morphological value, the test could give interesting clues in the dynamic study of hydrocephalus.

Value of Routine Cerebral Radionuclide Angiography in Pediatric Brain Imaging. Philip O. Alderson, David L. Gilday, Michael Mikhael and Arnold L. Wilkie[5] performed cerebral radionuclide angiography (CRAG) as a routine part of nuclide brain imaging in a prospective evaluation of 1,051 children at two institutions. Doses of pertechnetate of about 215 μCi ^{99m}Tc per kg were used, with oral pretreatment with perchlorate, 10 mg/kg. The minimal nuclide dose for neonates was 2 mCi. A saline-flush injection technique was

(5) J. Nucl. Med. 17:780–785, September, 1976.

used to ensure a compact bolus. Sequential 1-second images of the cranial transit of the bolus were followed by a 400,000-count blood pool image, and four-view static images were obtained immediately or an hour after nuclide injection and sometimes at 2–4 hours as well.

Abnormal nuclide images were obtained in 293 (28%) of the children studied. The CRAG was essential to the diagnosis in 60 children (5.7%), increasing the number of confirmed positive studies by 20%. The CRAG was more often "essential" in patients with a high probability of neurologic disease, in whom it increased the rate of confirmed positive studies by 21%. Displacement of convexity activity in the middle cerebral arterial territory provided the only definite evidence of a subdural collection in 22 children, 11 of whom had normal static images. The CRAG did not detect hydrocephalus well. It revealed nine moderately large intracranial cysts, but a small cyst was not detected and one false-positive study was obtained. The CRAG provided additional information in 16 of 244 children who presented with focal neurologic signs. The CRAG was also helpful in the 37 children who had abnormal cranial transillumination. The yield of the CRAG in 592 children with low-probability presentations was only 1.9%, but this still represented an 18% increase in the number of positive studies.

For maximum diagnostic yield, a CRAG should be performed with all pediatric brain-imaging studies. Where camera or technologist time is limited and selective use of the CRAG is warranted, it should be restricted to children with a high *a priori* probability of having detectable neurologic disease.

▶ [Raskin et al. (J. Neurol. Neurosurg. Psychiatry 39:424, 1976) found prominent paracentral lucent zones in the dynamic scintigrams of patients with hydrocephalus along with lateral displacement of the proximal middle cerebral vessels. These changes are obvious in cerebral angiograms, and I thought they were well known to all who use the radionuclide angiographic technique. – Ed.] ◀

Lumbar Epidural Venography in Diagnosis of Disk Herniations is discussed by Raziel Gershater (North York Genl. Hosp., Willowdale, Ont.) and Richard C. Holgate[6] (Univ. of Toronto). In patients with strong clinical evidence of lumbar disk herniation and "negative" myelograms, the

(6) Am. J. Roentgenol. 126:992–1002, May, 1976.

nerve root presumably is compressed after it leaves the sub-arachnoid space. Epidural venography is a means of clarifying problematic lumbar disk herniations.

Lateral intervertebral branches connect the anterior internal vertebral veins to the paravertebral channels above and below each pedicle, and cross-connections exist between the anterior internal vertebral veins as they course between the pedicles (Fig 10). The posterior elements are drained by a smaller chain of longitudinal veins, the posterior internal vertebral veins. The ascending lumbar veins may be rudimentary. The epidural venous plexus is opacified by transfemoral injection of contrast medium into the ascending lumbar or internal iliac veins. A No. 5 F endhole catheter and a straight 0.038-in. guide wire are used, with 30–40 cc of Renografin 76 or 60. Frontal views contain most of the diagnostic information but lateral films sometimes can be helpful. All the epidural veins proximal and distal to an unfilled vein must be well opacified.

Only one minor complication occurred in 227 patients. The most important signs of lumbar disk herniation are abnormal curvature of an anterior internal vertebral vein, which is usually bowed laterally on the anteroposterior venogram, and unilateral or bilateral occlusion of the ante-

Fig 10.—Diagrammatic (A) and angiographic (B) demonstration of epidural venus plexus. The inserts in A show common variations. Ascending lumbar vein, *alv;* anterior internal vertebral vein, *aiv;* suprapedicular vein, *spv;* infrapedicular vein, *ipv.* (Courtesy of Gershater, R., and Holgate, R. C.: Am. J. Roentgenol. 126:992–1002, May, 1976.)

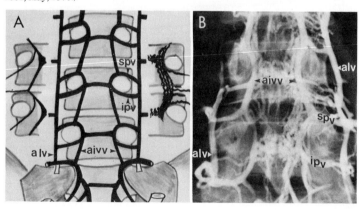

rior internal vertebral vein as it crosses the disk interspace. Suprapedicular vein occlusion is a frequent secondary feature. Supplementary findings include localized dilatation of epidural and extravertebral veins and opening of collateral channels around obstructed veins.

The usefulness of epidural venography is well established in patients with a good clinical picture of herniated disk and nondiagnostic myelographic findings. Patients tolerate the procedure well. Venography is useful in diagnosing extreme lateral disk herniations. Myelography was not necessary in two thirds of the 227 patients examined. Most studies were done on an outpatient basis. Eight venograms were inadequate and 152 were positive for disk herniation. Five extradural and two intradural neoplasms were found. There has been 1 false finding among 130 surgically explored patients.

▶ [Following the original of this article is one by Miller et al. based on 107 patients with normal or nondiagnostic myelograms (Am. J. Roentgenol. 126:1003, 1976). They report 92% correct preoperative diagnosis with herniated disk and 50% with nerve root compression without herniation. Confusing findings include flow defects, extravertebral veins and occlusion of radicular veins by the catheter. These authors believe venography is valuable when myelography has not been diagnostic of herniated disk.

An article by Drasin et al. (ibid., p. 1016) presents 5 illustrative cases. The authors have not always been able to catheterize the ascending lumbar veins, but the epidural plexus has always been seen after small sacral branches of the hypogastric veins have been catheterized. Accuracy has been 88.2% in detection of lesions proved by surgery. Included are cases of herniated disk, obstruction of medially buckled and hypertrophied joint facet and intradural and extradural fibroma at L5.

Comparisons of venography with Dimer-X myelography have been made by Roland et al. (J. Radiol. Electrol. Med. Nucl. 57:175, 1976). They advise diazepam-pentazocine sedation with transfemoral catheterization (usually on the left) of the ascending lumbar vein. The contralateral vein may need to be shown in some cases, and sacral catheterization is often needed to show veins at the L5–S1 space. Lateral views rarely are needed. In all 40 patients, venography was done after water-soluble contrast myelography. Some cases had normal tests by both techniques and some had abnormal findings by both; 3 patients had normal myelography but had defects due to disks in venograms. Two failures of venography were encountered—one due to duplication of the inferior vena cava and one due to inability to catheterize either ascending lumbar vein. One of 40 patients developed phlebitis a week after catheterization. The authors believe venography to be indicated when myelography fails to reveal the cause of clinical disorder, and the former is especially faithful if the dural sac is enlarged.

Sackett et al. (Surg. Neurol. 7:35, 1977) contend epidural venography will not replace myelography in evaluation of lumbar disk disease, because there are too many suboptimal studies, especially in patients operated on previously. Midline disk herniations were missed more often than the lateral herniations. Venography is most valuable, they say, when a patient has clinical evidence of nerve root compression in the face of a normal myelogram.

Kistler and Pribram (ibid. 5:287, 1976) use transfemoral epidural venography as a complement to, not a competitor of, myelography. The latter is used primarily to disclose a spinal tumor masquerading as a herniated disk, they say. Experience in 87 cases suggests epidural venography is superior at L5–S1 and at least as good as Pantopaque myelography at other lumbar levels. It is especially useful when oil study is normal but the clinical consideration is protruded disk. – Ed.] ◄

Nerve Rootlet Avulsion as a Complication of Myelography with the Cuatico Needle. The Cuatico needle has facilitated greatly the often tedious and occasionally painful withdrawal of Pantopaque at the end of myelography. Thomas F. Kennedy and John R. Steinfeld[7] (Meml. Mission Hosp., Asheville, N.C.) report a case of nerve rootlet avulsion occurring during use of the Cuatico needle.

Patient L. M. had myelography for the evaluation of neck pain. A midline lumbar puncture was done at the L3–L4 interspace, under fluoroscopic control with the patient prone. An 18-gauge Cuatico needle was used. A dose of 12 ml Pantopaque was introduced; most was removed easily by gentle aspiration. With about 2 ml Pantopaque remaining, flow ceased and the patient noted pain in the left gluteal area. The aspiration cannula then was introduced and a few more drops were aspirated before pain was reported in the left hip and coccygeal region. The assembly was advanced gently and rotated one-half turn but the radicular discomfort persisted and no contrast material could be aspirated. About 1 ml Pantopaque was left behind. The assembly was withdrawn, causing severe radicular discomfort. A 7-cm fibrous strand, a nerve rootlet, was wedged at the midportion of the assembly between the sleeve of the puncture needle and the inner aspiration cannula. The pain subsided immediately and there were no neurologic sequelae.

This is the first report of this complication involving the Cuatico needle. Presumably the rootlet became wedged when the assembly was advanced; withdrawal of the assembly resulted in shearing of the filament on either side of the point of fixation of the needle. Over 450 myelographic studies have been done during the past year using this needle and technique. This case presents a possible hazard of myelography, even when what is commonly considered to be the least traumatic of available needle designs is used.

► ↓ Dimer-X has often been used for myelography with relatively few side effects. This was true in the 6 patients described by Dullerud and Mørland (Radiology 119:153, 1976), but each of 15 patients who received Depo-Medrol in addition to Dimer-X exhibited adhesive arachnoiditis. The authors believe that it has not been shown that Depo-Medrol combined with *any* contrast material slows or prevents adhesions. They would not add steroids to Metrizamide, a new material, until it can be shown that the combination does not produce adhesions.

On the other hand, Perrigot et al. (Nouv. Presse Med. 5:1120, 1976) describe 4 cases of cauda equina syndrome after myelography with Dimer-X. No effective therapy has been found.

Bagchi (Surg. Neurol. 5:285, 1976) remarks on the use of meglumine iothalamate 280 (Conray-280) for myelography despite the manufacturer's caution not to use this material for this purpose. His patient had convulsions and subarachnoid hemorrhage and died (without postmortem study). The injection was made with the patient sitting — but the radiography was done with the patient prone, which is contraindicated for Conray and for Dimer-X, both of which are epileptogenic and can cause spinal cord "seizures" as well. The obvious point is that the patient should be in a foot-down position if circumstances dictate use of these materials. Metrizamide should be a preferable material for myelography — when and if it is released for general use in the United States. — Ed.] ◄

► ↓ Iophendylate is also not always innocuous, as is reported in the following article. — Ed. ◄

Reactions to Iophendylate in Relation to Multiple Sclerosis. Peter Kaufmann (Bristol Royal Infirm.) and W. D. Jeans[8] (Univ. of Bristol), after observing a severe reaction to iophendylate myelography, reviewed the data on a consecutive group of 26 male and 31 female patients, aged 20–79, who had myelography. The review was done to determine whether reactions might be related to underlying diseases. Studies were done with 5–6 ml iophendylate, which usually was left in place. Each patient had had 5–6 ml iophendylate injected into the lumbar subarachnoid space. Nine patients had clinically definite, 2 had early probable and 6 had latent multiple sclerosis (MS). Fourteen patients had multiple spondylosis or disk prolapse and 5 had noncompressive spastic paraplegia; 2 each had syringomyelia and cord tumors. The others had a wide variety of disorders.

Moderate and severe reactions occurred in 7 patients (12%), 5 of whom had MS; the number of reactions in the

(8) Lancet 2:1000–1001, Nov. 6, 1976.

group with MS was significantly increased. The most severe reaction was in a man aged 55 with spastic paraparesis and some obstruction to flow at myelography. Fever and obtundation developed after examination and meningism was present, with increased lower-limb spasticity. Reactive meningoencephalitis was diagnosed and hydrocortisone was given as contrast material was aspirated. The reaction resolved 8 days after myelography, although the EEG showed some generalized dysrhythmia with paroxysms of theta activity at this time. The EEG was normal 7 months later, when the patient's clinical state was unchanged. The underlying diagnosis for this patient is uncertain.

Reactions associated with myelography may be related to lumbar puncture, to the contrast medium and syringe, or to the contrast medium itself. The finding of an increased incidence of more severe reactions in patients with MS may suggest that myelography should not be done if this diagnosis is suspected. Potentially treatable conditions affecting the cord still must be excluded, however, and there is no evidence in current cases that the course of the disease has been adversely affected.

► ↓ The obvious answer to these problems is to use gas for myelography, as noted in the following article. To be sure, tomography is really essential for best results. — Ed. ◄

Diagnosis of Thoracic and Lumbar Disk Disease by Gas Myelography. Senichiro Komaki and Ritsuko Komaki[9] (Med. College of Wisconsin) obtained gas myelograms on 344 occasions over 2 years. Disk disease was found in 39 patients, 22 of whom had diskectomy and 2, laminectomy. Gas myelography is combined with tomography; tomograms are taken at 2.5-mm intervals. The amount of oxygen injected should exceed the amount of cerebrospinal fluid removed (about 10 ml). Tomograms are obtained in a lateral projection through the entire spinal canal, with the use of hypocycloidal movement. The subarachnoid space is demonstrated in over 95% of studies. When lumbar problems are suspected, tomograms of the lumbar spinal canal and of the low thoracic spinal canal, including the conus medullaris, are obtained. If a high-level lesion is suspected, the entire thoracic level is visualized.

---

(9) Wis. Med. J. 75:S 29–32, April, 1976.

Gas myelograms showed herniated disks in all 22 patients having diskectomy, 8 of whom had multiple disk protrusions. Five patients also had Pantopaque myelography within a short period, and in 2 cases there was extremely good correlation between the two studies. Pantopaque studies gave negative results in the other 3 cases in which disk lesions were present at the thoracic level. The 2 patients with positive results of Pantopaque studies had lesions at the lumbar level.

Gas myelography is indicated for studies at the cervical and thoracic levels. Lumbar disk disease also can be diagnosed by gas myelography easily and accurately if part of the disk is centrally located, but a sophisticated tomographic unit is needed. When the unit is available, gas myelography is recommended, especially in cases where thoracic disk disease is suspected.

► [A cisternal approach for avoidance of anomalies in suspected spinal dysraphism has been used by Cook (Br. J. Radiol. 49:502, 1976). A mixture of air and oxygen permits a number of films to be taken without excessively rapid disappearance of oxygen, and yet avoids much of the discomfort when air alone is used. The excellent correlation between the myelographic findings and the findings at operation leads Cook to propose this technique for preoperative assessment of patients suspected of having occult spinal dysraphism.

On the other hand, Elwyn and colleagues (see article earlier in this chapter) use nitrous oxide for encephalography. — Ed.] ◄

Simple Myelographic Maneuver for Detection of Mass Lesions at the Foramen Magnum. The diagnosis of lesions in the region of the foramen magnum often is delayed because of both confusing clinical manifestations and technical radiographic difficulties. M. Theodore Margolis[1] (Seattle) describes a simple maneuver added to routine prone myelography that can demonstrate these lesions more easily than the supine technique usually considered necessary. Forty patients aged 19–77 who were suspected of having a demyelinating process or a mass lesion involving the high cervical cord had positive contrast myelography with Pantopaque. The procedure is illustrated in Figures 11–14. With the table tilted to a 5- to 10-degree head-up position and the neck slightly hyperextended, the head is maneuvered into a lateral position with the occiput slightly dependent and the table is tilted head down about 10 degrees or in

---

(1) Radiology 119:482–485, May, 1976.

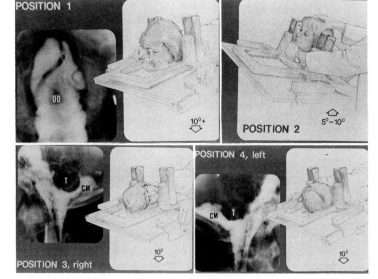

Fig 11 (top left). – Normal anteroposterior 90-mm spot film with the neck hyperextended and the table tilted downward. Contrast medium flows readily onto the clivus, outlining the basilar artery *(B)* and odontoid *(OD)*.

Fig 12 (top right). – Table is reversed into a slightly head-up position and, with the neck still hyperextended, the head is turned into either lateral position, as in following figure.

Fig 13 (bottom left). – Head is turned slightly past the true lateral position with the nose upward and the occiput slightly dependent. In this position, with the table tilted 5–10 degrees head-down, contrast medium readily fills the normal cisterna magna *(CM)*, outlining the dependent cerebellar tonsil *(T)*.

Fig 14 (bottom right). – Head is turned to the opposite lateral position. The occiput is slightly down and contrast medium fills the dependent portion of the cisterna magna *(CM)*, outlining the tonsil *(T)*. The transition from position 3 to position 4 should pass through position 2 to avoid flowing contrast medium into the middle cranial fossa.

(Courtesy of Margolis, M. T.: Radiology 119:482–485, May, 1976.)

some instances less, for contrast to flow into the cisterna magna. The opposite side of the cisterna magna is then filled to visualize the dependent tonsil.

Abnormalities in the vicinity of the foramen magnum were found in 10 of the 40 patients examined. Eight had low-lying tonsils compatible with a Chiari malformation; 3 of these had associated radiographic evidence of a syrinx. One patient had a meningioma at the C1–C2 level and 1 had what seemed to be a low biventral lobule or tonsil at the level of the foramen magnum on one side, but could not be studied further. The other patients had normal myelograms and were thought to have demyelinating or degenerative disorders. Vertebral angiography showed low-lying tonsils in all 6 patients thought to have a Chiari I malformation who were examined; these were subsequently confirmed operatively.

This method is reliable in detecting mass lesions in the foramen magnum region and cervicomedullary junction. Even minimal tonsillar herniation has been easily demonstrated and it seems unlikely that any lesion large enough to cause symptoms would escape detection. Routine supine studies may no longer be necessary for the evaluation of suspected foramen magnum lesions.

Computed Tomography of the Spinal Canal. Steven B. Hammerschlag, Samuel M. Wolpert and Barbara L. Carter[2] (Tufts-New England Med. Center Hosp., Boston) reviewed early experience with computed tomography (CT) of the spinal column. Scans were made with the Delta Scanner that obtains 8- or 13-mm slices in a scan time of $2\frac{1}{2}$ minutes. The 13-mm collimator was used for spinal studies. The x-ray generator is operated at 130 kv and 30 mA. The image is displayed on a 256×256 matrix. Examinations are greatly facilitated by use of the magnification mode. The area scanned is delineated by use of radiopaque catheter-markers applied to adhesive tape.

Computed tomography scanning is useful in spinal dysraphism. Roots of the cauda equina extending into a meningocele are demonstrated. It is expected that CT of the spine will become the chief modality in the diagnosis of spinal stenosis. The usefulness of CT in assessing the size of the spinal canal was evident in a case of metatrophic dwarfism. The irregularly expanded spinal canal produced by tumor may be demonstrated by CT. The value of CT scanning in the study of bone texture abnormalities is uncertain.

Computed tomography of the spinal canal is of considerable help in evaluating such lesions as spinal dysraphism, abdominal masses of a neurologic nature and spinal stenosis. It may justifiably be considered to be as valuable as CT scanning of the head. The success of DiChiro in the identifi-

(2) Radiology 121:361–367, November, 1976.

cation of syringomyelia has not been duplicated but the spinal cord might be visualized routinely with higher-kilovoltage techniques. Instillation of a water soluble contrast medium to demonstrate the subarachnoid space may also be helpful.

Cervical Analgesic Diskography: New Test for the Definitive Diagnosis of the Painful Disk Syndrome. A cervical disk can be a source of chronic pain without protrusion, nerve root compression or neurologic deficit. The discogenic syndrome is the most common cause of neck, shoulder and arm pain. David A. Roth[3] (Harvard Med. School) developed a new test, the analgesic diskogram, which locates the painful disk with great accuracy. Diskography was performed in 71 consecutive patients who had a clinical diagnosis of medically intractable cervical discogenic syndrome in 1973–74 and had operations. They had anterior cervical disk excisions and interbody dowel fusions aided by magnification and fiberoptic illumination. Diskography was done after recovery from all other tests only if the usual symptoms were present. A no. 22 spinal needle was inserted into the nuclear center of the disk thought to be producing the pain, with no sedation and under fluoroscopic image-amplification, and 1 ml of 2% local anesthetic was injected and the patient placed upright. If previous studies were not informative, the lower 3 cervical disks were studied sequentially.

Virtually immediate and complete relief of pain and paresthesias and a return of full neck mobility followed injection into a pain-producing disk. Seventy-one patients had positive results and only 21 of them had had diagnostic findings at previous contrast diskography. Only patients having positive analgesic diskograms had operations. Surgical recovery was excellent in 43 cases, good in 23, fair in 1 and poor in 4. Recovery was not related to the degree of degenerative disk disease or the myelographic appearances. Some of the most gratifying results were obtained in patients with normal myelograms and cervical spine roentgenograms, who had gone undiagnosed and suffered seemingly inexplicable pain for long periods.

Analgesic diskography leads to useful recovery nearly three times as often as with the use of plain roentgenograms

(3) J.A.M.A. 235:1713–1714, Apr. 19, 1976.

and myelograms. It also results in a substantial increase in good or excellent recoveries over those obtained with contrast-saline diskography.

► [We have found it convenient often to combine positive contrast diskography with analgesic diskography. We believe it important to use a 25- or 26-gauge needle in the disk center (passing through a 21-gauge shorter spinal needle to go through the soft tissues). Injection of iodinated contrast material usually reproduces the pain in the affected disk; anesthetic material (lidocaine) then makes this pain go away. — Ed.] ◄

Techniques

▶ Although the editors of *Advances and Technical Standards in Neuro-surgery* state that English is on the way to becoming the international medium of European scientific conferences (preface, Vol. 3 [New York: Springer-Verlag, New York, Inc., 1976]), this has not spread to scientific articles, and hence the large segment of American neurosurgeons who write in English often neglect the articles not written in English. Statements abound concerning "Search of the English-language literature reveals. . . ." Hence, one of the many values of the series of small monographs edited by Krayenbühl et al. is the collection of articles on recent advances written by prominent European neurosurgeons and appearing in English. This volume contains an article on surgical problems of pituitary adenomas by Guiot and Derome, one on management of aneurysms by Troupp and one on extracranial intracranial arterial anastomosis by Yonekawa and Yasargil.

The second half of the volume is devoted to details of techniques of operative procedures. Luyendijk details operative approaches to the posterior fossa. Brihaye writes of the approaches to orbital tumors, with special reference to those used by neurosurgeons (temporal and transcranial routes). Methods of percutaneous spinothalamic tract section are described by Lorenz. I would have appreciated more operative detail in this portion, perhaps with radiographs or drawings of the landmarks for lateral, ventral and posterior approaches.

Nevertheless, these articles have intrinsic value in helping the neurosurgical technician, as well as introducing him to some of the leading neurosurgeons of Europe. The series has merit and, with a cumulative index after 5 or 10 volumes, will constitute an ongoing manual of neurosurgery which can show new advances from time to time and thus act in place of a long-awaited loose-leaf multivolumed neurosurgical encyclopedia. — Ed. ◀

Lateral Microsurgical Approach to Intraorbital Tumors. Joseph C. Maroon and John S. Kennerdell[4] (Univ. of Pittsburgh) describe a combined neurosurgical-ophthalmologic preoperative evaluation of orbital tumors and a microsurgical lateral orbital approach to the tumors. Patients are seen jointly by an ophthalmologist and a neurosurgeon and have polytomography and skull film study with special views of the optic canal and orbit. A brain scan may be included as well as carotid angiography and orbital ve-

---

(4) J. Neurosurg. 44:556–561, May, 1976.

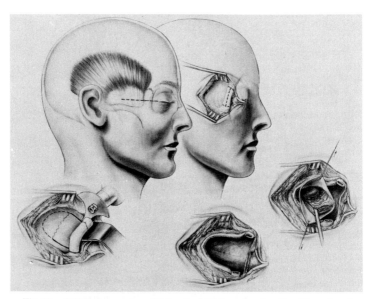

Fig 15. — Artist's impression of lateral orbitotomy showing the skin and periosteal incision, the saw cut through the lateral orbit, the bone removed and the lateral rectus muscle retracted to expose an orbital tumor. (Courtesy of Maroon, J. C., and Kennerdell, J. S.: J. Neurosurg. 44:556–561, May, 1976.)

nography, if indicated. Currently computerized axial tomography (CAT scanning) is used routinely before any contrast studies. The lateral orbitotomy is illustrated in Figure 15. General anesthesia is administered. The operating microscope is used in incising the periorbital fascia and retracting the lateral rectus muscle. Microdissection is carried out through the orbital fat with use of saline irrigation to prevent charring when small vessels are coagulated. Exposure of tumors is facilitated by dissection and retraction on small cottonoid strips. Complete hemostasis must be obtained after tumor removal. A firm pressure dressing is used for 24 hours, and a less bulky but firm dressing is then reapplied. Sutures are removed in 5–7 days.

Seven patients with solitary intraorbital tumors have had this operation. Five hemangiomas, one neurofibroma and one epidermoid cyst were treated. No patient had intracranial tumor extension. All patients had positive ultrasonograms, and all three CAT scans gave a correct diagnosis.

Complications included one postoperative orbital hematoma and slow resolution of lateral rectus palsy over 3–18 weeks. Conjunctival and lid edema is routine. In only 1 patient was visual acuity affected. The cosmetic results were quite satisfactory in all cases.

A team approach is recommended for the management of patients with intraorbital tumors. If there is a serious question concerning the medial aspect of the tumor, a transcranial approach should be used. Circumscribed tumors superior, lateral or inferior to the optic nerve can be safely and completely removed through a 30 to 35-mm lateral skin incision, with use of microsurgical dissecting techniques.

► [Pia (Acta Neurochir. (Wien) 35:243, 1976) advises sterilization of the operating microscope (not the stand!) and its attachments, including still and cine cameras, in a specially developed 52×58×42-cm container. It is airtight, and into it is placed 10 gm formaldehyde. After 10 hours, the materials are sterile (deliberate inoculation with pathogenic bacteria was carried out, and no organisms found at the end of that period). The formaldehyde exposure, unlike previously used sterilization with ethylene gas, did not affect the lens coatings or optic apparatus adversely.

However, Bernouilli et al. (Lancet 1:478, 1977) report that exposure of silver macroelectrodes to 70% alcohol and formaldehyde failed to prevent transmission of Creutzfeldt-Jakob (C-J) virus from a woman, aged 61, with C-J disease to 2 younger patients, aged 23 and 17, respectively, in whom the same electrodes (after presumed sterilization) were used for study prior to temporal lobectomy for epilepsy. Only later was it found that exposure to formaldehyde (which prevents bacterial infection transmission) does not inactivate C-J virus or scrapie. The electrodes in question were heat sensitive and hence chemical sterilization was used. The source of the infection was proved by biopsy and autopsy to be C-J disease.—Ed.]

Monitoring of Visual Function during Parasellar Surgery. Damage to the visual system is a major concern during surgery in the area of the optic chiasm. W. B. Wilson, W. M. Kirsch, H. Neville, J. Stears, M. Feinsod and Ralph A. W. Lehman[5] attempted to determine if the visual evoked response is sensitive and dynamic enough to detect premorbid changes in visual function. Studies were done in 4 patients having parasellar surgery. The visual evoked response to flashes of light from light-emitting diodes was recorded. The diodes were embedded in a plastic shell that was inserted under the eyelids of each eye. A record was obtained by averaging 100 3-per-second flashes, and the patterns were photographed for a permanent record.

---

(5) Surg. Neurol. 5:323–329, June, 1976.

The procedure was found to be a practical and simple one. The surgical routine was not altered significantly. The responses became disorganized and of extremely low amplitude with manipulation of the optic chiasm and returned to baseline levels soon after manipulation was stopped, usually in 2–3 minutes. Inconsistent relationships were noted between the response pattern present at the end of surgery and changes in vision after the operation.

Further study should show whether an improved visual evoked response pattern during surgery will correlate with improved visual function afterward, whether a stable pattern will correlate with comparable preoperative and postoperative vision or whether a prolonged abnormal pattern during surgery will correlate with decreased visual function postoperatively.

Lateral Sitting Position for Neurosurgery has been used satisfactorily for operations in the posterior fossa and upper spine for 20 years. Francisco Garcia-Bengochea, Edwin S. Munson and James V. Freeman[6] (Univ. of Florida) describe the technique for the anesthesiologist as it presently is carried out.

TECHNIQUE. — The patient is placed supine on the operating table for induction of anesthesia and tracheal intubation. The skull clamp is fixed to the patient's head and the operating table is maximally "flexed" while the seat is kept almost horizontal. The back section is elevated further to about 80 degrees from the horizontal and, while the patient's head is held, the patient is rotated to be perpendicularly oriented to the long axis of the table. A special backrest (Fig 16) is attached and the table is tilted about 5–10 degrees toward the dorsum of the patient. The skull clamp is then connected to the table attachment and the head fixed in the desired position. The regular foot section of the table is flexed completely. The operation can be completed in the lateral horizontal position or, if conditions permit, the head can be elevated toward the vertical position.

The lateral sitting position can be converted to the lateral horizontal position by simply manipulating the T handle. In patients with lateralized lesions, there may be advantage in reversing the patient's position on the operating table so that the operative side is uppermost.

More than 300 neurosurgical procedures have been done

(6) Anesth. Analg. (Cleve.) 55:326–330, May–June, 1976.

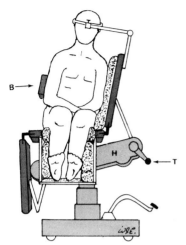

Fig 16. — Left lateral sitting position as seen from left side of operating table. *H,* main movable frame of table; *T,* handle for moving in Trendelenburg direction and reverse; *B,* backrest. (Courtesy of Garcia-Bengochea, F., et al.: Anesth. Analg. (Cleve.) 55:326–330, May–June, 1976.)

with patients in the lateral sitting position. About half were suboccipital craniectomies and the others were cervical and upper thoracic laminectomies. No mortality or serious morbidity was attributed to use of this position. In 9 cases where patients were placed in the lateral horizontal position for the treatment of hypotension, the arterial pressure was restored to adequate levels. Each operation was completed satisfactorily with the patient kept either in the lateral horizontal position or with the head subsequently raised 35–80 degrees from the horizontal plane.

Repair of Denuded Cranial Bone by Bone Splitting and Free-Skin Grafting. Denuded cranial bone defects with avascular floors may heal by epithelialization from surrounding skin or may require sliding grafts or rotation flaps. Distant-flap procedures may be considered in extreme cases. Finn Jensen and Niles C. Petersen[7] (Aarhus) found that bone splitting followed by free-skin grafting is a useful procedure as an alternative to the use of pedicled skin flaps.

A bur drill is used to section the outer table into small squares, which are chiseled away, and a split-skin graft of medium thickness is taken from the thigh or upper arm and applied immediately if bleeding from the diploë is not exces-

(7)   J. Neurosurg. 44:728–731, June, 1976.

sive. The graft also may be stored until healthy granulation tissue is evident. One large graft is preferred to "stamp" grafts. The graft usually is left exposed.

CASE 1. — Woman, 61, had been treated for decades for multiple basal cell carcinomas and had a large recurrence on the scalp. She had excision down to bone, leaving a 12×7-cm defect. Stamp grafts were applied after a delay of 16 days and residual defects were regrafted after 12 days. The wound was almost healed 41 days postoperatively.

CASE 2. — Boy, 5, had multiple skull fractures; after operation, a necrotic area developed, measuring 8×10 cm. The outer table was removed and coverage was done with split-skin grafts.

CASE 3. — Woman, 57, with a benign skin lesion and diffuse radiation necrosis, had a 20×14-cm area excised over both parietal regions, followed by coverage with free-skin grafts and the application of stored grafts in some small areas. Complete healing resulted within 1 month.

One large skin graft is used in these cases unless healing conditions are extremely poor. The procedures are easy to perform and cause minimal discomfort. If the treatment fails, alternative reconstructive methods are still available; this is also true if the skin graft should prove to be vulnerable or esthetically unsatisfactory.

Repair of Recurrent Osteomeningeal Gaps in the Cranial Base is discussed by J. Brunon, J. L. Sautreaux, G. Fischer and L. Mansuy[8] (Neurologic Hosp., Lyons, France). Despite correct treatment, $5 - 30\%$ of the cerebrospinal fluid (CSF) fistulas from osteomeningeal fracture of the base of the skull recur after operation. Among more than 70 patients operated on for the first time during $1967 - 75$, there have been 6 reoperations. Three of them occurred after failure of 1 or several reoperations.

In 4 cases, operation was done for posttraumatic osteomeningeal gap. Two cases involved fronto-orbitoethmoidal wounds. Obliteration of the opening was attempted at the time of the first operation or in the days following. In 1 patient, the fistula recurred 22 years after trauma and caused formation of a pneumatocele. In the other, recurrence was early and led to 4 episodes of purulent meningitis and necessitated 2 reoperations before placement of a bony graft.

CASE 1. — Man, 38, sustained a serious head injury with cranio-

(8) Neurochirurgie 22:455 – 467, Sept. – Oct., 1976.

cerebral, right fronto-orbitoethmoidal and right eyeball wounds, traumatic coma and left hemiplegia. During the initial operation, the craniocerebral wound was treated, the osteomeningeal break was closed, and the right eye was enucleated. There was progressive improvement of consciousness with practically complete recovery of the hemiplegia in 1 year. Medical treatment effected stabilization of a posttraumatic seizure. There were no clinically visible CSF fistulas.

Two years later, a generalized seizure followed untimely barbiturate weaning. Two months later, an episode of rhinopharyngeal infection was complicated by sinusitis and discharge of CSF from the right nostril. The rhinorrhea stopped within a few weeks, but there was progressive obnubilation with left hemiparesis. The x-rays showed a large right frontal intracerebral pneumatocele and an osteomeningeal gap in the ethmoidal region, with visualization of a clinically silent CSF fistula on cisternography.

During the second operation, the osteomeningeal break was closed by iliac corticospongy graft and plastic repair with fascia lata. There was clinical recovery.

In 2 cases, operation was performed because of postsurgical osteomeningeal tear. In 1 case, there was a fistula of the middle fossa that appeared after removal of a nasopharyngeal fibroma, complicated by several episodes of purulent meningitis. Two former procedures had failed to close the opening.

The goal of surgery is simultaneous obliteration of the meningeal tear with an aponeurotic graft and of the bony gap with an autograft of corticospongy bone. It is hoped that the latter will be incorporated into the base of the skull and form a tight barrier against increasing infection. A good radiologic identification of the break and, if possible, an isotopic one of the fistula are indispensible. The principal cause of failure of the initial operation was unfamiliarity with the topography of the lesions.

Surgical exploration should be extensive. For lesions of the anterior fossa, an overlapping bilateral frontal flap centered on the midline should be made. For lesions of the middle fossa, a temporal flap flush with the cranial base and centered on the external acoustic meatus should be carried out. Closure of the meningeal tear should not be attempted until its limits have been defined. This is done with a piece of fascia lata or epicranial aponeurosis.

In the 6 cases, the immediate result was excellent, with

disappearance of all CSF leakage. Long-term results (possible for only 5 patients) were more difficult to interpret considering that certain CSF fistulas can reappear many years after the initial trauma. Nevertheless, in certain cases, a good permanent result after bony grafts can be expected.

Oblique Muscle-Splitting Incision for Cervical Laminotomy. Timir Banerjee (Univ. of North Carolina) and William E. Hunt[9] (Ohio State Univ.) have found that a muscle-splitting incision produces less morbidity and a better scar than the conventional midline incision in operations for unilateral lower cervical disk disease. The technique has eliminated deep wound dehiscence and has reduced postoperative pain greatly. No complications of the wound itself have resulted. Patients can turn themselves and do not need a figure-of-eight bandage.

TECHNIQUE. — With the patient's head flexed in the forward oblique position, the head of the table elevated 30–45 degrees and the interspace localized by x-ray if necessary, an oblique line is drawn through a point over the root to be explored parallel to the trapezius fibers, laterally for 6–8 cm, and the incision is carried to the deep fascia. The serratus posterior superior muscle also is split and an incision is made directly onto the 2 adjacent spinous processes (3 if 2 interspaces are to be explored) just below their tips. Further lateral dissection exposes the fibers of the joint capsule. The technique of Scoville is followed, with a partial hemilaminotomy and hemifacetectomy with a Hudson bur. The extradural sleeve is cut after bipolar coagulation and the disk or osteophyte is removed or decompressed. One or two sutures may be placed in the serratus posterior superior aponeurosis and a few 4-0 silk sutures are placed in the trapezius aponeurosis. Four or five sutures are placed in the deep layer of the superficial fascia.

This muscle-splitting incision for cervical disk operations is based on sound surgical principles. No wound complications have occurred in the last 60 patients treated surgically. The surgeon using this technique must be familiar with the anatomical planes to be certain of the level of exploration.

Laminotomy and Total Reconstruction of Posterior Spinal Arch for Spinal Canal Surgery in Childhood. Anthony J. Raimondi, Francisco A. Gutierrez and Concezio

(9)   Am. Surg. 42:326–329, May, 1976.

Di Rocco[1] (Northwestern Univ.) present an alternative to laminectomy for complete exposure of the spinal canal, which allows anatomical reconstruction of the vertebral arches and reinsertion of interspinous ligaments and paravertebral masses. Patients under age 1 year have a laminotomy even if only one level is to be exposed. Children aged 1–15 are operated on for two or more levels and older patients when three or more levels are to be exposed. All patients with trauma, syringomyelia, hydromyelia and tuberculosis undergo laminotomy but it is not performed in patients with extensive epidural metastases.

TECHNIQUE. – Exposure extends from one full vertebra above to one below the planned extent of the laminotomy. The dissection is carried laterally to just beyond the articular facets. The laminar osteotomy is made with a high-speed drill along a line separating the pedicle from the lamina. The laminotomy is best made using the bur in brushlike strokes along the laminar surface in the direction of the planned line. Sharp dissection of the loose connective tissue minimizes stretching in removal of the laminar flap. After interspinal surgery and closure of the dura, the flap is brought into anatomical position and symmetric drill holes are made at either side of the incision for the placement of suture material in an inferosuperior direction.

Postoperatively the patient is immobilized appropriately and x-rays are obtained at monthly intervals. The reflection of a free laminar flap over the intraspinal lesion allows as complete an access to the spinal canal as the most extensive laminectomy. Multiple-level laminotomy flaps provide access to the entire spinal canal, permitting removal of the most extensive lesions without permanently weakening the spine or destroying growth centers in the posterior spinal arch. Considerably more time is necessary to remove multiple laminae than to perform a laminectomy but the procedure is not dangerous. Appropriate immobilization is important to assist bone bridging and minimize the risk of pseudarthrosis developing.

Angiographic Study of the Effect of Laminectomy in the Presence of Acute Anterior Epidural Masses. Proponents of anterior decompression of acute anterior epidural masses suggest that laminectomy may not decompress the cord adequately in the presence of a large mass. John L.

(1)   J. Neurosurg. 45:555–560, November, 1976.

Doppman and Mary Girton[2] (Natl. Inst. of Health) evaluated the effects of laminectomy on spinal cord displacement and blood flow in monkeys with simulated acute anterior epidural masses. Spinal cord lateral view arteriograms were obtained of 16 rhesus monkeys before and after a 4 F Fogarty balloon catheter was placed in front of the cord percutaneously and inflated to diameters of 3.4 – 6.2 mm. All the masses were large enough to cause paraplegia without operative intervention. A 3-level laminectomy centered over the balloon was done to decompress the cord 1 – 2 hours after balloon inflation.

Laminectomy appeared to influence the recovery of cord function favorably in the 11 evaluable animals when the mass was less than 4.5 mm in diameter. Larger masses could not be decompressed adequately by a posterior approach. Posterior migration of the cord was minimal after decompression but filling of the posterior veins returned to normal. Microangiography showed normal perfusion of the intrinsic cord vasculature at the level of the balloon in 2 animals without a deficit. Posterior venous filling improved but not to normal in 4 animals with postlaminectomy paraparesis. Microangiography showed decreased perfusion of the sulcocommissural arteries in 1 of these animals. Microangiographic findings were abnormal in all 5 animals with persistent postlaminectomy paraplegia, with poor sulcocommissural artery perfusion at and below the level of the balloon.

Surprisingly little posterior migration of the cord was seen after decompression in this animal study. Acute anterior epidural masses can be too large to be decompressed adequately by laminectomy. When a mass obstructs the anterior spinal artery, laminectomy does not restore normal cord hemodynamics. Whether or not deflation of the balloon after 1 hour, equivalent to an anterior decompression, would result in better functional recovery than with laminectomy is under study.

▶ [The questions raised by the authors concerning the lack of posterior migration of the spinal cord after 3-level laminectomy had, I thought, been long since answered for human subjects by the French surgeons who decompressed the entire cervical spinal canal from behind for cervical spondylosis and showed migration of the entire thecal canal backward.

(2) J. Neurosurg. 45:195 – 202, August, 1976.

Shorter areas of laminectomy frequently did not permit much migration, and it is for this reason that those who operate from behind for spondylosis anterior to the spinal cord insist on long laminectomies. It would be interesting to have the authors' experiments repeated with enlargement of the dural sac by incision and grafting — and by sectioning the dentate ligaments when only 3 segments are to be decompressed. — Ed.] ◄

Microsurgical Anterior Cervical Myelotomy. Hemorrhagic infarction occurs in the central gray matter of the spinal cord after a nondisruptive injury, resulting in paraplegia or quadriplegia. Whether removal of this necrotic material increases the possibility of neurologic recovery is unclear. Franklin C. Wagner, Jr., and Stephen E. Rawe[3] (Yale Univ.) describe a microsurgical procedure for performing an anterior cervical myelotomy and evacuating an intramedullary hematoma.

Man, 44, fell two stories and landed on the vertex of the skull when he struck the ground. A complete sensory and motor paraplegia and a fracture-dislocation of C5 on C6 were noted. The intercostal muscles were paralyzed, but the patient was not in respiratory distress. Skeletal traction with Crutchfield tongs was instituted, and air myelography and polytomography showed a complete obstruction in the central subarachnoid space at the C5 level with the patient in a 45-degree head-down position. Additional skeletal traction was applied, but the dislocation could not be reduced, and the patient was transferred to a Foster turning frame.

Under general anesthesia, the anterior cervical spine was approached as described by Cloward, and the fractured anterior part of the body of C5 was removed, with the cartilage plates and disks between C4 – C5 and C5 – C6. The rest of the body of C5 was then removed with an air drill, along with a large fragment of extruded disk material from between C5 and C6 and the remaining lacerated posterior longitudinal ligament. The dura and arachnoid were incised under the operating microscope, and an area of subpial ecchymosis measuring about 1×3 mm was found over the anterior quadrant on the left side. The pial surface was coagulated and the cord incised to release several drops of liquified hematoma. Remaining hematoma in the gray matter was removed with a suction tip, leaving a 1-cm-long cavity in the cord. No active bleeding was seen within the cord substance. The dura was closed, and the fractured spine was fused with a strut graft between C4 and C6.

When last seen, 4 months after injury, the patient had antigravity movement in both carpi radialis longus muscles, and pain perception was normal over the left thumb and index finger.

(3) Surg. Neurol. 5:229 – 231, April, 1976.

This case shows how easily the injured spinal cord can be approached anteriorly and how readily the necrotic, hemorrhagic gray matter can be identified and removed, leaving the normal gray matter and surrounding white matter intact. The operating microscope and bipolar coagulating forceps are essential for this purpose.

Simplified Percutaneous Lumboperitoneal Shunting. Communicating hydrocephalus poses a special problem in management in that it is difficult if not impossible to determine if a patient will respond favorably to surgical shunt procedures. Robert Spetzler, Charles B. Wilson and Rudi Schulte[4] (Univ. of California, San Francisco) recently described a lumboperitoneal shunt that can be inserted into the lumbar subarachnoid space through a 14-gauge Touhey needle. The catheter is tunneled subcutaneously around the flank and connected to a reservoir, and a peritoneal catheter is attached to the reservoir, tunneled subcutaneously to the abdomen and introduced into the peritoneal cavity. The two catheters have now been incorporated into a single shunting unit, which opens at 100–120 mm water, for use in treatment of active hydrocephalus.

The modified shunt consists of an 80-cm spring-reinforced Silastic catheter having a multiperforated tip for subarachnoid insertion and three pairs of slit valves on the opposite end for peritoneal insertion. The opening pressure of the slit valves is tested in saline before insertion of the shunt. The catheter tip is inserted through the Touhey needle into a 1-cm skin incision made between the spinous processes of L4–C5 or L5–S1. A tunneling instrument is passed through a skin incision in the flank to the lumbar incision and the catheter is then passed from the flank to the abdomen, where the shunt can be inserted into the peritoneal cavity either under direct vision or through an abdominal trocar. The trocar is inserted through a small stab incision in the superficial layer of the aponeurosis. Any slack tubing is inserted into the peritoneal cavity. A sleeve is placed about the catheter at all incision sites and sutured into the subcutaneous tissues. Shunt function is easily checked by injecting pertechnetate-albumin into the cervical subarachnoid space.

(4)   Surg. Neurol. 7:25–29, January, 1977.

This procedure gave generally good results in the first 11 patients treated. Complications included single instances of shunt blockage, shunt tubing migration into the peritoneal cavity and postoperative rupture of an aortic aneurysm. The patient's clinical response is used to determine the efficacy of the procedure. Patients who clearly improve after shunting require no further treatment. When clinical benefit is not apparent, the tubing can easily be removed under local anesthesia. Ease of insertion makes this shunt useful in the diagnosis and treatment of communicating hydrocephalus.

Congenital Malformations

▶ Concentrations of α-fetoprotein (AFP) can be determined in amniotic fluid by an electroimmune diffusion technique or by an antibody radioimmune assay. Measurements reported by Weiss et al. (Obstet. Gynecol. 47: 148, 1976) indicated gradual decrease in AFP values with increasing gestational age. Before 26 weeks of gestation, AFP was elevated markedly in pregnancies associated with confirmed neural tube defects. Other nonneurologic fetal disorders (duodenal atresia, nephrosis, omphalocele, teratoma) also may give elevated AFP values. The authors believe a single elevated AFP reading should be supplemented by sonography and amniography before elective termination of pregnancy is undertaken.

Among the malformations discoverable by this means are myelomeningoceles. Those that protrude laterally through defects in the neural arches are rare. In the 3 cases reported by Reddy et al. (Aust. N. Z. J. Surg. 46:69, 1976), there was scoliosis, hemivertebrae and absence of neural arches on the affected side. Another case is reported briefly by Das et al. (Int. Surg. 61:239, 1976).

Anterior sacrococcygeal meningocele usually is diagnosed by the typical scimitar-shaped sacral defect and can be confirmed by myelography. Monteverde and Russo (Rev. Inst. Nacl. Neurol. (Mex.) 10:108, 1976) described a case with approach via a transperineal, retroperitoneal technique, with incision of the skin horizontally just anterior to the tip of the coccyx. This route appears superior to a transabdominal one and should be considered when a retrosacral approach is not feasible.

In the 1976 YEAR BOOK (pp. 349 and 350), there are two articles on early operation for meningomyelocele, and reference is made to Lorber's scheme for selection of children for operation. In general, these articles deal with criteria for early operation and appear to indicate the uselessness of operation in some instances. Rickham (Med. J. Aust. 2:743, 1976) discusses at some length the indication for operation on myelomeningoceles, based on his own long experience as a pediatric surgeon with cases apparently dismissed by others: "The neurosurgeons of the period refused to do anything at all about these children and advised that they should be left to die." He contends that the pendulum against operation has swung too far and gives his medical, ethical, eugenic and legal understandings of the problem. He concludes that doctors ask the wrong questions about selection, that they should ask only how to relieve suffering and restore health as far as possible. The decision not to treat an infant should be made, he says, for only two reasons: (1) inability of the infant to benefit from treatment (with extremely wide open myelomeningoceles that are virtually impossible to close) and (2) probability of death, as in those with other severe malformations, extensive thoracic myelomeningoceles or extensive kyphoscoliosis. The article is obviously an extremely personal one (without references) and gives one side of a vexing problem that should be pondered by those who disagree. — Ed. ◄

Experience with Arnold-Chiari Malformation, 1960– 70. Ruben J. Saez, Burton M. Onofrio and Takehiko Yanagihara[5] (Mayo Clinic and Found.) reviewed the data on 22 male and 38 female patients (mean age, 38) treated for symptoms associated with the Arnold-Chiari malformation in 1960– 70. In all cases the diagnosis was confirmed surgically and no patients had complicating neurologic problems. The average duration of symptoms before admission was 4.5 years. Pain was the most common complaint and usually involved the occiput, cervical area and arms. Weakness of the hands and a stiff-legged gait were also common complaints. The most common neurologic findings were lower extremity hyperreflexia and upper extremity atrophy. Over half the patients had sensory abnormalities. A foramen magnum compression syndrome was present in 23 patients, paroxysmal intracranial hypertension in 13, and a central cord disturbance in 12. Cerebellar dysfunction predominated in 6 patients, spasticity in 4 and bulbar palsy in 2. Pantopaque myelography and pneumoencephalography invariably showed abnormalities.

All patients underwent cervicomedullary decompression by suboccipital craniectomy and upper cervical laminectomy. The dura was left open or a homologous graft was applied. In 38 patients, arachnoidal adhesions bound the tonsils to the upper cervical cord. The exposed cervical cord was grossly distended in at least 14 patients. There were no operative deaths and only 2 patients had morbidity after surgery. Follow-up for up to 14 years showed that 39 of the 60 patients (65%) benefited from surgery, 12 becoming asymptomatic; 11 of the patients continued to deteriorate. Over 80% of patients with paroxysmal intracranial hypertension or cerebellar dysfunction had a favorable outcome, but only 33% of those with central cord disturbance improved. Of the 14 patients with a grossly widened cervical cord, 5 improved and 5 became worse. Benefit was not always sustained and many patients had progression of the neurologic deficit.

Early surgical treatment aimed at restoring normal cerebrospinal fluid dynamics at the foramen magnum may be

---

(5) J. Neurosurg. 45:416–422, October, 1976.

indicated for patients with Arnold-Chiari malformation and associated hydromelia. In some patients, severe adhesive arachnoiditis enveloping the cerebellar tonsils precludes a vigorous, direct operative approach without risk of irreparable ischemic damage to the medulla and cervical cord occurring.

► [Angiography has not been wholly supplanted by computerized tomography and may be useful in evaluation of displacement of the pons in adult Arnold-Chiari malformation. Weinstein and Newton (Am. J. Roentgenol. 126:798, 1976) use the anterior pontomesencephalic vein as a delineator of the position of the pons. They determine its position in relation to a line tangent to the floor of the sella and perpendicular to a line from the posterior clinoid to the anterior foramen magnum. Normally the superior aspect of the pons lies 4 mm below to 20 mm above the sellar tangent line. In 9 patients with Arnold-Chiari malformation, the pons was more than 5 mm below the line. In 5 others, the measurement was within normal limits, although in 3 of these, the measurement was 1–3 mm below the line. – Ed.] ◄

Microsurgery of Arnold-Chiari Malformation in Adults with and without Hydromyelia. Hydromyelia often accompanies Arnold-Chiari malformation in the adult. Albert L. Rhoton, Jr.[6] (Univ. of Florida), concluding that Gardner's mechanical concept of a pressure-distention origin of syringomyelia cord syndrome is correct, based treatment on this concept. Microsurgical exploration of 15 adults with Arnold-Chiari malformation, 11 of whom had hydromyelia, indicated that the associated hydromyelia is a progressive mechanical disorder causing cord deficits by pressure distention of the cord, whereas Arnold-Chiari malformation causes progressive bulbar dysfunction by impaction of the malformation in the foramen magnum. The age range of patients was 19–64. All 4 who were followed without surgery had an increase in deficit and had surgery within a year of initial diagnosis. Both lesions can be decompressed by a suboccipital craniectomy and upper cervical laminectomy, establishing an outlet from the 4th ventricle and opening the distended cord in the thinnest exposed area, usually along the dorsal root entry zone. A wick was used to maintain patency of the outlet of the 4th ventricle. Shunting from the lateral ventricle is indicated only if the ventricles are large or the intracranial pressure is increased.

Only 1 patient had an increased deficit as a result of sur-

(6) J. Neurosurg. 45:473–483, November, 1976.

gery, a mild proprioceptive sensory loss in the thumb. Otherwise no complications occurred. Most patients noted some subjective improvement in sensory and motor deficits, but the neurologic signs remained about the same as before operation. No patient has shown progression of deficits during follow-up for 1–6 years, except 1 with an Arnold-Chiari malformation alone who subsequently had classic amyotrophic lateral sclerosis.

Most syringomyelic cord syndromes are caused by treatable conditions, and an active investigational approach should be taken for early treatment as patients have little likelihood of recovery beyond a certain stage of disability.

▶ [Oil myelography was carried out by Peserico et al. (J. Neurosurg. 45: 576, 1976) in a woman, aged 27, suspected of having syringomyelia. There was a Chiari type I deformity, oil droplets in the C1–C3 area suggesting an open central canal, and marked widening of the cord from T9 upward. Gas myelography showed collapse of the cervical spinal cord. Ventriculography with ^{111}In showed a narrow line of uptake along the spinal cord, widening at the cervicothoracic level. Lumbar myelocisternography with the same material showed a wider uptake along the spinal cord than on ventriculography, with slowed upward flow presumed due to the swollen cord. Myodil ventriculography showed a droplet within the cord at T4. Operation permitted placement of a muscle plug into the opening of the central canal into the 4th ventricle.

It appears that even in Italy, multiple diagnostic techniques are being used; one wonders what the medical malpractice situation is there. The authors suggest the combined use of radionuclide ventriculography and lumbar myelocisternography as a safe and valuable way to verify communicating syringomyelia. – Ed.] ◀

"Noncommunication" Syringomyelia: Nonexistent Entity. W. James Gardner and Fred G. McMurry[7] (Cleveland Clinic) indicate that encroachment by man's overlarge forebrain is responsible for the anatomical substrate of syringomyelia, i.e., a hindbrain hernia developing in fetal life with persisting hydromyelia. Communication between the syrinx and 4th ventricle is readily disclosed at operation but, because of postmortem shrinkage, almost never at autopsy. At operation for syringomyelia, the herniated hindbrain pulsates vigorously because the increased crowding at the level of the foramen magnum in systole interferes with the free escape of the intracranial pulse waves of the subarachnoid fluid; in diastole, the block is relieved. Spinal puncture in the syringomyelic patient reveals pulse waves.

---

(7) Surg. Neurol. 6:251–256, October, 1976.

Syringomyelia developing in 16 of 864 posttraumatic paraplegics was classed as noncommunicating, but the syrinx, its fluid and the ultimate clinical picture were the same as in nontraumatic cases. Surgical exposure disclosed the communication. Symptoms develop when the traumatic subarachnoid block exaggerates the causative intracranial fluid pulse waves by eliminating the damping effect of the yielding dural sac below. A nontraumatic spinal block also may result in syringomyelia.

Syringomyelia is treated surgically to relieve obstruction by causing freer communication with the subarachnoid space. This may be accomplished at craniovertebral decompression by separation of the impacted tonsils, with or without plugging the funnel-shaped central canal at the obex, by syringotomy or by its equivalent in the patient with permanent posttraumatic paraplegia, using local excision of the irreparably damaged portion of the cord. An alternate treatment method is to reduce the exaggerated pulse waves of the ventricular fluid by introducing a low-pressure ventricular shunt.

Every syrinx communicates with the 4th ventricle. Although the anatomical substrate is laid down during early development of the cerebrospinal spaces, the symptoms usually do not become manifest until adulthood. The substrate is much more likely to become symptomatic if the ventricular pulse waves are further amplified by the development of a spinal subarachnoid block, traumatic or otherwise.

Management of Scaphocephaly. Premature fusion of the sagittal suture with scaphocephaly is the most common form of craniosynostosis referred for surgical correction. The standard operation involves the creation of artificial sagittal sutures by bilateral parasagittal craniectomies. Embryologic and anatomical evidence, however, suggests that growth of the fetal and infantile brain is solely responsible for skull growth and that fibrous dural bands determine the directions in which this growth occurs. Sutural changes are merely secondary or compensatory.

Sherman C. Stein and Luis Schut[8] (Univ. of Pennsylvania) have used an operation that involves extending the cra-

---

(8) Surg. Neurol. 7:153–155, March, 1977.

niectomy to the skull base. A bicoronal skin incision is made midway between the nasion and inion and bur holes are placed behind the coronal sutures 2 cm from the midline so parasagittal craniectomies may be performed along the entire length of the sagittal suture. The craniectomies are carried across the coronal and lambdoidal sutures. Craniectomies are carried along the coronal sutures to the skull base. Bilateral lambdoidal craniectomies are carried down to the squamosal sutures and then forward for about 2 cm. Bone over the sagittal sinus is cut across at its anterior margin and removed; its removal is often followed by immediate shortening of the cranium.

Fifty consecutive patients with premature sagittal synostosis had operations in the first 15 months of life in 1968–74 and were followed for up to 5 years. There was no postoperative mortality. Seven patients required transfusions postoperatively; 1 patient had transient hemiparesis and 1, a wound infection. Cosmetic results were considered optimal in 96% of patients; 2 patients with optimal appearances had radiologic evidence of residual scaphocephaly. Regrowth of excised cranial bone was rapid. Ossification arose in islands of new bone within the craniectomy defects, not from the skull edges.

This operation deals directly with the disorder of growth pattern originating at the skull base and allows the immediate assumption of a more normal shape of the skull and maintenance of this shape despite inevitable bony fusion of the craniectomy. This and other operations for craniosynostosis are always more successful if done early in life. The best results are obtained with operation at age 4–6 weeks. Even in the absence of intracranial hypertension there is little to be gained from merely observing the child with severe scaphocephaly.

▶ [I am not sure I know exactly what is meant anatomically by carrying a craniotomy along the coronal suture to the skull base. However, a 96% success rate in reshaping an elongated skull, associated with a low complication rate, seems worthwhile, even if the operation is considerably more extensive that the more widely used linear craniectomies. The lack of a need for plastic material to line the bone or for Zenker's solution to paint the dura mater is extremely appealing. — Ed.] ◀

New Surgical Approach to Treatment of Coronal Synostosis is described by Anthony J. Raimondi and Francisco A. Gutierrez[9] (Northwestern Univ.). Premature unilateral coronal synostosis, or plagiocephaly, is a congenital abnormality of the skull for which early surgery has been advised to prevent visual loss, cosmetic deformities and brain damage. The frontal region is flattened and the orbits are asymmetric. The sphenoid is displaced frontally, causing sagittal shortening of the orbit and exophthalmos. At times the temporal lobe may be both lateral and inferior to the orbit. Early repair of the deformity, especially when it is bilateral or associated with the Crouzon deformity, may release the maxillae and allow them to develop normally, thus minimizing the need for subsequent total craniofacial reconstruction.

The frontal lobe and orbital contents are decompressed by freeing the pterion from the zygomatic process of the frontal bone and the lesser wing of the sphenoid and by freeing the superior orbital rim. A coronal incision is made with the child supine and the periosteum over the supraorbital region is dissected to place bur holes over the glabella, behind the zygomatic process and lateral to the sagittal suture. A free bone flap is lifted, incising or excising the coronal suture, and the bones at the pterion are removed with a rongeur. The lateral third of the lesser sphenoid wing also is removed. Periosteum is dissected from the orbital roof and the roof is freed. The zygomatic process is then detached from the malar bone. The greater sphenoid wing on the lateral surface of the skull is then removed and the supraorbital ridge is anchored loosely into position.

This operation has been done on 16 children aged 2–12 months. None have required reoperation. The orbital contour generally became nearly symmetric and physiologically normal. Ten patients had optimal results, 5 had suboptimal results and 1 improved only slightly. The average follow-up is 20.5 months. All children required needle aspiration of a subdural fluid collection shortly after the frontal flap was lifted.

This procedure allows the orbital contents and the frontal and temporal lobes to expand normally. Maxillary recession apparently is avoided. Normal expansion of the frontal lobe

(9) J. Neurosurg. 46:210–214, February, 1977.

occurs with early operation and the orbital contents are provided with adequate space.

Congenital Anomalies Associated with Thoracic Outlet Syndrome: Anatomy, Symptoms, Diagnosis and Treatment are discussed by David B. Roos[1] (Univ. of Colorado). Personal experience in evaluation of over 2,300 patients for possible thoracic outlet syndrome (TOS) and operating on 776, 204 of them bilaterally, has led to the conviction that patients with TOS have an underlying anatomical abnormality that predisposes them to develop symptoms of TOS under particular circumstances. Several distinct types of congenital fibrous or muscular band anomalies have been distinguished, including a fibrous ligament attached to the anterior tip of an incomplete cervical rib, a muscular band passing from the 1st thoracic rib across the thoracic outlet, an anomalous muscle connection between the anterior and middle scalene muscles, and bands representing the scalenus minimus muscle. The most common bands are associated intimately with the brachial plexus. Symptoms of venous insufficiency, made worse by limb exercise, are more frequent than those of arterial insufficiency.

Subclavian artery compression has little to do with the symptoms in about 99% of patients with TOS. Pulse obliteration with the arms and head in various positions is a normal finding in most asymptomatic persons. If certain test positions reproduce the usual symptoms of the patient, the response suggests only that the symptoms are arising from the thoracic outlet. Reproduction of symptoms by shoulder bracing and the 3-minute elevated-arm stress test will usually delineate TOS from other problems with similar symptoms. Testing for tenderness over the brachial plexus will indicate whether the symptoms emanate from the plexus itself. Appropriate tests must always be done for clinical states that may produce similar symptoms, such as the carpal tunnel and cervical disk syndromes and cervical or shoulder sprain. Electromyography and nerve conduction velocity tests have been of little help in the specific diagnosis of TOS or the selection of patients for operative intervention.

Mildly symptomatic patients may respond well by avoid-

(1) Am. J. Surg. 132:771–778, December, 1976.

ance of the activities or positions that precipitate symptoms. When surgery is indicated, a transaxillary approach is used with the patient in the lateral position for resecting the 1st thoracic rib, and cervical rib if present, and removing all anomalous fibromuscular tissue. Congenital bands must be totally excised for complete neurovascular decompression. If patients are appropriately tested and highly selected for surgery, gratifying relief will be obtained in over 90% of patients, if the correct operation is performed with meticulous technique.

▶ [In the elevated arm stress test, the brachium is at right angles to the thorax and the forearm is flexed 90 degrees. The patient is instructed to open and close the fist at moderate speed for 3 minutes, with the elbows braced somewhat posteriorly. In the series reported by Roos, this has been found to be the most reliable test for thoracic outlet syndrome if the usual symptoms of the patient are reproduced within 3 minutes. — Ed.] ◀

Infections

Brain Abscess in Congenital Heart Disease: Twelve Surgical Cases and Review of the Literature are presented by J.-E. Paillas, J.-C. Peragut and S. Ugarte[2] (Marseilles, France). Among abscesses of the brain in neurosurgical series, cardiogenic abscesses represent a little less than 10%. In the authors' experience, 12 of 130 patients had cardiogenic abscesses. All age groups were affected, but 4 patients were under age 20 years, and 5 were aged 20–40 years. Ten patients were male.

The cause of heart disease in 8 patients was cyanosis. Cardiac malformations were classified according to the actual functional disorders, but there were various associated malformations. The most typical malformation was tetralogy of Fallot (5 patients), which has been reported in more than half of the known cases. All abscesses were supratentorial, with a slight predominance in the frontorolandic region, and most often appeared singly. Two patients had multiple abscesses.

Intracranial hypertension was the most frequent initial manifestation (10 times). Torpor often prevailed and was associated always with headaches and sometimes (5 times) with a high fever. In the initial stage, diagnosis was often difficult because obnubilation and heaviness of the head voluntarily occurs in heart patients. Inversely, the syndrome could develop in three steps, induced by antibiotics in some cases. Diagnosis was further confirmed by EEG, radiology, cerebral angiography and gamma encephalography.

Surgical techniques were those generally used for patients with brain abscesses, but adapted to the patient's weakness due to the heart condition, his age and stage of development.

Operation effected cure in 9 of the 12 patients. There were 3 operative deaths, 2 from major cerebral edema with tem-

---

(2) Sem. Hop. Paris 52:1129–1138, May 9–16, 1976.

poral involvement and 3 from cardiac arrest in diastole. Two others patients died of cardiac failure 1 and 3 months, respectively, after removal of the abscess. The operative mortality of 25% and the mobidity are high, but no higher than for abscesses of other origins. Surgical treatment of the heart condition postoperatively is needed to maintain the patient in good condition. If the patient and his advisors consented, he was entrusted to a cardiosurgeon.

Transthoracic Approach for Pott's Disease. Spinal tuberculosis with paraplegia remains a major health problem in most underdeveloped countries and continues to occur in certain areas of the United States. J. David Richardson, Donald L. Campbell, Frederick L. Grover, Kit V. Arom, Kaye Wilkins, John P. Wissinger and J. Kent Trinkle[3] (Univ. of Texas, San Antonio) reviewed experience with 16 male and 12 female patients treated for spinal tuberculosis on a thoracic surgical service in 1967 – 75. The average age of patients was 25; 9 were under age 12. The common features were back pain, gibbous spinal deformity and neurologic symptoms in the lower extremities. Nine patients were paraplegic and 3 of them became paraplegic while hospitalized; 8 patients were febrile. Most were healthy apart from the spinal disease. Only 3 patients had signs of active pulmonary tuberculosis. Bone involvement was most often in the mid-lower thoracic spine, 2 or 3 vertebrae showing destruction. Antituberculosis chemotherapy was given for 4 – 6 weeks before operation.

Twenty-two patients had thoracotomy. Removal of the rib one level above the abscess gave optimal exposure. All involved bone was curetted out. The collapsed vertebral space was opened for curettage and placement of a rib strut. Three rib struts were wedged into grooves cut in the normal vertebrae, and bone fragments were packed into the remaining defect. Most patients were placed in a bivalved jacket cast postoperatively for 6 – 12 weeks. All 22 patients had a paravertebral abscess drained. Rib grafts were used in 20 patients and iliac bone grafts in 2. Excessive bleeding occurred in 1 patient. All patients had prompt spinal fusion but 2 have a minor persistent gibbous defect. All 9 formerly paraplegic patients can now walk and 6 are totally asymptomat-

---

(3) Ann. Thorac. Surg. 21:552 – 556, June, 1976.

ic. The average hospital stay was 2.4 months. All 21 survivors are improved and 20 are greatly improved. The 1 operative death was due to aortic bleeding. Of the 6 patients treated medically, 3 patients achieved spinal fusion in an average of 14 months; 2 others had progressive neurologic changes in the lower limbs and 1 died of tuberculosis and heart failure before spinal fusion.

Operative treatment of Pott's disease provides excellent reversal of even long-standing paraplegia and markedly shortens the hospital stay.

Control of Shunt Infection: Report of 150 Consecutive Cases. Infection is a major complication of cerebrospinal fluid (CSF) shunting procedures. Joan L. Venes[4] (Yale Univ.) reviewed 150 consecutive placements of venous and peritoneal shunts. Nonelective revisions were done within 12 hours of admission when possible. Elective revisions of ventriculoatrial shunts were done when the distal catheter reached the T4 – T5 level. Ventriculoperitoneal shunts were revised electively when the catheter was thought to be too short to allow free mobility with peristalsis.

A ventriculoperitoneal shunt was the initial procedure in 36 infants, and a ventriculoatrial shunt was the initial procedure in 18 older patients. Three intravenous doses of oxacillin were given, starting at anesthetic induction and totaling 100 mg/kg. Surgical preparation was with pHisoHex and 2% Amphyll (now replaced by povidone iodine). No more than 3 – 5 cc ventricular fluid was lost during operation. A Hakim medium-pressure valve was used in all cases. Bacitracin was used for irrigation. Shunt tubing was not allowed to touch the patient's skin. Most children were discharged on the 2d postoperative day.

No infections followed the initial placement or revision of ventriculovenous shunts in patients followed for up to 2 years. One patient had primary *Staphylococcus epidermidis* infection after placement of a ventriculoperitoneal shunt early in the series and 2 others had secondary infections. The other infections were due to gram-negative organisms (4) or *S. aureus* (2). Three children were treated before a cellular response appeared in the CSF. Cultures of the CSF, blood and urine are obtained from children with fever of no

(4)   J. Neurosurg. 45:311 – 314, September, 1976.

apparent cause and CSF cultures are obtained from children treated for infection at other sites who do not respond to antibiotic therapy within 48 hours. Children with positive culture findings receive intraventricular and intravenous antibiotics for 7 days, followed by 1 week of oral or intramuscular administration of antibiotics. Shunt replacement is done within 24 hours of the start of intraventricular therapy. Three infections caused by gram-negative organisms required ventricular drainage for control.

Intraventricular oxacillin should be used in cases of infection with gram-negative organisms. Infection by gram-negative organisms occurring in peritoneal shunts continues to be a problem.

Trauma

Value of Repeat Cerebral Arteriography in Evaluation of Trauma. Eugene J. McDonald, Jr., David P. Winestock and Julian T. Hoff[5] (San Francisco) have been impressed by the value of repeat cerebral angiography in trauma patients whose clinical condition does not improve satisfactorily. Arterial narrowing or spasm may occur after severe trauma. Contributing factors include increased intracranial pressure, subarachnoid hemorrhage, vascular stretching and sympathetic discharge at the time of impact. Spasm may develop after the initial negative angiographic studies, or it may be present initially and then resolve spontaneously. The demonstration of spasm is helpful, because the resulting cerebral ischemia can explain a patient's failure to improve.

Trauma to an artery can cause intimal disruption or partial transection with pseudoaneurysm formation. The intimal tear may lead to subintimal dissection, complete obstruction and profuse bleeding of the pseudoaneurysm. Pseudoaneurysms may be demonstrated by angiography as a delayed result of trauma. Repair of an accessible aneurysm may be attempted.

Intracerebral hematoma, extracerebral hematoma and hygroma are well-known sequelae of trauma. They may develop or enlarge many days after injury and cause clinical deterioration. Subdural hygroma and intracerebral hematoma have been demonstrated initially on repeat angiograms, and the patients have improved after appropriate surgical treatment.

▶ [For those who do not have access to a computerized tomography scanner for immediate posttrauma investigation (or if the machine is temporarily inactivated), isotopic angiography and scan may yet be useful. Buozas et al. (J. Nucl. Med. 17:975, 1976) found an area of decreased activity superiorly in the arterial phase and downward displacement of the sinus in the venous phase, indicative of epidural hematoma. A rim of activ-

---

(5) Am. J. Roentgenol. 126:792–797, April, 1976.

ity in the delayed scan in this case is ascribed to uptake in compressed underlying brain tissues. Another case of rim sign in epidural hematoma, this time over one hemisphere, is reported by Zilkha and Irwin. It is somewhat surprising to read of "a well-organized membrane" found with a large epidural membrane a week after injury. — Ed.] ◄

Definitive Treatment of Chronic Subdural Hematoma by Twist-Drill Craniostomy and Closed-System Drainage. Access to the subdural space at the patient's bedside by twist-drill perforation of the skull was originally proposed as a temporary emergency measure in subdural hematoma. Kamran Tabaddor and Kenneth Shulman[6] (Albert Einstein College of Medicine) felt that a twist-drill craniostomy and slow continuous drainage of the collection would be a rational approach to chronic subdural hematoma. Twenty-one consecutive patients with chronic and subacute subdural hematomas have been treated this way in the past 1½ years. A twist-drill hole is placed in the rostral part of the subdural collection under local anesthesia to make

Fig 17. — Diagram illustrates the direction of the drill in relation to skull and subdural space. (Courtesy of Tabaddor, K., and Shulman, K.: J. Neurosurg. 46:220–226, February, 1977.)

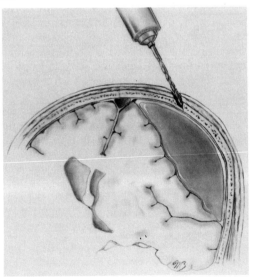

(6) J. Neurosurg. 46:220–226, February, 1977.

the hole at a 45-degree angle to the bone surface (Fig 17). A large Scott cannula with multiple side holes is cut to the length of the diagonal diameter of the subdural capsule and inserted and the collection is drained slowly by gravity. The patient is kept recumbent for about 24 hours, after which the drain is removed.

The 1 mildly symptomatic patient was the only technical failure in the series. All 12 patients with lethargy and variable neurologic deficit recovered completely. Three of 5 stuporous patients had bilateral subdural hematomas and all made essentially complete recoveries; 2 patients had mild hemiparesis. Two of the 3 patients who were comatose and had decerebrate or decorticate posturing died, whereas 1 recovered to the extent that he could be cared for in a nursing home. No complications or deleterious effects were noted. Many untoward effects of conventional surgical treatments were avoided in these patients.

Twist-drill craniostomy and closed drainage of subacute or chronic subdural hematomas constitute a simple, efficient approach, superior to conventional treatment. The method permits steady, more complete evacuation of the subdural collection and a smoother reexpansion of the compressed brain. A clotted component of the collection will resolve in a short time and will not interfere with clinical recovery of the patient.

▶ [Van der Werf (Clin. Neurol. Neurosurg. 18:162, 1975) has followed Ransohoff's procedure for hemicraniectomy for *acute* subdural hematoma after 16 of 17 patients who had only bur holes died. He emphasizes access to the base of the temporal fossa, exposure of the entire brain surface, excision of macerated brain, section of the tentorial margin and closure of the dura only if there is adequate room. The bone flap may be autoclaved and stored for replacement after a few weeks. In 1 patient, bilateral hemicranial flaps were replaced after several weeks. At times, swelling is so marked as to make closing the skin extremely difficult. Osteoplastic bone flap procedures were done in 13 cases and hemicraniectomies in 14. Of these 27 patients, one-third survived; 2 remain disabled. Those with good results (7 cases) include patients able to return to their former activities, and 1 is in fair state. The author's single patient with bifrontal decompression (Kjellberg ånd Prieto) died. – Ed.] ◀

Unoperated Subdural Hematomas: Long-Term Follow-up Study by Brain Scan and Electroencephalography is presented by John Lusins, Robert Jaffe and Morris B. Bender[7] (Mount Sinai School of Medicine, New

(7) J. Neurosurg. 44:601–607, May, 1976.

York). Of over 100 patients with subdural hematoma treated successfully without surgery since 1958, 9 with angiographically proved subdural hematoma who had multiple scans and EEGs and were available for follow-up were evaluated. Two patients who underwent surgery were studied for comparison. Nine of the 11 patients had a history of head injury 2–4 weeks before hospitalization. Nine had significant lateralizing signs and 7 had evidence of a depressed level of consciousness. All patients improved in the hospital. Six of the patients not operated on received steroids parenterally and orally. The average follow-up was 4 years. Eight patients had uneventful courses. The 5 patients who had been employed returned to their previous work. One patient had a subdural hematoma on the opposite side after 3 years, treated nonsurgically; 1 had chronic alcoholism and a moderate organic mental syndrome and 1 acquired a convulsive disorder.

All patients had abnormal nuclide uptake on the side of the hematoma on admission, appearing as a "crescent sign" on the anterior view. All but 1 had EEGs showing dysfunction on the side of the hematoma, with marked unilateral slowing and some evidence of underlying diffuse dysfunction. Brain scans gave positive results 3–6 weeks later but the EEG findings were normal in 7 cases and showed distinct improvement in 2. All patients were markedly improved clinically, most having only minimal dysfunction. After 3–4 years, all patients had normal findings on EEG and all but 1 had normal brain scan findings; this patient had a small amount of increased activity on the side that previously had shown a large area of increased uptake. Repeat angiogram showed no evidence of residual subdural collection. The scan and EEG findings were diagnostic in a patient who acquired another subdural hematoma on the opposite side. One patient operated on had positive scan findings over the area of the previous hematoma after 5 years; the second patient operated on had positive scan findings at 8 months.

The EEG is a more reliable indicator of clinical dysfunction in the presence of subdural hematoma than is the radiographic appearance of the lesion. Nuclide scanning and a practical method of long-term follow-up of the resolution of the hematoma may be reliable indicators of the presence of a subdural collection; however, the scan is no more reliable than the angiogram in indicating whether the lesion is likely to be causing clinical cerebral dysfunction.

► [I cannot give a scientific reason for a feeling of dismay that comes over me whenever I read of Doctor Bender's work with hematomas not treated surgically. Perhaps it is from the autopsies of patients with subdural collections not operated on; perhaps it is from the acquired "instincts" of a neurosurgeon who wishes to remove that which presses on the brain if it can be done. The angiograms in this article certainly indicate the presence of a subdural collection that subsequently vanished. To be sure, not every patient with an empty space has a subdural hematoma; certainly a number, especially after trauma, have collections of yellowish cerebrospinal fluid, and I could understand such collections disappearing. Not all patients with radionuclide crescents have subdural collections; a number have cervical vascular disease with normal angiograms — but the article in question deals with 11 cases with angiographic evidence of "proved subdural hematoma." It would be well, it seems to me, to have a report from these authors giving the criteria whereby 2 of the 11 patients were selected for operation, or, indeed, a general lesson in diagnosis whereby one might hope to select the patient who may be followed without operation from the one who may not.

S. Galbraith, of Glasgow, analyzed 3,147 case histories of patients with head injury; 2% of whom developed hematoma. Of these 51, 11 (22%) were undiagnosed until autopsy. Ten of these had skull fractures. In 6, a depressed level of consciousness was ascribed to cerebrovascular accident and in 5, to excess alcohol. Galbraith says that alcohol levels less than 200 mg/100 ml are unlikely to produce altered consciousness alone. If a patient who is suspected of having a cerebrovascular accident has a skull fracture, his condition is likely to be due to a traumatic intracranial hematoma. Emphasis is again placed on the progressive deterioration of consciousness as a sign of traumatic intracranial hematoma.

Perhaps the increasing use of the computerized tomography scanner with head injury will permit better diagnosis and follow-up, both in the acutely ill patient and in the patient with chronic subdural collections. — Ed.] ◄

Management of Intracranial Calcified Subdural Hematomas. Certain patients might derive benefit from the surgical removal of calcified subdural hematomas. Clark Watts[8] (Univ. of Missouri) describes 4 patients with intracranial calcified subdural hematomas. One case was found incidentally and 1 each during study for acute, progressive, chronic neurologic disorders.

In 1 case, the intracranial calcifications were not clinically significant and there was nothing to be gained by operation. One patient, with a long-term problem in seizure control culminating in status epilepticus, was seizure-free on

(8)   Surg. Neurol. 6:247–250, October, 1976.

phenytoin postoperatively. One patient was seen with a progressive neurologic deficit and may have had a calcified postmeningitic subdural effusion, an entity similar to calcified subdural hematoma. A chronic subdural hematoma with calcification was seen in a man aged 50 who had been in a mental institution for several years; he died postoperatively of pneumonia and septicemia.

All calcified subdural hematomas should not be ignored surgically; those found in patients with acute or progressive neurologic disorders should be evaluated and their removal considered, while those found incidentally or in patients with long-standing nonprogressive deficits should be left alone. Consideration of removal is particularly appropriate when no other condition explains the neurologic disorder.

EMI Scan in Management of Head Injuries. J. Ambrose, M. R. Gooding and D. Uttley[9] (London) attempted to define the role of EMI scanning in the management of head-injured patients. Comparison was made between 100 head injury patients admitted before the EMI scan became available in 1971, a group seen just after the technique was established and a group evaluated in 1975, when the method was being used in routine investigations. There were 100 patients in each group. A dramatic fall in the number of other studies done was observed—from 61 in the earliest group to 16 in the latest. The number of invasive studies done fell from 39 to 8 over the period of the survey. This has largely freed patients from the risks associated with both the tests themselves and with the attendant anesthetic. Exploratory surgery was done in 33 patients in the earliest group and in 2 in the latest, but the overall mortality has not changed. No false positive EMI scan results were recorded during the study.

The EMI scanning has drastically reduced the number of brain scans and of invasive neuroradiologic studies required in head-injured patients. It affords a considerable savings of medical and technical manpower. The results are obtained rapidly and are not ambiguous. A significant hematoma produces a definite scan appearance. Extradural and subdural hematomas can be distinguished, and both can be dif-

(9) Lancet 1:847–848, Apr. 17, 1976.

ferentiated from traumatic intracerebral hematoma. Contusion and edema are seen as an area of low density. Multiple lesions in different brain regions can be elucidated during a single comprehensive study, and the contribution of such secondary pathologic factors as edema and ventricular shift can be assessed with great accuracy. Sequential EMI scan studies can be done in patients who fail to improve or who deteriorate after operation or during medical management. Repeat studies permit the evolution of atrophy or communicating hydrocephalus to be detected.

▶ [Although Ambrose and his colleagues remark on the freeing of the patient from risks, including those of anesthesia, sedation and general anesthesia may well be needed for computerized tomography (CT) scans of good quality, as pointed out by Merine-de Villasaute and Taveras (Am. J. Roentgenol. 126:765, 1976). The evaluated CT scanning in 100 consecutive patients with head injury, 36 of whom had operation before scanning. With increasing experience, the value of scanning has become so impressive that 24-hour emergency coverage has been provided. The authors believe that CT and plain skull survey should be the first neuroradiologic procedures performed. Sequential scans are extremely helpful and will provide many observations on the natural history of tissue changes induced by trauma, as in their cases in which edema developed 48 hours after trauma with initially unremarkable CT scans. They also report several cases of bilateral subdural hematomas in which diagnosis was not made on CT scans.

In a series of 97 CT scans taken after head injury, there were 46 without hematoma. Two neurosurgeons without knowledge of the clinical findings agreed about the presence or absence of hematoma in all but 2 instances, and here the neurosurgeon who thought there was a hematoma was correct. At present, Galbraith et al. (Br. Med. J. 2:1371, 1976) have their patients anesthetized to avoid movement artifacts in the scanning for hematoma. They have extended their investigation recently to patients with posttraumatic neurologic dysfunction but without deteriorating clinical state. A surprising number have had positive scans, but have not required operation (see article by Lusins et al. in this chapter). Close monitoring of clinical state and intracranial pressure has permitted conservative therapy until the pressure progressively increased. It would be interesting to find out if these patients had scans that showed hematoma or hygroma, which surely should have differing densities.

Because subacute subdural hematomas often are now shown by CT scan, Messina (Radiology 119:725, 1976) uses contrast enhancement and delays scanning for 4–6 hours. The hematoma may then be seen because the iodinated material passes into it.

A patient of Kobrine et al. (J. Neurosurg. 46:256, 1977) was examined within 3–4 minutes after head injury and had CT scan within 20 minutes. This showed massive right cerebral swelling without intracranial hemorrhage. Some resolution was seen in the scan done at 24 hours, and almost all the edema had receded by 15 days. The basic treatment was with dexamethasone and mannitol drip. — Ed.] ◄

Cerebral Vascular Thrombosis after Closed Head Trauma. H. Reisner, W. Profanter and Th. Reisner[1] (Univ. of Vienna) present data on 6 patients, in 5 of whom thrombosis of the carotid artery was diagnosed after closed craniocerebral trauma; the posterior cerebral artery was involved in the sixth patient, as confirmed by autopsy.

Clinical signs in a man, aged 62, suggested thrombosis of the right carotid artery with subsequent massive neurologic symptoms 1 day after an automobile accident in which he sustained a cranial concussion. No remission of symptoms was achieved and he died 4 months after injury. Autopsy confirmed occlusion of the left internal carotid artery by an organized thrombus; arteriosclerotic alterations were noted in several other cerebral vessels. Although it could not be clearly stated that the thrombosis was not present prior to the accident, it is possible that the trauma resulted in damage to the vessel wall, with resultant stress on the carotid artery, and thus triggered the thrombosis.

In a patient, aged 33, with hemiparesis 1 day after an automobile accident, the occlusion of the internal carotid artery was suggested by a hematoma on the left side of the neck. Thrombectomy and subsequent symptoms confirmed the traumatic etiology of the thrombosis.

In a man, aged 46, the neurologic symptoms appeared 2 weeks after cranial trauma. Histologic investigation revealed traumatic intramural hematomas with intimal tears and establishment of thrombi. The patient fell on the ice, landing on his chin; this action caused a brusque shift in cranial content and resulted in an intimal injury. This case indicates the even relatively slight cranial trauma, without unconsciousness, may cause serious parietal vascular injury. A similar course is described in the fourth patient, in whom the interval between cranial trauma and clinical manifestation of carotid occlusion was 6 weeks. This patient had also fallen on ice without becoming unconscious.

In the fifth patient, aged 52, the first manifestation of thrombosis had occurred as a transient sensory disturbance in the right arm and a flickering of the left eye 2 months af-

(1) Wien. Klin. Wochenschr. 88:162–165, Mar. 5, 1976.

ter the accident. The subsequent period brought cerebral symptoms of vacillating intensity until the carotid occlusion could be demonstrated 4 months after the initial trauma. In this patient an almost total remission occurred.

The course of the thrombosis in the sixth patient, aged 49, could be followed by two angiographic examinations. Four weeks after the accident a narrowing of the left internal carotid artery was noted, with complete occlusion 20 months later. The clinical picture, with left cerebral signs of deficit, had worsened accordingly during this period.

Traumatic origin can be proved only by macroscopic or microscopic demonstration of a parietal lesion, although several additional factors are significant in the development of a consecutive thrombosis. The various forced torsion, stretch or shock motions of the head and neck may cause the injury, particularly a "slingshot" type of trauma. Massive cerebral shifts (countercoup effect) may lead to vascular lesions just as easily as direct alteration of large cervical vessels by blows to the neck region. Vulnerability is influenced by the patient's age and possible presence of arteriosclerosis and predisposing factors such as hypertension, diabetes, gout, obesity and disturbance of fatty metabolism. Preexisting vessel wall damage is assumed more easily in the elderly patient. However, data on the second and fourth patients show that even younger persons may have a traumatically triggered cerebroarterial thrombosis.

▶ [A compilation of 100 references with a review of the literature on cerebral thrombosis after closed head injury by Reisner and Reisner has also been published recently (Wien. Klin. Wochenschr. 88:158, 1976). – Ed.] ◀

Harrington Instrumentation in Fractures and Dislocations of the Thoracic and Lumbar Spine was evaluated by Kenneth M. Hannon[2] (Mobile, Ala.). In the United States, injuries of the thoracolumbar spine are treated most widely by laminectomy to "decompress" the spinal cord. Laminectomy and fusion frequently are combined, but without adequate internal fixation the combined procedure is no better than laminectomy alone. The indications for laminectomy are to debride compound wounds, to remove an identifiable bone fragment impinging on a nerve root and possibly to treat a worsening neurologic picture. Anterior decom-

(2)   South. Med. J. 69:1269–1273, October, 1976.

pression with bone grafting does not produce the stability gained by strong posterior internal fixation, but is a more rational approach than laminectomy. Harrington instrumentation may be used for instability of the thoracic or lumbar spine secondary to injury or laminectomy, or both. Two Harrington distraction rods are used as a spinal traction system. A padded Taylor spinal brace or Jewett brace is applied a few days postoperatively.

Harrington instrumentation was used to treat 23 patients with thoracolumbar spine injury and neural damage in 1966–75; 16 of the patients were males. All patients but 2 were in the 2d through 4th decades of life. Twelve were injured in automobile accidents and 7 were struck by falling objects. Three patients had stable injuries. Twelve had incomplete spinal cord lesions and 1 had a cauda equina lesion. All but 1 of these 13 patients improved postoperatively. None of the 10 complete lesions was altered but no patient was worse after operation. Eighteen patients had laminectomy. Nine patients had serious concomitant injuries and 7 had serious complications recorded during the acute hospital stay. The total acute stay averaged 51.1 days; follow-up averaged 31.2 months. Only 1 patient had a complication from the instrumentation itself, pseudarthrosis of the spinal fusion.

Harrington instrumentation for the treatment of injuries in the thoracic and lumbar spine offers the strongest system of internal fixation available today. It also offers the only system of internal fixation that permits active correction of nearly all traumatic deformities of the spine at the time of surgery.

▶ [The French and other European neurosurgeons are much more prone than Americans to use metal plates and screws to hold together vertebrae, especially after posterior decompression. This is illustrated by Blahavitch et al. (Neurochirurgie 21:447, 1975), whose thesis deals with return of pain perception as an indicator of return of motor function. They claim the latter never occurs without return of pain sensation.

Similar internal fixation is useful for stabilization of the spine after decompressive procedures on tumors of the spine (Brunon et al.: ibid., p. 435).

Not only is the anterior approach increasingly being used for chronic protrusions of disks and infections, but Weiss et al. (Bull. Los Angeles Neurol. Soc. 40:112, 1975) have found it helpful in 6 cases of acute spinal cord compression in the area from T1 to L1. Three cases were of disk protrusion due to trauma and 1 each was due to tuberculosis, coccidioidomy-

cosis and neuroblastoma. A right-sided approach is used above the car-
diophrenic level and a left-sided one, below that level. — Ed.] ◄

Local Cooling in Spinal Cord Injury. Complete destruction of cord segments, responsible for irreversible paraplegia or tetraplegia, often does not occur at the moment of
impact but is related to a type of self-destructive process in
the cord that may be evolutionary in nature. Experimental
local hypothermia has proved effective in reducing neurologic impairment from acute cord injury. A. Bricolo, G. Dalle
Ore, R. Da Pian and F. Faccioli[3] (Verona, Italy) evaluated
hypothermic stabilization of the injured spinal cord in 8 patients with acute cord injuries at different levels. Early laminectomy was done and the subdural space was irrigated
with saline at 5 C for about 2 hours. Five patients received
local epidural cooling for a few days after the surgical
wound was closed. Subdural irrigation was with a 50% solution of ethyl alcohol in water.

All patients initially had a complete loss of cord function
below the injured segment. Four had cervical, 2 had upper
dorsal and 2 had lower dorsal injuries. Cervical dislocations
were managed by skull traction and all patients received
dexamethasone, antifibrinolytic agents and reserpine. The
interval from injury to the start of cooling ranged from 7 to
26 hours. Two of the 3 patients who died had cervical lesions
and severe pulmonary complications and 1 had severe cerebral lesions. Four patients did not improve but 4 positive
results were obtained; 1 patient recovered completely. All
clinical recoveries were associated with an improvement in
sensory cortical evoked potentials from segments below the
level of injury. In the patients with permanent paraplegia,
somatosensory evoked responses were definitely absent
from the 2d day on.

These results agree with experimental observations and
appear to justify the use of this procedure in human beings.
Results of the evoked response studies support the view that
the presence of a response after injury excludes complete
transection of the spinal cord.

► [The use of steroids and hypothermia in experimental spinal cord injury in dogs, reported by Kuchner and Hansebout (Surg. Neurol. 6:371,
1976), reemphasizes the value of this combination of therapies, neither of
which is thought to be superior to the other. I am amused at their state-

(3) Surg. Neurol. 6:101–106, August, 1976.

ment, "An evaluation of the efficacy of a combination of these two modalities has not been previously reported"; their own 1975 article on this subject, with C. Romero-Sierra as a co-author, appeared in the 1977 YEAR BOOK (p. 352).

Caccia et al. (J. Neurol. Neurosurg. Psychiatry 39:962, 1976) describe spinal evoked responses recorded extradurally after stimulation of mixed limb nerves in 22 subjects. In all the cases of noncompressive systemic myelopathy, the evoked potentials were normal; in those with cord compression, they were depressed or absent. — Ed.] ◄

Spectrum of the Hangman's Fracture. The hangman's fracture, a bilateral avulsion fracture of the C2 arch and an anterior fracture-dislocation of the axis through the C2 – C3 interspace, is believed to be due to acute hyperextension of the mandible and skull on the upper cervical spine, but casual study of lateral x-rays may erroneously indicate a fracture in flexion. Edward L. Seljeskog and Shelley N. Chou[4] (Univ. of Minnesota) treated 26 cases of hangman's fracture during 1966 – 74. The injuries were sustained mainly from automobile accidents. Many associated injuries were present, including mandibular fractures and contusions about the mandible and face. Only 1 acute postfracture death occurred, presumably related to respiratory failure. Two patients had an incomplete cord injury and both recovered almost completely. The radiographic appearances ranged from the classic avulsion fracture of the C2 arch and significant anterolisthesis of the C2 vertebral body to an isolated C2 laminar-pedicle fracture without arch avulsion or vertebral subluxation; several subtypes were seen.

Most patients had reduction and immobilization with skeletal traction, followed by a period of bracing or, more recently, halo casting. More unstable fractures required longer immbolization. Patients with significant subluxation and avulsion of the C2 arch generally were immobilized for 4 – 6 weeks in skeletal traction and then supported for several months by a heavy brace. Halo-cast stabilization was used for 4 – 6 weeks. Avulsion fractures of the C2 arch alone are well managed by the halo cast without previous skeletal traction. Stable, isolated laminar-pedicle fractures probably are best managed by direct immobilization by a heavy brace. One patient with significant instability had posterior fusion. Twenty-two patients have had spontaneous, solid

(4)   J. Neurosurg. 45:3 – 8, July, 1976.

fracture healing with little or no postinjury morbidity. Cervical spine motion has been adequate except in 2 patients with mild limitation of rotatory movement. There have been no neurologic sequelae. One patient died before treatment was begun and 2 died of unrelated causes.

The halo cast, where applicable, is useful because prolonged bed rest and hospitalization are avoided and early ambulation is possible once the fracture has been reduced by more conventional methods. It also provides excellent fracture immobilization, allowing earlier and more solid bone union.

The authors did not use an anterior route to stabilize C2–C3 subluxations associated with these fractures, for fear of accentuating problems by mandibular retraction and cervical hyperextension, mimicking the original type of injury.

Disk Disease and Spondylosis

A Neurosurgeon Looks at Spinal Conditions. Harold Schaeffer[5] (Adelaide, Australia) discusses a number of spinal conditions from a neurosurgeon's viewpoint. The many "failures" of back surgery or other treatment seen in practice generally relate to basic errors of judgment in patient selection, errors that usually are a result of a tendency to concentrate on the back area itself and to ignore the person as a whole. Many patients have psychosomatic illnesses and tend to see their essentially psychologic problems in physical terms. Patients with genuine back conditions, especially those with acute lumbar disk herniation, nearly always present in a classic manner. The interpretation of clinical signs and a general assessment of the patient's personality are extremely important. Diskography is not recommended in evaluating these patients since many degenerating disks are asymptomatic. Physiotherapy can help only when the diagnosis is not one of ruptured lumbar disk. The occasional indifferent results of lumbar disk surgery can often be ascribed to lengthy conservative treatment, since a nerve root can become bound up with scar tissue. There is no logical basis for treating back pain by percutaneous denervation of spinal joints.

Late symptoms of "whiplash" injury are presumably nonorganic in type and arise in part from psychosomatic factors, compensation claims and a sense of grievance. The author has not seen genuine radicular brachialgia arising from a "whiplash" type of injury. True brachialgia is managed by removing the disk and osteophytes to decompress the nerve root. Severe brachialgia disappears after a radical Cloward operation, and this operation is also valuable in cases of cervical myelopathy where cord compression is caused by central osteophytes. The Cloward procedure can also be used to stabilize cervical fracture-dislocations. Diskography is

(5) Med. J. Aust. 1:267–269, Feb. 28, 1976.

valueless in the cervical area as well as in the lumbar area. Benign intradural spinal tumors often present in elderly patients and surgical extirpation may give good results. The use of magnification techniques has helped in the surgical treatment of certain arteriovenous malformations of the spinal cord. Extradural abscess is a neurosurgical emergency; management is by urgent myelography and spinal decompression, which often must include many laminae. Whatever the cause of spinal compression, once paraplegia is total it is irreversible; if treatment is possible it must be instituted before paraplegia becomes complete.

▶ [Schaeffer's opinions are not such as to leave the reader in doubt. Whether or not they are all based on logical grounds is another matter. It is true, for instance, that plain x-ray films are of little value in the diagnosis of lumbar disk herniations; however, they help rule in or out conditions (such as metastatic carcinoma or spondylolisthesis) that may mimic disk herniation. Rest and repeated observation are certainly basic to treatment; the uselessness of physical therapy in patients with lumbar disk hernia is moot, because Schaeffer does not define what is meant by physical therapy and refers to manipulation as a possible source of adverse results (with which I agree—but some of my patients proclaim that acute attacks have been overcome by chiropractic manipulation—temporarily, or else they would never have come to see me). Schaeffer's views on operations on spinal gliomas, "There is still little that can be done for spinal cord gliomas," are obviously subject to much contradiction from those who have successfully removed ependymomas with good results (or have given radiation therapy). Nonetheless, the article is worthwhile, if only to induce renewed thinking about ancient problems. — Ed.] ◀

Double-Blind Evaluation of Intradiscal Chymopapain for Herniated Lumbar Disks: Early Results. Successful results of intradiscal chymopapain injection have been reported in 50–80% of patients treated for lumbar disk disease, but the method has not been evaluated in carefully controlled trials. P. Robert Schwetschenau, Archimedes Ramirez, James Johnston, Elnora Barnes, Charles Wiggs and Albert N. Martins[6] (Walter Reed Army Med. Center, Washington, D. C.) assessed the effects of chemonucleolysis in 130 patients hospitalized during 1974–75 with a diagnosis of herniated lumbar disk. No patient had previously had surgery or chemonucleolysis. The age range was 18–65 years. Symptoms had been treated conservatively for at least 3 weeks without significant improvement. All patients had myelographic abnormality and signs of disk herniation.

(6)   J. Neurosurg. 45:622–627, December, 1976.

Patients with acute paralysis or loss of sphincter control were excluded from the study, as were those with compensation claims pending.

Hydrocortisone and Benadryl were administered before local anesthesia and chemonucleolysis under image intensification fluoroscopy. Discography was performed with 60% Conray to verify the position of the needle within the disk. The level indicated as abnormal by the myelogram was injected in all cases. Either 20 mg chymopapain or placebo in cysteine and disodium edetate solution was injected in a volume of 1 ml. Of the 66 patients in the study, 31 received chymopapain and 35, placebo. The groups were comparable in age, duration of complaints, previous treatment and the levels injected. Follow-up ranged from 2 to 11 months. There was no significant difference in success rates with the active treatment and placebo. The overall success rate was 49% for active-duty personnel and 57% for civilians. No complications or adverse reactions were observed.

Chymopapain was no better than placebo in relieving symptoms of herniated lumbar disk in this study. Most, if not all, of the apparent efficacy of chemonucleolysis may be due to a placebo effect. The criteria for laminectomy may be too liberal, and proper controls are needed to assess accurately the value of any treatment for symptomatic disk disease. Any new enzyme advocated for disk dissolution should be part of a controlled double-blind therapeutic trial initially.

► [Chymopapain is not yet a dead issue. Patients still ask for it, and some are being sent to Mexico and to Canada for injections. The discussion in this article implicates placebo and double-blind technique as essential items in the beginning of any future study of enzymes for disk dissolution. The success of epidural steroid injections in symptomatic relief of patients with disk syndromes is another cause for wonder as to what injections into the back really do. – Ed.] ◄

Lumbar Thermography in Discogenic Disease. Michael M. Raskin, Manuel Martinez-Lopez and Jerome J. Sheldon[7] (Univ. of Miami) evaluated lumbar thermography as a potential means of screening patients with clinical lumbar disk symptoms. Thermograms were obtained using a commercial unit in 82 consecutive patients who underwent myelography immediately afterward.

There were equal numbers of men and women aged

(7)   Radiology 119:149–152, April, 1976.

20–82 in the study. Sixty patients had clinical lumbar disk symptoms and 12 had cervical symptoms. Six had vertebral body metastases in the thoracic area. Normal lumbar thermographic patterns were determined in 85 asymptomatic subjects aged 18–75. Twelve patients with cervical symptoms but normal lumbar myelograms were also examined. Studies were done in a temperature-compensated room kept at 20 C. The erect patient was examined from the lower thoracic spine to the midportion of the buttocks at two different sensitivity settings.

Constant areas of increased infrared emission on normal thermograms included the spinous processes, the upper sacroiliac joints, an area between the lower lumbar and sacroiliac areas and an area just medial to the sacroiliac area (Fig 18). Twenty-four of 38 patients with lumbar disk symptoms had a herniated lumbar disk confirmed at surgery; 14 had spinal stenosis. A positive thermogram showed a focal area of increased infrared emission in the lower lumbar spine. Myelograms were accurate in 88% and thermograms in 71% of the patients with proved herniated lumbar disk. Thermograms were positive in 3 of the 14 patients with proved spinal stenosis and myelograms were diagnostic in 10 of these

Fig 18.–**A,** lumbar thermogram shows focal area of increased infrared emission (*arrow*) on right. **B,** lumbar myelogram shows effacement of nerve root on right by herniated intervertebral disk at L5–S1. (Courtesy of Raskin, M. M., et al.: Radiology 119:149–152, April, 1976.)

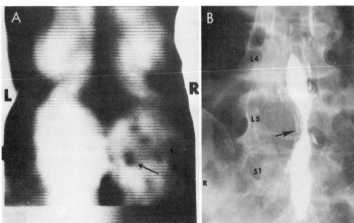

patients. Thermography was nearly as accurate at myelography in determining levels of herniated disks at the L4–L5 interspace but it was decidedly inferior at the L5–S1 interspace. Positive thermogram rates in patients not operated on were essentially the same as in the surgically confirmed group.

Lumbar thermography may be a useful procedure for patients with clinical disk symptoms. If the thermogram is positive, the probability of a normal lumbar myelogram is small; however, the myelographic findings cannot be predicted by a negative thermogram.

Challenge of Arteriovenous Fistula Formation Following Disk Surgery: Collective Review. Sixty-eight cases of arteriovenous fistula formation secondary to disk operations have been reported in the English-language literature. Bruce S. Jarstfer (Brooke Army Med. Center) and Norman M. Rich[8] (Walter Reed Army Med. Center) add 5 cases to those previously reported and review the 73 reported cases. The L4–L5 disk space was involved 35 times in the 48 evaluable cases and the L5–S1 interspace 13 times. Four patients (8.7%) had had reoperation on the incriminated interspace. There were 49 common iliac artery and 5 aortic injuries. The inferior vena cava was injured in about 30% of cases and the common iliac vein in about 70%.

Nearly 30% of patients bled from the disk space during operation; 10 patients became hypotensive. Symptoms of fistula appeared within a month of diskectomy in over 50% of the cases and within 6 months in 70%. Cardiorespiratory problems occurred in about half the patients. Only 3 patients were asymptomatic. Only 2 had significant lower-extremity pulse abnormalities. Venous injury was most often repaired by lateral suture of the defect. Numerous methods of arterial repair were used. Six patients died of arteriovenous fistula secondary to surgery (8.2%) and 5 postoperatively, for an operative mortality of 6.9%. Twelve survivors (18%) had complications of operation.

Intraoperative injury usually was not associated with significant hemodynamic changes suggesting its presence in this series of patients. The right common iliac artery was injured most frequently. Cardiorespiratory symptoms or

(8)   J. Trauma 16:726–733, September, 1976.

findings were the most common presentation leading to diagnosis. The overall mortality was 8.2%. Early repair of an arteriovenous fistula resulting from disk surgery is indicated and both arterial and venous lesions should be repaired. It may not be possible to determine the location of the fistula accurately until operation is carried out.

► [In some of these cases, review showed other injuries, including those to the ureter, ileojejunum and other areas of the small bowel, including complete transsection of the ileum; in 1 case, the base of the transsected appendix was found in the margin of the disk space! A biting instrument, such as a pituitary rongeur, was most often implicated. Hiccuping with arching of the back sometimes caused the instrument to go too deep. Placing items under the abdomen potentially increases compression of the great vessels and increases the likelihood of injury. The proximity of the right iliac vessels, inferior vena cava and left common iliac vessels to the L4–L5 disk space suggests the reason for most injuries occurring to these vessels (89.9%) and at that disk space (72.9%). – Ed.] ◄

Division of the Piriform Muscle for the Treatment of Sciatica: Postlaminectomy Syndrome and Osteoarthritis of the Spine. In 1937, Freiberg advocated sectioning the piriform muscle to treat sciatica where the cause could not be found. Principally, this muscle is one of external rotation of the hip when in extension and of abduction with the hip in flexion. Its division is intended to relieve impingement on the sciatic nerve. The efficacy of pain relief is directly proportional to tension relief on the nerve itself, which depends largely on the degree of compression or adhesions of the nerve roots in the spine. Tomoji Mizuguchi[9] (VA Hosp., Des Moines, Ia.) performed division of the piriform muscle at its tendinous insertion on the greater trochanter in 14 patients during 1974–75. Six patients had sciatica after laminectomy and 8 had sciatica associated with spinal osteoarthritis; 3 of the latter patients also had narrow spinal canals. The average age was 48.5 years; average duration of low back pain was 9.5 years in the first group and 14.6 years in the second. Neurologic manifestations were quite variable. Eight laminectomies had been done previously in the first group. A posterior modified Osborne approach was used in the 16 operations.

Four postlaminectomy patients and 6 with osteoarthritis had excellent results and 1 in each group had good results. Immediate pain relief was obtained in all patients but 1.

(9) Arch. Surg. 111:719–722, June, 1976.

One patient with a poor result had had 2 laminectomies and showed a complete block on myelography at the L2 – L3 level; after piriform muscle division, pain was relieved from the buttock to the knee, but pain recurred and was relieved by a decompression laminectomy at L5. The second patient with a poor result had advanced osteoarthritis with a narrow spinal canal and also needed decompression laminectomy after piriform muscle division to relieve recurrent pain. The average follow-up has been 12 weeks, with a range of from 5 to 40 weeks.

The early results of piriform muscle division have been gratifying, though follow-up is short. This is a simple and safe procedure that causes minimal functional loss; it might also be beneficial in some well-selected patients with sciatica due to herniated lumbar disks, especially at the L4 – L5 and L5 – S1 levels.

► [The modified Osborne approach referred to in this article has to do with the patient in the lateral position leaning 10 – 15 degrees forward. Incision is made 5 cm distal and lateral to the posterior superior iliac spine and is carried to the superolateral portion of the greater trochanter, then curved distally for 2 cm. The gluteus maximus is separated parallel to the line of the skin incision and the pyriform muscle is isolated under the inferior margin of the gluteus medius. After the sciatic nerve is exposed, the muscle is divided at the trochanter and freed to the sciatic foramen to release impingement on the sciatic nerve. Stauffer's editorial comment (Arch. Surg. 111:722, 1976) printed with this article expresses interest, caution and hope for long-term follow-up. Cases to be considered include those with seemingly true radicular pain in the leg, without objective findings and with negative myelogram (and presumably with negative epidural venogram). – Ed.] ◄

Narrow Lumbar Spinal Canal. The significance of a narrow lumbar spinal canal has been relatively neglected. Rhondda M. Williams[1] (Prince Henry Hosp., Sydney) describes a simple method of assessing the approximate size of the lumbar spinal canal.

The Jones and Thomson method of determining the relative size of the canal was used. The anteroposterior (AP) diameter and interpedicular distance are measured and are related to vertebral body size on plain lumbar spine x-rays. Correction for magnification is unnecessary. Slight errors in estimating the posterior margin of the canal do not alter the ratio much. The AP canal measurement is multiplied by the

(1) Australas. Radiol. 19:356 – 360, December, 1975.

interpedicular distance and used as a ratio with AP×transverse diameters of the same vertebral body.

Measurements were made on the plain films of 100 consecutive myelograms made during 1973–74. The range was between 1:2.5 and 1:8. The mean ± 1 SD was 1:3 to 1:6 for L3 and L4 and 1:3.2 to 1:6.5 for L5. A canal was significantly narrow if the ratio was above 1:6 for L3 and L4 and above 1:6.5 for L5. Three patients had significantly narrow canals at all three levels. The normal range of Jones and Thomson was 1:2.5 to 1:4.5; different patient selection may account for the difference from the present findings.

Primary narrowing of the lumbar spinal canal is important, since any further slight decrease in capacity of the canal will cause significant cauda equina compression. It is important to recognize a narrow canal before myelography, because lumbar puncture and removal of contrast medium usually are quite difficult. Long-term conservative management of the narrow canal is unrewarding. If operation is contemplated, a more radical approach with multiple laminectomies should be planned; these alone often are difficult because of thickened laminae and encroachment of the posterior joints on the midline.

► [Salibi reviewed the syndromes of neurogenic intermittent claudication and stenosis of the lumbar canal (Surg. Neurol. 5:269, 1976). He found 13 instances of the postural form of claudication, 3 of the ischemic form and 2 of both types in a series of 20 consecutive cases of lumbar spinal stenosis. Operation done in 16 patients was wide bilateral laminectomy and partical facetectomy; in 3 with unilateral myelographic deformities, unilateral laminectomy was done. One woman refused operation. Full return to premorbid activities occurred in 14 and partial return in 4; 1 patient was more comfortable but not rehabilitated.

We anticipate that further improvements in computerized tomography will yield accurate pictures of the cross-sectional anatomy of the lumbar spine and help clarify the role of such abnormalities as have been described already.—Ed.] ◄

Influence of Laminectomy on the Course of Cervical Myelopathy was studied by K. Gorter[2] (Univ. of Groningen). Cervical myelopathy resulting from spondylarthrosis of the cervical spine still presents a pathogenetic and surgical problem. Cord compression in a narrow canal can occur intermittently by a "pincers" mechanism as the posterior spinal artery circulation is impaired by bulging of the liga-

(2) Acta Neurochir. (Wien) 33:265–281, 1976.

menta flava and dura. In a narrow canal, the slowly expanding disk protrusion may eventually compress the feeding radicular arteries. In a normal-sized canal, multiple disk protrusions can cause flexion of the cord over the hard bars and overstretching of the long-tract axons. Extension injury to a spondylotic cervical spine compresses the radicular arteries and precipitates myelopathic lesions.

Review was made of the surgical results obtained in 75 patients having operations in 1957–71, 54 men and 21 women with a mean age of 53.9 on admission. A history of trauma was obtained in 20 patients. Thirty-eight patients had limited laminectomy and 37 the Aboulker procedure. Improvement occurred in 51.4% and 66.6% of patients, respectively. Paresis of the lower extremities had predominated in both groups, and in both groups the upper extremities recovered more than the lower. Micturition disorders responded better after limited laminectomy. Overall improvement was comparable after the two procedures. In both groups, a narrow canal was related to improvement and younger patients showed more improvement than older ones. In the Aboulker group, a shorter history of symptoms was associated with better results of decompression. Pain relief was more evident in men than in women.

Limited laminectomy and total laminectomy by the Aboulker procedure gave comparable improvement in this series of patients with cervical myelopathy. Surgery should be considered as soon as possible after neurologic signs appear if conservative treatment fails. Where localized spinal canal narrowing is present at one level, limited laminectomy at this site is preferable. Only if extensive spondylosis with disk protrusions at several levels is present along with narrowing of the canal is total laminectomy indicated. If there is no evidence of a subarachnoid block, ventral or anterolateral fusion of the appropriate segments is preferred to laminectomy. Older patients should not be operated on unless they are close to becoming totally incapacitated by paresis of the lower extremities.

▶ [The Aboulker technique (1965) includes an extensive laminectomy from C1 to T1, with the dura remaining unopened. – Ed.] ◀

Late Results of Cervical Disk Surgery. William Beecher Scoville, George J. Dohrmann and Guy Corkill[3]

(3)   J. Neurosurg. 45:203–210, August, 1976.

(Hartford, Conn.) reviewed the late results of operation for cervical disk disease in 383 patients operated on since 1941. Follow-up was possible in 296 cases, and in 208 it ranged from 5 to 33 years. Thirty patients were followed for 20 years or longer and 76 for 10–20 years. Lateral disk protrusions were present in 83% of cases, the central bar ridge spondylosis type in 13% and the central soft disk type in 4%. Fracture-dislocations with disk protrusion were excluded from study.

Lateral disk lesions were treated by partial facetectomy and separation and retraction of nerve root sleeves. Osteophytes were removed only if extremely large. Lateral disk protrusions were of the soft type in 72% of cases and were hard osteophytes in 28%. One third of the patients were active within 2 weeks; the average time was 4.2 weeks. Continuing complaints were minor and included paresthesias and mild pain. Older patients did somewhat better than younger ones. Other disk herniations requiring operation developed in 19% of these patients.

Either an anterior or posterior approach can be used in cases of central cervical spondylosis. Spondylosis occurred at the midcervical spine. The results were not as good as in patients with lateral disk lesions but 64% of the patients had good-to-excellent results and 3 were clinically cured. Five patients had minor adverse effects from operation. Operation revealed central or paracentral ruptures in 11 patients; all but 1 of these patients had good results. The ideal approach should be via an anterior diskectomy, but diagnostic operations often are done from a posterior approach. The preferred posterior procedure consists of limited laminectomy with unilateral facetectomy and combined intra- and extradural removal of a soft central disk.

There were no recurrences or serious complications in this series, although 20% of patients acquired other cervical or lumbar disk herniations. More recently, the first catastrophic air embolism in 37 years of surgery occurred, without a fall in blood pressure.

Anterior Cervical Diskectomy with and without Interbody Bone Graft. Some studies have shown that cervical disk disease can be treated adequately by anterior diskectomy alone, questioning the need for a bone graft to be inserted at the diskectomy site. Albert N. Martins[4] (Walter Reed Army Med. Center) attempted to resolve this issue in a series of 51 patients with symptomatic cervical disk disease refractory to conservative management.

Neck pain alone generally was not an indication for operation. The patients had disk disease at one or two levels between C4 and C7; long tract signs did not lead to exclusion from the series. Patients were allocated at random to treatment by the Cloward anterior approach as modified by Kempe or to radical diskectomy and foraminotomy. Twenty-five patients had the Cloward procedure and 26, diskectomy; the respective average ages were 48.8 and 44 years. Signs, radiographic findings and the distribution of operated disk levels were comparable in both groups. Twenty-three patients have been followed for 1 year or longer after operation.

Diskectomy was as successful in relieving symptoms as the Cloward procedure for patients with two-level disease. No patient was made worse by operation. Hospitalization periods were similar for both surgical groups. Bone bridged the site of disk removal in all 12 Cloward cases and in 7 of 11 diskectomy cases 1 year postoperatively. Cervical spine alignment was better after the Cloward procedure, but the alignment obtained was not consistently related to the clinical results and alignment tended to improve with time in the diskectomy group. The 1 major complication was a prevertebral *Staphylococcus aureus* infection at the diskectomy site. Diskectomy was technically more difficult than the Cloward procedure in patients with advanced spondylosis. In patients with minimal spondylosis, diskectomy generally was completed more quickly than the Cloward procedure.

Anterior cervical diskectomies with and without interbody bone grafting are safe and effective procedures for relieving recalcitrant symptoms of cervical disk disease at one or two levels between C4 and C7. Diskectomy is more suitable for patients with soft disk herniations and the Cloward procedure for patients with advanced spondylosis.

► [Long-term follow-up is still the key to the problem in anterior cervical disk operations: to fuse or not to fuse. With Cloward's operation, active

――――――――――

(4)   J. Neurosurg. 44:290–295, March, 1976.

people may develop apparently new spondylosis at the levels above and below the fused region. With the nonfusion operation, I am concerned about the decreased diameter of the intervertebral foramen and the anticipated slipping of the zygapophyseal joints to produce a true degenerative arthritis—if fusion does not take place in a reasonable length of time.

Although the subject of the article on the superior laryngeal nerve by Droulias et al. is concerned with thyroidectomy, I believe it is important for those who operate via an anterior approach to cervical spine disease to know about this nerve that passes medial to the carotid arteries and divides at the level of the hyoid bone into a large sensory internal laryngeal nerve and a smaller external nerve to the cricothyroid muscle. The latter passes with the superior thyroid vein and artery to lie outside the thyroid sheath close to the inferior pharyngeal constrictor muscle. Injury causes voice change due to loss of adduction and tension of the ipsilateral vocal cord. Added to this is the anatomical fact that the recurrent laryngeal nerve sometimes is not recurrent but comes off the vagus nerve and goes directly to the larynx; therefore, one can understand why (especially with high disk operations) one should warn the patient of the possibility of voice change (luckily usually transient). — Ed.] ◄

Tumors

▶ At the New York University-Bellevue Medical Center, from 1964 to 1973 there were 20 cases of chordoma. Firooznia et al. (Am. J. Roentgenol. 127: 797, 1976) describe 4 intracranial, 8 vertebral and 8 sacrococcygeal chordoma cases. In the last two groups, the striking feature is the presence of multiple asymmetric adjacent vertebral body destruction associated with involvement of the intervening disk spaces. Osteosclerosis is often seen, primarily in the periphery of the lytic lesion. Osteomyelitis is the most difficult diagnosis. The cranial chordomas are usually confused with pituitary tumor and craniopharyngioma unless there is erosion of the clivus, calcification and nasopharyngeal mass. Irradiation may lengthen survival, but the prognosis of cranial chordoma is poor (4 – 5 years). Sacrococcygeal masses are best treated by combined operation and irradiation.

Although it is common for neurosurgeons to approach intracranial chordoma by a frontal approach to the pituitary area, this does not appear to allow a definitive cure. Transpalatal approach also only permits partial removal, but has the merit, according to Tarshis and Briant (J. Otolaryngol. 5:243, 1976) of repeated decompressions without more dangerous craniotomy. – Ed. ◀

Stereotactic Investigations in Cerebral Tumors were carried out by J. M. Scarabin, J. Pecker, J. Simon and J. Fradin[5] (Rennes, France). Stereotactic explorations have numerous advantages: tridimensional analysis of different vascular pedicles, precise identification of structures with which the tumors and some cortical loops are related, early demonstration of minimal pathologic displacements, histologic diagnosis of space-occupying processes, elaboration of a detailed surgical procedure and, finally, radiologic control of such conditions in every operation.

Techniques have been perfected, especially in radiology. A type of craniograph called "Neurocentrix" with an isocentric chair is used. It is equipped with two film changers and an incorporated brightness amplifier: one is mobile and slides on a pulley for the frontal view; for the lateral view, the other is fixed to the center of the ring. Two fixed tubes (frontal and lateral views) are arranged 5 m apart; enlargement is thus negligible. All investigations included at least

---

(5)   Ann. Radiol. (Paris) 19:253 – 262, Mar. – Apri., 1976.

bilateral carotid arteriography and fractional gas encephalography.

Five cases illustrated the possibilities of this method.

CASE 1.—Woman, 34, had an intracranial hypertension syndrome and a bilateral cerebellar syndrome. Stereotactic investigation permitted complete angiographic screening by the femoral route (carotid and vertebral) and intraventricular measuring. The large epidermoid cyst of the vermis made remarkably modest displacements. Nevertheless, the existence of a bordering vessel, shown in the lateral view, delimited the anterior part of this lesion.

This case showed that it was possible, under rigorous stereotactic conditions, to investigate a tumor of the posterior fossa. It also demonstrated the advantages of superposition of the vascular and ventricular data.

The other cases were a pinealoma in a child aged 10 years, a noncommunicating cyst of the septum in a man aged 25, an astrocytoma of the lower rolandic region in a woman aged 25 and bilateral optic atrophy plus left hemiparesis, predominantly in the upper limb, in a child aged 2 years.

The great variability in form and size of the brain led Talairach to propose a nonmillimetric, proportional type of reference system for supratentorial structures. This system, using the line between the anterior and posterior commissures (CA-CP) and its perpendicular lines, allows gathering all information in a single reference unit. Two electronic systems were used to do this. With their aid, one can easily carry out a statistical study of different vascular courses and use the reference procedures described in the literature. Computerization of neuroanatomical and neuroradiologic images is being undertaken to permit comparison with one or several experimental models that could be set up as standards.

▶ [The three articles preceding this one in *Annales de Radiologie* also deal with stereotactic technique in relation to cerebral tumors. Sindou et al. (Ann. Radiol. (Paris) 19:227, 1976) describe multicontact electrodes to be inserted at right angles to the cortex, permitting total transcortical recording (from depth to surface), called "transcorticography," or recording from various layers of cortex between adjacent contacts, called "straticorticography." The latter is said to be of value in finding small tumors under a macroscopically normal cortex. In the immediate vicinity of a tumor, the cortex shows slow rhythms, sometimes of microvolt amplitude, produced by pyramidal intracortical generators. The closer the electrode is to the tumor, the less likely are alpha rhythms to be found.

Laitinen of Helsinki has carried out stereoelectroencephalography and also measurements of cerebral impedance (ibid., p. 237). These often are more accurate for intended cerebral biopsy than angiography, pneumography and scintigraphy. Biopsy specimens are taken with a thin forceps 25 cm long and 2 mm in diameter, using regions where the electric activity is absent.

Pneumography using a somersaulting chair is extremely valuable for Waltregny (ibid., p. 241), in conjunction with scintigraphy and electroencephalography by deep electrodes, to permit deep biopsies of brain tumors. Puncture of deeply lying cysts and differentiation of these from fleshy tumors are possible with stereotactic techniques. Injection of ^{32}P-colloid beta emitters can be used for cystic tumors, and ^{198}Au can be used for solid tumor irradiation. – Ed.] ◄

Lateral-Trigonal Intraventricular Tumors: New Operative Approach is described by L. G. Kempe and R. Blaylock[6] (Univ. of South Carolina). Truly intraventricular tumors are rare lesions. The clinical picture is

Fig 19. – Operative approach to removal of intraventricular tumors. (Courtesy of Kempe, L. G., and Blaylock, R.: Acta Neurochir. (Wien) 35:233 – 242, 1976; Berlin-Heidelberg-New York: Springer.)

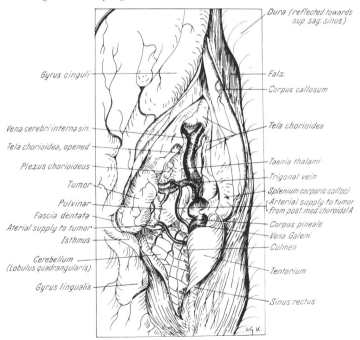

(6) Acta Neurochir. (Wien) 35:233 – 242, 1976.

not striking, symptoms may be extremely vague. The only symptom with localizing value that is not infrequently present is visual field defect or hemianopsia. The tumor is supplied by the choroidal arteries, especially the posterior median and lateral choroidal arteries. Extremely small intraventricular lesions may be discovered at computerized axial tomographic study. Three patients with tumors within the dominant left hemisphere have been treated.

A craniotomy is made over the parietal and occipital bones in the seated patient, under general endotracheal anesthesia and controlled ventilation. The craniotomy must reach over the sagittal sinus. The entire splenium and posterior corpus callosum are divided, either bluntly or by fine suction, and the arachnoid is opened posteriorly with the use of the surgical microscope or loops and 4-power magnification. The entire arachnoid paralleling the left internal cerebral vein should be opened before the brain retractor is readjusted (Fig 19). It is helpful to insert a silk suture through the exposed tumor to move it and identify its base. It may be necessary to divide the choroid plexus by clipping and bipolar coagulation, starting at the part of the choroid plexus leading over the thalamus. The tumor is moved medially and elevated to identify branches of the posterior lateral choroidal artery. Freeing the choroid plexus by tearing it bluntly may permit the tumor to be mobilized without making more than one adjustment of the retraction of the lateral hemisphere.

Use of this operative approach in 3 patients with atrial trigonal meningioma of the dominant hemisphere did not result in any neurologic deficit that was not present before surgery. The procedure abolished paroxysmal attacks of hemianopsia and severe headaches in 1 patient, who was believed to have had migraine for 2½ years.

Pulmonary Neoplasm with Solitary Cerebral Metastasis: Results of Combined Excision. In 1954, Knights suggested that a solitary cerebral metastasis of lung cancer may occasionally be removed successfully along with the primary, with prolongation of life resulting. Donald J. Magilligan, Jr., J. Speed Rogers, Robert S. Knighton and Julio C. Davila[7] (Henry Ford Hosp.) reviewed data on 22 patients

(7) J. Thorac. Cardiovasc. Surg. 72:690–698, November, 1976.

in whom a primary pulmonary neoplasm was resected and removal of a solitary cerebral metastasis attempted during 1960–75.

All patients but 1 had cerebral angiography, and 2 had bilateral studies. A solitary tumor was identified in 20 patients, whereas another had a cerebellar tumor and 1 with a cerebellar tumor was not examined. The EEG was abnormal in 19 of 21 patients and brain scan findings were abnormal in 17 of 19 patients. Pneumoencephalography localized cerebellar tumors in the 2 patients examined. The 15 men and 7 women had an average age of 54.8.

Seven patients lived longer than a year after craniotomy and had continued improvement in neurologic symptoms for at least this long. Three of them are alive and without significant symptoms after 25–42 months. Three patients had a second craniotomy for recurrence after several months, with subsequent symptom-free periods of at least 1 year. Five patients lived at least 9 months after craniotomy and were free of significant symptoms for at least 6 months. Three died of recurrent brain metastasis. Ten patients lived less than 6 months after craniotomy or were symptom free for less than 6 months and were considered to have had less satisfactory results. The average survival time after thoracotomy was 8 months; after craniotomy it was about 5 months. Half the patients were symptom free for at least 3 months. Four of 9 patients with stage I disease had good results from craniotomy. Radiotherapy to the brain, especially in conjunction with surgery, appeared to affect the prognosis favorably, as did a longer interval between pulmonary resection and the appearance of cerebral symptoms.

Excision of a solitary cerebral metastasis had a low operative mortality in this series and relieved severe neurologic symptoms for at least 3 months in 77% of the patients. Combined with pulmonary resection, the procedure prolonged life and improved the quality of life in most patients. The results encourage an aggressive surgical approach to pulmonary neoplasia with solitary cerebral metastasis.

▶ [Mosberg (J.A.M.A. 235:2745, 1976) removed a solitary metastasis from the left parietal region of a man, aged 42, in 1964. Right lobectomy removed pulmonary carcinoma of the same type as the metastasis. The patient is still doing well after 12 years.

Review of autopsies at the University of Michigan Hospitals allowed Teears and Silverman (Cancer 36:216, 1975) to collect 88 cases of carcinoma metastatic to the pituitary gland. These deposits were not grossly evident in about three fourths of the cases. Metastases most often occurred in the posterior lobe. Such hidden metastases might well account for the poor result of craniotomy in some patients with pulmonary carcinoma metastasis.

One would anticipate that brain tumor present at the same time as a mass in the chest would be a metastasis, or, less commonly, an independent lesion. In the case reported by Hulbanni and Goodman (ibid. 37:1577, 1976), the histologic appearance of the lung and brain tumors was the same—namely, glioblastoma multiforme! Invasion of cerebral vessels by tumor was demonstrable and embolizaton was presumably the mode of spread, because there was no surgical intervention.—Ed.] ◄

Cerebral Tumor with Intracranial Angioma. Ronald D. Fine and Alexander Gonski[8] (Sydney) report data on 2 patients in whom there was simultaneous occurrence of an arteriovenous vascular malformation and a primary brain tumor.

A woman, aged 43, with seizures for 6 years and headaches for 10 years, had markedly increased radioisotope uptake in two right-sided cerebral areas and carotid angiographic evidence of a large meningioma arising from the right parietal convexity. An arteriovenous malformation was present in the right midfrontal region that was supplied by frontal branches of the right middle cerebral artery. The meningioma and the 5×3-cm malformation were removed. No neurologic abnormality was present after surgery.

The second patient, a boy aged 15, presented with paroxysms of headache for 10 days and vomiting. Gross papilledema and neck stiffness were noted. Ventriculography showed a large midline mass that probably occluded the aqueduct and angiography showed an arteriovenous malformation in the right parietal region, fed by a middle cerebral branch. Craniotomy revealed the angioma, which was resected, and tumor which had the appearance of an oligodendroglioma, most of which was removed. Headache was relieved but a marked left hemiparesis developed postoperatively.

When regional perforating vessels of the brain participate in angiomatous malformations, important secondary changes will result in the cerebral parenchyma, though these are not malignant in nature. Meningiomas account for some 15% of cerebral tumors. They arise extraparenchymally, with their clinical manifestations stemming from dis-

(8) Med. J. Aust. 1:227–230, Feb. 21, 1976.

placement rather than from invasion. Vascular proliferation may be a feature of both oligodendrogliomas and meningiomas. It is concluded that the coexistence of lesions in
the present cases is no more than fortuitous.

▶ [I had reported a number of cases of concurrence of brain tumor,
aneurysm and arteriovenous malformation to the Society of Neurological
Surgeons a number of years ago, but did not publish them because I considered them as curiosities of not much particular significance. However,
since then, techniques for operating on vascular lesions have so greatly
improved that these lesions assume more importance, for many unrup-
tured aneurysms are now being operated on successfully. There will
still be room for decision making, especially when the vascular lesion
is far removed from the neoplasm and when the neoplasm is malignant.
— Ed.] ◀

**Suboccipital Removal of Acoustic Neuromas: Re-
sults of 125 Operations.** J. Thomsen[9] (Univ. of Copenhagen) reviewed the results of suboccipital surgery for
acoustic neuroma for 125 patients treated during 1957–72.
Large tumors were present in 105 cases and medium-sized
tumors in 20. Most patients were aged 30–60 years. Women
outnumbered men by 2:1. The initial symptom was hearing
loss in 85% of cases.

Seven patients had bilateral tumors and 4 of them were
less than age 30 years; all 4 had signs of Recklinghausen's
disease. Cerebellar signs were most frequent in patients
with large tumors (83%); choked disks were seen in 39% of
cases and brain stem features in 12%. All patients had an
increased cerebrospinal fluid protein content. A unilateral
suboccipital approach to the cerebellopontine angle was
used in all cases. Hyperventilation, intravenous urea and
positioning were used to induce brain skrinkage. Complete
tumor removal was possible in 94 cases.

Primary mortality was 22% and postoperative condition
was good in 27% of cases, acceptable in 33% and poor in 18%.
No difference between total and subtotal tumor removal was
seen. Facial paralysis was present in 84% of patients postoperatively. Of 45 cases, peroperative resection of part of the
cerebellum was necessary in one-third to one-fourth. More
patients in good condition postoperatively lacked brain stem
impression. Mortality was greater in cases of large tumors,
but facial paralysis was not significantly more frequent in

(9)   Acta Otolaryngol. (Stockh.) 81:406–414, May–June, 1976.

this group than in the group with medium-sized tumors. Brain stem thrombosis and malacia were the main causes of death. Mortality from 39 operations done with the operating microscope has been lowered to 13%.

The results of suboccipital removal of large and medium-sized acoustic neuromas generally have been unsatisfactory with respect to mortality, postoperative condition and facial paralysis. Closer neurosurgical-otologic cooperation is needed in treating acoustic neuromas with regard to diagnosis of the tumors and surgical treatment.

▶ [The exact definition of a small versus a large tumor is not given in the text. The more recent operations have been done with the patient prone; note the preference of Tarshis and Hunt for this position for cervical laminotomy now. Thomsen states that the only safe way to identify the facial nerve is by the translabyrinthine approach, but most of us are able to find it by taking off the posterior wall of the acoustic canal from behind. An operative mortality of even 13% with the use of the operative microscope would be considered unacceptable by most experienced neurosurgeons, even in association with large tumors. Reduction of volume in the posterior fossa by preliminary ventricular shunting was not mentioned.

A 0.9-cm schwannoma of the 8th cranial nerve was serially sectioned and examined by Neely et al. (Laryngoscope 86:984, 1976). It arose from the inferior vestibular nerve just medial to the internal meatus. Part of the tumor was continuous with nervous tissue, but part of it compressed remaining fibers of the nerve within the tumor capsule. – Ed.] ◀

Cerebellopontine Angle Tumors Other Than Acoustic Neuromas: Report on 34 Cases – Presentation of 7 Bilateral Acoustic Neuromas. J. Thomsen[1] (Univ. of Copenhagen) reports the findings in 34 cases of cerebellopontine angle tumors other than neuromas seen during 1957 – 72; 125 acoustic neuromas also were diagnosed. Data on 7 patients with bilateral acoustic neuromas also were reviewed.

Four of the 34 study patients were less than age 30 years and 10 were over age 60; most were aged 30 – 60 years. There were twice as many female as male patients. Only 15% of patients had had symptoms for over 5 years. Hearing loss and vertigo presented in less than half the cases; 20% of patients presented with headache and 15% with trigeminal neuralgia. About half the patients had hearing loss and canal paresis of varying degrees at diagnosis. Taste deficiency was identified in 26% of cases, a diminished nasolacrimal reflex in 38%, facial palsy in 12% and reduced corneal sensi-

(1) Acta Otolaryngol. (Stockh.)82:106– 111, July– Aug., 1976.

bility in 44%. Cerebellar features were present in 59% of cases, brain stem symptoms in 29%, mental deterioration in 15% and increased intracranial pressure in 24%. The cerebrospinal fluid protein level was elevated in 35% of cases.

There were 19 meningiomas, 4 epidermoid tumors and 4 arachnoid cysts; 8 endotheliomatous, 7 fibromatous and 4 transitional meningiomas were seen. Two patients with meningioma also had other associated intracranial tumors. Eight patients (24%) had operation for recurrent tumor; 6 of these had meningiomas. Five patients died during or after operation and 3 others died of recurrence or metastasis. Of the surviving patients, 19% had facial palsy. Four of the 7 patients with bilateral acoustic neuromas were relatively young and had signs of Recklinghausen's disease. Three patients had signs of other intracranial neuromas, especially trigeminal neuromas.

Age and sex distributions are similar for acoustic neuromas and "nonneuromas" but many patients with "nonneuromas" have normal hearing and vestibular function. The symptoms are much less uniform than in patients with acoustic neuromas, where 8th nerve features are dominant. A few patients with "nonneuromas" have elevated cerebrospinal fluid protein levels. Operative mortality is comparable in the two groups but postoperative facial palsy is much less frequent in patients with "nonneuromas" of the cerebellopontine angle than in those with acoustic neuromas.

Biologic Factors Involved in the Clinical Features and Surgical Management of Cerebellar Hemangioblastomas are discussed by Sixto Obrador and José Gerardo Martin-Rodriguez[2] (Autonomous Univ., Madrid). The estimated frequency of hemangioblastoma in the general population is 50 cases per million. The authors found 65 cerebellar hemangioblastomas in a series of 5,283 cases treated surgically for mass lesions, excluding traumatic processes. Clinical symptoms are most frequent in the 3d to 5th decades of life. Headache was the presenting feature in 76% of patients and papilledema was present in 70–90% of patients. The multiple nature of the condition is shown by the development of other vascular tumors within the central nervous system and also in the kidney, liver and pancreas.

(2) Surg. Neurol. 7:79–85, February, 1977.

The hemoglobin and red blood cell number are increased in cerebellar hemangioblastoma. Computerized axial tomography may give very useful information. Vertebral angiography is the most useful preoperative procedure at present. Cerebellar lesions have a predilection for the hemispheres; most of these tumors have a large cystic component.

Surgical excision is the best treatment for capillary hemangioblastoma of the posterior fossa. The average postoperative mortality in 523 cases reviewed was 17%. Mortality was greater for solid than for cystic tumors. Bipolar coagulation and microsurgical techniques have improved the radical removal of solid hemangioblastomas. Good long-term results were obtained in 73% of the patients, with an overall morbidity rate of 7%. The reported rate of recurrence is 9%. Three of the authors' patients had reoperation for known recurrences, in 2 due to incomplete removals.

Some workers believe that a dynamic process is superimposed on a heredofamilial developmental defect in these patients, whereas others postulate a blastomatous potential factor of differing degree that relates the angioreticulomatosis to the phakomatosis. Multicentric presentation is an unfavorable presentation of these tumors. Angiographic study of the kidneys is extremely important.

► [Cerebellar hemangioblastoma is now added to the list of tumors that may spread and seed into the spinal cord. Two cases are reported by Mohan et al. (J. Neurol. Neurosurg. Psychiatry 39:515, 1976). Radiotherapy tried in one case did not seem to have made any difference. The histologic appearance of the spinal tumors was the same as of the original tumor, and the reasons for the spread are unclear. — Ed.] ◄

Efficacy of Cryohypophysectomy in the Treatment of Acromegaly: Evaluation of 54 Cases. Michael V. DiTullio, Jr., and Robert W. Rand[3] (Univ. of California, Los Angeles) reviewed the results of cryohypophysectomy in 54 acromegalic patients seen in 1963–74, 28 men and 26 women with respective average ages of 43 and 46. The most common acromegalic features were acral and facial enlargement. Skull x-rays showed an abnormal sella in 70% of patients. The definitive endocrinologic diagnosis was made by radioimmunoassay of human serum growth hormone. Transsphenoidal cryohypophysectomy was indicated for all patients except those with evidence of pituitary apoplexy,

(3) J. Neurosurg. 46:1–11, January, 1977.

sudden or marked visual acuity or field loss or significant suprasellar tumor extension associated with cranial nerve palsies or obstructive hydrocephalus. A liquid nitrogen-cooled cryoprobe was used, with stereotactic manipulation and fluoroscopic control. Several overlapping cryogenic lesions were produced on either side of the midline at cryoprobe tip temperatures of −170 to −180 C for 10–15 minutes. Except for extremely large tumors, an average of five lesions was made. Patients were awake under local anesthesia and sedation.

Acral enlargement diminished in 63% of patients and facial enlargement in 61%. Improvement occurred during the first 24 hours and progressed for several months. Little or no change in the osseous abnormalities was observed. Body weight returned to premorbid status in half the patients and headaches resolved in over a third. Blood pressure levels became more normal after operation; fasting blood sugar and glucose tolerance rapidly decreased. The growth hormone level was below 10 ng/ml an average of 5 years postoperatively in 77% of patients. There was no postoperative evidence of residual visual deficit. Complications were infrequent and transient. Three patients had inflammatory, noninfectious meningitis, which usually resolved within 1 week. In 26 patients treated solely with cryosurgery, only 7 required postoperative exogenous hormones.

Cryohypophysectomy is the procedure of choice for acromegalics with intrasellar tumor exhibiting only minimal extension. In the near future, as acromegaly is recognized in progressively earlier stages, this technique will become the most commonly used surgical procedure.

▶ [Of 62 women with pituitary tumors (without Cushing's disease or acromegaly), 36 (58%) presented with amenorrhea and galactorrhea, and 15 more (24%) had amenorrhea only. Nader et al. (Clin. Endocrinol. (Oxf.) 5:245, 1976) found hyperprolactinemia in 79% of those in whom pretreatment prolactin levels were available. They also found 12 pituitary tumors in 25 women with unexplained galactorrhea. The authors suggest assay of serum prolactin in all patients with apparently functionless pituitary tumors. All patients with unexplained galactorrhea should be investigated for possible pituitary tumor.

Cerebrospinal fluid analysis for adenohypophyseal hormones permits diagnosis of suprasellar extensions of pituitary tumors, according to Jordan et al. (Ann. Intern. Med. 85:49, 1976). The levels drop again when the tumor is successfully treated.

In the opinion of van Alphen (Clin. Neurol. Neurosurg. 78:246, 1975), the microsurgical, frontotemporal approach to chromophobe adenomas is the best current one even though current authorities seem to prefer the transsphenoidal route. He maintains that the intracranial extensions cannot always be predicted, other lesions may coexist with the tumor and other tumors may mimic pituitary tumors and not be amenable to operation through the nose. He believes direct exposure is safest for preservation of vision, because one can see the lesion better by the suprasellar approach.

Tortuous carotid vessels may give great trouble in some attempts at transnasal hypophysectomy. They may also cause sellar erosion that, according to Anderson (Am. J. Roentgenol. 126:1203, 1976), may mimic pituitary adenoma. Angiography thus becomes necessary before treatment of such a neoplasm. Medial position of the carotid sulci may be demonstrated on tomography. — Ed.] ◄

Craniopharyngioma: Based on 160 Cases. Craniopharyngiomas constitute an estimated 13% of all intracranial neoplasms in children. M. Banna[4] (Newcastle upon Tyne) reports a retrospective study of the clinical and radiologic manifestations of 160 cases of craniopharyngioma from 5 neuroscience centers in the United Kingdom. About half the tumors were cystic and about one-third were partly cystic; 14% were solid. Cysts usually were multilocular. About 96% of all cystic craniopharyngiomas are lined by stratified squamous epithelium; 4%, the cysts of Rathke's cleft, are lined by cuboidal or columnar epithelium.

Calcification of craniopharyngiomas usually involves the suprasellar region and occurs about midline. Almost any type of sella may be seen in craniopharyngioma. Conventional carotid angiography showed findings consistent with suprasellar tumor in 57% of 56 adults and 74% of 19 children examined. Nearly all the children had abnormalities on plain skull x-rays. Over half the angiograms showed no elevation of the horizontal segment of the anterior cerebral artery, including some with 3d ventricular filling defects. No pathologic tumor circulation was seen. Vertebral angiograms showed posterior extensions of the tumors.

Air studies showed tumor growth occurring in various directions in all age groups, though massive lesions were more frequent in children and often seemed to arise above the sella. The inner lining of a cystic craniopharyngioma can be outlined by air or steripaque, 0.1- to 0.5-μ barium particles. Only large and solid craniopharyngiomas can be

(4) Br. J. Radiol. 49:206–223, March, 1976.

detected by radionuclide scanning. Computerized tomography with contrast enhancement may reveal a dense tumor "capsule" in cases of cystic tumor. Solid, uncalcified lesions seem infiltrative and cannot be distinguished from invasive tumors in the hypothalamus. It is only the suprasellar extension of the lesion that can be detected by computerized tomography.

▶ [Interesting historical details concerning Rathke, Mihalkivics and Erdheim, whose investigations led to the current concepts of origin of these lesions, are given in this article. Considerable additional clinical material is available, along with more histopathologic detail in the review of 245 cases from the Armed Forces Institute of Pathology by Petito et al. (Cancer 37:1944, 1976). The clinical data are skewed by the high percentage (65%) of military personnel, with 72% males. Under age 10, the ratio of males to females is 1:1.2. Mean survival from diagnosis to last known status was 4.8 years (34% had a 5-year survival). Suprasellar calcification occurred in 25% (more in the younger patients) and enlarged or eroded sella in 44%. Headache and visual difficulties were the presenting symptoms in 75% patients. Cystic tumors were much more common than solid ones. Survival rates were greater with no calcification, normal cerebrospinal fluid, tumor under 3 cm diameter, diagnosis after 1955 and radiotherapy. The authors could not often distinguish "epidermoid inclusion cysts" from "craniopharyngiomas." They often found both squamous and adamantinomatous areas within the same tumor, and transitions could be seen. Cysts were ascribed to maturation of squamous epithelium, degeneration of stellate nests or degeneration of stroma. Squamous-lined cysts rarely contained kerotohyalin granules, in contrast to epidermoid cysts that occur elsewhere.

Banna did not include data on the relative merits of various treatments of craniopharyngiomas. This can be found in other sources (including 1976 YEAR BOOK, p. 439; and Sweet, W. H.: Radical surgical treatment of craniopharyngiomas, Clin. Neurosurg. 23:52, 1976).

The exact techniques used in radiation therapy are indeed important, as shown by Harris and Levene (Radiology 120:167, 1976). A linear accelerator was used to deliver 4,500–5,000 rad in 4–5 weeks to pituitary tumors and 5,500 rad in 5–6 weeks to craniopharyngiomas. Five of 55 patients showed visual loss compatible with radiation damage to the optic nerve. No patient who received doses less than 250 rad per day showed this effect, which when present, appeared 5–34 months after therapy. The absence of tumor regrowth or empty sella syndrome was assured by operation, postmortem study or pneumography. The authors suggest fraction size should not exceed 200 rad per day. – Ed.] ◀

Treatment of Meningiomas in Childhood. Recently, it has been suggested that postoperative irradiation may be beneficial for incompletely removed meningiomas. Steven A. Leibel, William M. Wara, Glenn E. Sheline, Jeannette J. Townsend and Edwin B. Boldrey[5] (Univ. of California, San

(5) Cancer 37:2709–2712, June, 1976.

Francisco) reviewed the treatment results in 13 patients less than age 20 who were seen with intracranial meningoma during 1942–72; initially 213 patients were found. Only 1 patient was less than age 12. Total removal was done when possible; otherwise, the maximum amount of tumor was removed consistent with minimal operative damage. Irradiation sometimes followed incomplete removal; megavoltage irradiation was given in total doses of 4,500–5,500 rad with daily increments of 180 rad, over about 5½ weeks.

One study patient had a diffuse meningioma and 1 had an intraventricular tumor. Two patients had presumed complete excision of meningioma; 1 is alive 4 years later, but 1 with concurrent Recklinghausen's disease and bilateral 8th nerve sheath tumors died of intracranial bleeding 3 years after resection. Eight patients had subtotal resection without postoperative irradiation; 1 died postoperatively and 7 had recurrences after 1–12 years and had further removal. Four patients with recurrences received no subsequent radiotherapy and died 1–9 years after the second operation with active disease, while 2 of the 3 patients irradiated survived. Three patients had radiotherapy immediately after subtotal tumor resection; 1 died of postoperative complications, 1 had a minimal response and died 4 months after treatment and 1 is alive with persistent tumor at 9 years, after a second subtotal resection of recurrent tumor.

Better salvage was obtained in these children with recurrent meningioma when radiotherapy was given at recurrence. Preoperative irradiation may increase the potential resectability of certain highly vascular tumors. Doses of 5,000–5,500 rad are well tolerated by children but the risk of hormonal deficiencies from hypothalamic-pituitary irradiation must be weighed against the risk of recurrent tumor. It is unclear whether preoperative irradiation might increase the chances of total resectability by sterilizing peripheral microscopic tumor cells that might contribute to the high recurrence rate.

► [Even when one does not have an experienced catheter technician available, it is possible to carry out external carotid embolizaton, as reported by Pandya and Nagpal (Neurol. India 24:182, 1976). In their case of recurrent convexity meningioma in a man aged 19, they used 11 units of blood, 3 units of Dextraven and 1,000 ml glucose to maintain blood volume the first time operation was done. Somewhat over 2 years later, recurrence was treated by preliminary exposure of the external carotid, which was ligated, then opened a few mm distal to the ligature to allow passage of a vinyl catheter tapering from 14 F to 5 F. Through this, 3×8-mm Gelfoam pieces bearing a silver clip were forced into the artery. The removal of the angioblastic meningioma was much more easily accomplished, with only 3 units of blood needed. The ligation has the merit of preventing reflux of the spongy material into the internal carotid artery, as reported by Manelfe in *Advances in Cerebral Angiography,* edited by Salamon (Springer Verlag Berlin, Inc., 1975). — Ed.] ◄

► [The Fifth European Congress of Neurosurgery was held in Oxford, England, in September, 1975; its major papers appear in volumes 34 and 35 of *Acta Neurochirurgica,* pages 1 – 303 and 3 – 219, respectively, in 1976. The first segment deals with classification, assessment and treatment of coma. The second half of the first volume deals with tumor of the pineal body. An excellent "survey" (ibid. 34:109) by Ariëns Kappers emphasizes the endocrine function of this gland, which, developing as a part of the brain, is innervated by peripheral autonomic nerve fibers. In general, it functions to inhibit the function of other organs or systems, especially producing materials that are antigonadotropic. Many enzymes involved with indoleamines show a circadian rhythm, and the pineal activity of these enzymes is controlled by photic stimuli, via visual and sympathetic pathways.

The treatment of pineal region tumors varies. Direct attack is believed to be so dangerous that Pertuiset et al. (ibid., p. 151) prefer to relieve pressure by shunting and then give cobalt therapy. Diagnosis of pineoblastoma (sic!) is made by pneumoencephalographic demonstration of shrinkage of tumor size after irradiation. If the tumor does not get smaller, operation is indicated. Sano (ibid., p. 153) prefers to reduce the bulk of the tumor by direct approach via a parietal-occipital approach with division of the tentorium; pinealomas are then treated with radiotherapy. Other views of surgical management are given in the following article. — Ed.] ◄

Surgical Management of Tumors of the Pineal Region is discussed by S. Obrador, M. Soto and J. A. Gutierrez-Diaz[6] (Univ. of Madrid). Tumors of the pineal region and posterior 3d ventricle represent 0.5 – 1% of all intracranial tumors and are rare events in neurosurgical practice. Many tumors in this region may invade and infiltrate the structures near the posterior 3d ventricle or occupy the cistern of the velum interpositum and tela choroidea, compression of the roof of the posterior 3d ventricle and midbrain. A series of 262 verified tumors of the pineal region included 103 pinealomas, 60 gliomas, 28 atypical teratomas (germinomas), 31 teratomas and 21 meningiomas. About one-fourth of the tumors were benign histologically and could be removed surgically. From 10 – 25% of tumors of the pineal region are circumscribed, encapsulated or cystic.

(6) Acta Neurochir. (Wien) 34:159 – 171, 1976.

Many patients with tumors in the pineal region and posterior 3d ventricle have palliative operations to reduce increased intracranial pressure. At least 35% of the patients undergoing palliative surgery and radiotherapy have lived for 2–20 years. In a series of 200 tumors treated by direct surgical attack, postoperative mortality was 38% for partial removal and 36% for total removal. The Brunner-Dandy approach was used in 133 cases. Most pineal tumors are soft and can be partially removed by suction. Typical teratomas, however, are hard and should be enucleated after intracapsular removal. Complete removal of meningiomas, epidermoid tumors and cysts is usually possible. Use of the operating microscope is extremely helpful in dissection and in preserving the large deep veins. The surgical risk may be lower with the transtentorial and supracerebellar approaches. In 78 patients mainly operated on in the past 10–15 years, the postoperative mortality after 54 partial removals was 31%. It ranged from 14% with the supracerebellar approach to 45% with the Brunner-Dandy transcallosal approach. No deaths occurred in 7 total removals by the transventricular, transtentorial and supracerebellar approaches. Of 16 patients undergoing total removal by the transcallosal approach, 25% died postoperatively.

Histologic verification of tumors of the pineal region should be obtained. These tumors can be approached now more safely than in the past.

Results of Irradiation of Tumors in the Region of the Pineal Body. Radiotherapy usually has been an integral part of the planned management of tumors in the pineal region. N. J. Smith, A. M. El-Mahdi and W. C. Constable[7] (Univ. of Virginia) reviewed the records of 20 previously untreated patients who were seen during 1950–69 with tumors in or about the pineal body. There were 15 male patients, aged 2 months to 65 years, and 5 women, aged 22–58 years. The most common presenting symptoms were those of increased intracranial pressure; 76% of patients presented within 6 months of the onset of symptoms. Five patients had diagnostic exploration. Treatment was by decompression and, if necessary, ventricular shunting, followed by radiotherapy; 2 patients did not need shunting and 14 received

(7)   Acta Radiol. [Ther.] (Stockh.) 15:17–22, February, 1976.

a planned course of radiotherapy. A tumor dose of 4,000 rad or more was delivered, most recently with cobalt teletherapy with parallel-opposed or three fields. Retreatment with doses of 1,000–2,000 rad was tried in 5 cases.

Eleven of the 14 study patients (79%) had significant improvement from radiotherapy. Signs of brain stem involvement were relieved in 7 of 8 cases and cerebellar signs improved in 1 of 3 patients. Eight patients lived for over 3 years with minimal residual neurologic deficit; in 1 a spinal metastasis developed 3½ years after treatment and caused death, whereas the other 7 lived for 5 years or longer. Only 1 of 8 patients presenting with cerebellar signs is a long-term survivor. One of the 2 patients in whom metastases developed is alive at 5 years without evidence of disease. Retreatment was successful in 1 of 5 cases and palliative in 2.

Half the patients in this series lived 5 years or longer after radiotherapy for tumors in the pineal region. The similarity of most pineal tumors to radiosensitive testicular and ovarian tumors may explain the radiotherapeutic success. A dose of about 5,000 rad, using conventional fractionation, seems to be indicated. The incidence of spinal metastasis is low enough to justify treating patients with small fields, sparing as much normal tissue as possible.

► [Mincer et al. (Cancer 37:2713, 1976) reviewed records of 12 patients with pinealoma or ectopic pinealoma irradiated at Montefiore Hospital from 1961 to 1971. Eight patients show no evidence of active disease 4–14 years after receiving 5,000–6,000 rad. One patient developed cerebrospinal spread. Diagnosis was made clinically except in 1 patient with a pretreatment biopsy showing dysgerminoma. Posttreatment excision of one tumor revealed cystic teratoma. Autopsy in another showed medulloepithelioma. Eight patients had decompression or bypass for relief of pressure. The challenge to radiotherapy is to select those patients who need large fields of radiation, because fields that are too small may permit regrowth. – Ed.] ◄

Radiation Therapy in the Treatment of Glioblastoma. Yasuto Onoyama, Mitsuyuki Abe, Eizo Yabumoto, Tsutomu Sakamoto, Takehiro Nishidai and Sumio Suyama[8] (Kyoto Univ.) report a retrospective study of the survival of 127 patients treated for glioblastoma (astrocytomas, grades III and IV) during 1955–72 by radiotherapy; 116 cases were referred after surgical resection, 5 after biopsy and 6 after shunt operation. There were 84 male and 43 female pa-

(8) Am. J. Roentgenol. 126:481–492, March, 1976.

tients, aged 4–72 years; average age was 35.4. The incidence of glioblastoma among all brain tumor patients was 10.5% for children under age 15 and 27.1% for adults. Tumor was in the midbrain or brain stem in 13 patients, 8 of them children, and in the cerebrum in 114 cases. Thirty-seven patients received 200-kv x-ray therapy before 1962 and 90 received cobalt therapy. The planned tumor dose was 5,000–6,500 rad over 5–8 weeks in most cases, but in 27 cases the therapy was discontinued before 5,000 rad was given. The average tumor dose was 5,285 rad and the nominal standard dose was 1,501 ret. Most patients were treated by 210-degree arc therapy with field widths of 6–8 cm.

Eleven patients were alive at the end of 1974 and 6 of them survived 5–13 years after radiotherapy. The overall survival was 52% at 1 year, 19% at 3 years and 12% at 5 years after therapy. Children had the most unfavorable prognosis, with a 6-month survival rate of only 47%. Symptom duration was inversely related to survival. No patient with a deep or bilateral tumor lived 3 years after radiotherapy. Among patients with hemispheric tumors, those with right-sided lesions did better. Higher tumor doses resulted in longer survival but irradiation with a higher dose through a larger field was not associated with a better 3-year survival rate. Six 5-year survivors died of recurrent tumor 5.2–7 years after treatment; 4 other long-term survivors have returned to normal and useful lives.

Radiotherapy can prolong the survival of patients with glioblastoma but a tumor dose of over 6,000 rad or 1,700 ret is needed to improve the prognosis significantly. Treatment should be given through generous fields according to the extent of the tumor.

▶ [Electron microscopic analysis of delayed radiation necrosis has been made by Llena et al. (Arch. Pathol. Lab. Med. 100:531, 1976). Usually the affected brain is a firm mass, but the parenchyma may be waxy yellow. Prominent changes are seen in blood vessels, with necrosis and gliosis of the parenchyma. Perivascular changes and endothelial proliferations as well as flattening are described. Ultramicroscopic changes are compatible with increased permeability of the endothelium. The significance of the conspicuous increase in filaments, microtubular and tubular bodies is unclear.

Biochemical abnormalities of endocrine function were present in almost all of 17 patients receiving cranial irradiation for extrasellar intracranial tumors who were studied by Harrop et al. (Clin. Endocrinol. (Oxf.) 5:313, 1976). They believe endocrine assessments should be made prospectively, especially concerning growth hormones in children. In the same journal (ibid., p. 373), Perry-Keene et al. describe 3 cases of panhy-popituitarism and 5 of isolated growth hormone deficiency found 1–9 years after irradiation of tumors distant from the adenohypophysis. They refer to other studies showing evidence of endocrine dysfunction 5–20 years after external irradiation for nasopharyngeal cancer. Recognition of this syndrome is important so replacement therapy can be instituted. Damage is believed to be at the hypothalamic level.

Late brain necrosis may occur after radiation for brain tumor–or for scalp neoplasm as in the case reported by Queiroz and da Cruz Neto (J. Neurosurg. 45:581, 1976). The patient, a man aged 68, had 6,800 rad delivered in 4 weeks to a right preauricular ulcerated basal cell epitheliomia. Two years later he had headache, a clumsy left hand and lethargy. Right temporal lobectomy was done and dexamethasone was given for edema, but he died 2 months later of gastrointestinal hemorrhage. The mass removed showed ischemic changes, coagulation necrosis, demyelination and gliosis typical of radiation necrosis. The authors believe the radiation was given too rapidly and individual doses were too high (340 rad).

Radiation injury was found to be the cause of neurologic symptoms in a man, aged 45, treated for carcinoma of the maxillary sinus and adjacent areas and in a woman, aged 43, given irradiation with a linear accelerator for chromophobe pituitary tumor. Kusske et al. (Surg. Neurol. 6:15, 1976) suggest that possible improvement may follow excision of the necrotic material.

Delayed effects of radiation mimicking temporal lobe glioma are reported by Diengdoh and Booth (J. Neurosurg. 44:732, 1976). This time, fast-neutron therapy (dose unknown) was given for adenocarcinoma metastatic to the parotid gland.

Besides changes in the brain proper, radiation appears capable of evoking new neoplasms. In the case reported by Gonzales-Vitale et al. (Cancer 37:2960, 1976), a man underwent radiotherapy (3,600 rad) after subtotal removal of a pituitary chromophobe adenoma. Eleven years later, visual symptoms recurred and hydrocephalus was shunted, but the patient died of *Klebsiella* sepsis. Autopsy showed a fibroxanthosarcoma of the base of the skull and brain without metastasis. The tumor is classed as a malignant fibrous histiocytoma. – Ed.] ◄

Computerized (Axial) Tomography in the Serial Study of Cerebral Tumors Treated by Radiation: Preliminary Report. Richard J. Carella, Norman Pay, Joseph Newall, Anthony T. Farina, Irvin I. Kricheff and Jay S. Cooper[9] (New York Univ.) have used computerized tomographic (CT) scan routinely to follow patients with brain tumor treated by radiotherapy since 1974. The routine examination uses a 160×160 matrix and consists of four pairs of tomographic cuts, 13-mm thick, overlapping by 3 mm. Adults receive 300 cc 30% Hypaque by intravenous drip and

(9) Cancer 37:2719–2728, June, 1976.

scanning is begun while the last 100 cc is being infused. Ninety-four patients with cerebral tumors treated by radiotherapy had CT scanning before and after treatment over a 20-month period during 1974 – 75.

Both metastatic and primary cerebral lesions regressed and metastatic lesions disappeared. Primary lesions shrank in some cases, developed central necrosis in others and disappeared in a few instances. Clinical symptoms may improve considerably despite the persistence of a significant mass lesion. Contrast studies differentiated tumor from surrounding edema in many cases. Dilated ventricles were found in many patients after radiotherapy; this requires further study.

Currently, differentiation of edema from necrosis is difficult. Hopefully, increased experience will make differentiation of the two conditions possible and allow a more accurate determination of normal cerebral tissue tolerance.

► [Presumably the same patients (but now increased to 100) are studied in the report by Pay et al. (Radiology 121:79, 1976). Computerized axial tomography (CAT) scans help in depiction of regression of primary and metastatic tumors and recognition of radionecrosis and edema and permit the study of changes in tumor density and ventricular size as a result of radiation therapy.

Spiegel et al. (Ann. Intern. Med. 85:290, 1976) have used CAT scans to diagnose lesions consistent with intracranial atypical teratoma of the hypothalamus (endocrine abnormalities were obvious). Radiotherapy was instituted without craniotomy, and the efficacy of treatment was documented objectively by serial scans. This technique of follow-up of lesions in the hypothalamus would appear superior to iodized oil ventriculography. – Ed.] ◄

Trial of Treatment of Glioblastomas in the Adult and Cerebral Metastases with a Combination of Adriamycin, VM 26 and CCNU: Results of a Type II Trial are reported by P. Pouillart, G. Mathé, M. Poisson, A. Buge, P. Huguenin, H. Gautier, P. Morin, H.-T. Hoang Thy, J. Lheritier and R. Parrot.[1] Forty-three patients with inoperable glioblastomas and 30 patients with cerebral metastases were given intermittent cyclical sequential chemotherapy. The regimen for each 5-day treatment cycle was as follows: day 1, adriamycin, 45 mg/sq m by intravenous injection; days 2 and 3, VM 26 (4 dimethyl-epipodo-phyllotoxin D-thenylidene), 60 mg/sq m in isotonic glucose given by rapid

(1) Nouv. Presse Med. 5:1571 – 1576, June 19, 1976.

perfusion; and days 4 and 5, CCNU (1-(2 chloroethyl)-3-cyclohexyl-nitrosourea), 60 mg/sq m orally. Each treatment cycle was given only after complete hematologic restoration.

Clinically objective improvement was obtained in the 2d month of treatment in 31 (72%) of the 43 patients with glioblastomas. In 3 patients, temporary stabilization was observed; in 9 others, the clinical state worsened despite treatment.

Twenty-five of the 33 patients who improved with treatment underwent regular cineradiography every 3 months. Objective regression of the pathologic picture was established in 14 cases; the regression was complete 5 times and incomplete 11 times. In all, chemotherapy had an objective effect in 21 of the 25 patients studied. Agreement between the objective clinical effect and scintigraphic improvement was not perfect because 5 apparently clinically improved patients showed progression in the site visible by scintigraphy.

With combination chemotherapy, median survival was 180 days. Of 22 patients who survived longer than 6 months, 12 are alive and well and 10 are apparently in remission at 180–510 days.

Of the 30 patients with cerebral metastases, 13 who had bronchial epidermoid cancer received 1–3 cycles of treatment. Three showed objective regression of neurologic signs in 2 months, 1 was stabilized, and 9 were failures. Of 8 patients with metastases of mammary origin, 6 were improved, 1 was stabilized, and 1 was a failure. Of the 9 patients with metastases of other origins, 3 were improved, 1 was stabilized, and 5 were failures. Survival time was 72 days, 240 days and 109 days, respectively, for the three categories. There is a low sensitivity of cerebral metastases to the action of the drug combination studied except in cases of breast cancer.

▶ [Virtually the same material also appears in another article by Pouillart et al. (Cancer 38:1909, 1976).

Chemotherapy of brain tumors continues to be investigated, with confusing results. A 5-year review of single agents has been made by Wilson et al. (Arch. Neurol. 33:739, 1976). Response rates were 44–47% with carmustine (BCNU), lomustine (CCNU) and procarbazine but only 38% with BIC. Combined drug therapy did not appear worthwhile with the agents tried thus far. Brisman et al. (ibid., p. 745) found no prolongation of quantity or quality of survival with BCNU, CCNU or methyl CCNU (semustine). All the patients also had surgery and radiation therapy for gliomas.

Mithramycin was given in addition to operation and, sometimes, radiation, in a controlled, prospective, randomized study carried on by the Brain Tumor Study Group. Details of this evaluation are given by Walker et al. (J. Neurosurg. 44:655, 1976). Mithramycin was not an effective agent. Radiation did permit significant improvement in survival. – Ed.] ◀

Lymphoma of the Spinal Extradural Space. Paul Haddad, John F. Thaell, Joseph M. Kiely, Edgar G. Harrison, Jr., and Ross H. Miller[2] (Mayo Clinic) report data from a retrospective study of patients treated surgically who had histologically proved lymphoma in the extradural space with extrinsic compression of the spinal cord or cauda equina. Ninety-four such patients were encountered in 1907–69. The 59 men and 35 women had a median age of 48. Seventy-two patients had non-Hodgkin's lymphoma and 22, Hodgkin's disease.

Clinical evidence of neurologic involvement preceded the diagnosis of lymphoma in 71% of patients and 52% appeared to have "primary" or localized extradural lymphoma. Pain was the most common initial symptom and had been present for a median of 6 months. Forty patients had essentially complete paralysis in one or both lower extremities, and 29 of these were paraplegic. A sensory level was detectable in 54 patients. Spinal x-rays showed compression fractures in 18 patients, pedicle erosion in 10 and a paraspinal mass in 6. All 71 myelograms showed obstruction to contrast flow. The cerebrospinal fluid protein was elevated in 71 of 77 instances. Operation showed paraspinal involvement in 28 patients and direct involvement of vertebral bone by tumor in 27. Only 13 patients received preoperative treatment for lymphoma. All but 7 received radiotherapy postoperatively and 2 of these patients received systemic chemotherapy. Only 13 of 40 patients with leg paralysis had significant improvement in gait; nearly half of 28 patients regained voluntary control of bladder function. The actuarial survival was 50% at 27 months and 40% at 5 years. Survival at 5 years of patients with apparently localized extradural lymphoma was about the same as for those with more readily detected tumors in other sites at the time of operation.

Patients with extradural spinal cord compression by malignant lymphoma have a relatively good prognosis both for functional recovery and for survival, in contrast with most

(2) Cancer 38:1862–1866, October, 1976.

patients with metastatic carcinoma. The present data do not establish the superiority of initial surgical treatment over conservative management alone.

► [Radiation applied to meningeal or cerebral spread of lymphoma appears more successful. Methotrexate was used by Herbst et al. (Cancer 38:1476, 1976) after radiation therapy produced only temporary remissions. Thio-TEPA was used intrathecally for meningeal neoplasia by Gutin et al. (ibid., p. 1471).

In the past 30 years, there have been only 8 cases of Hodgkin's masses in the hemispheres found in a search by Truelle et al. (Rev. Neurol. (Paris) 132:494, 1976). They add another case, one producing an avascular right frontal cerebral lesion. It was removed and radiation therapy given thereafter.

In 13,500 consecutive autopsies, Gonzalez-Vitale and Garcia-Bunuel (ibid. 37:2906, 1976) found 18 cases of meningeal carcinomatosis (without metastasis elsewhere in the central nervous system). The malignant cells are thought to reach the leptomeninges via neural and perivascular lymphatics through intervertebral and cranial foramina. In 40% of the reported cases of "pure" meningeal carcinomatosis, no other spread in the body was found. Hence, radiation or local chemotherapy may well be effective; it would need to be all along the subarachnoid spaces, cranial and spinal. — Ed.] ◄

Microsurgical Removal of Intramedullary Spinal Hemangioblastomas: Report of 12 Cases and Review of Literature. Von Hippel-Lindau disease is a heredofamilial disorder characterized by vascular tumors of the retina and the central nervous system, most often of the cerebellum but also of the spinal cord, cerebrum and brain stem. About 2–3% of the primary cord neoplasms are hemangioblastomas. M. G. Yaşargil, J. Antic, R. Laciga, J. de Preux, R. W. Fideler and S. C. Boone[3] (Univ. of Zurich) reviewed 150 cases of intramedullary spinal hemangioblastoma from the world literature, including 12 personal cases.

More than half the patients were male. The mean age at evaluation was 37. The lesion occurred extradurally in 17 patients, extramedullarly in 38 and intramedullarly in 95. They were located mainly in the cervicodorsal and dorsolumbar regions. The symptoms are those of cord compression, usually progressing fairly slowly to paraplegia or quadriplegia. Syringomyelia is present in about 70% of the patients, pial varices in about 40% and root involvement in about 15%. Visceral involvement is present in about 30% but is usually not symptomatic.

(3) Surg. Neurol. 6:141–148, September, 1976.

Among 23 patients having exploration alone, cyst puncture or partial removal, 12 died, 5 were much worse after surgery, 5 deteriorated slowly and 1 was unchanged. Among 30 patients having radical removal of intramedullary lesions, 1 died, 2 were unchanged, 5 improved slightly, 14 improved substantially and had only slight symptoms and 8 were normal neurologically.

The authors' patients were operated on with microsurgical technique. The tumor may be compressed or displaced during operation but should not be opened. Eleven total removals were done but one operation had to be ended because an attempt was made to extirpate the angioma from the center of the tumor. Ten patients were improved after surgery, 1 was unchanged and 1 was worse. Two patients had persistent arm pain postoperatively.

Total microsurgical removal of intramedullary spinal hemangioblastoma is the treatment of choice. Selective angiography is of great value in the management of these patients. Use of the operating microscope and the bipolar cautery is essential.

▶ [The microsurgical treatment of 12 patients with intramedullary spinal hemangioma is described by Yaşargil and de Preux (Neurochirurgie 2: 425, 1975). Three were at the bulbocervical junction; 5 involved the cerebellum and medulla and 4 involved the spinal cord alone. Eleven patients had total removals, with the surgeons working on afferent vessels in the periphery first. Four patients are in excellent condition; 5 are independent and able to do part-time work. One has permanent tracheotomy with deficits of cranial nerves 9, 10, and 11, and 1 died of cardiac causes, with recurrence of cerebellar tumor, 12 months after operation. – Ed.] ◀

Benign Encapsulated Neurilemoma: Report of 76 Cases. Neurilemoma, although the most common tumor of nerve trunks, is quite rare. William G. Whitaker and Constantine Droulias[4] (Emory Univ.) reviewed case reports of 76 patients encountered in about 1,500,000 general hospital admissions in six hospitals in Atlanta. Tumors primarily involving bone, the spinal cord or intracranial nerves and those arising in the thoracic cavity were excluded, as were the plexiform neurilemomas often seen in association with Recklinghausen's disease. Neurilemoma may arise in any nerve where Schwann cells occur. It typically produces few symptoms, grows slowly and rarely causes significant neurologic disturbances. It is often fusiform and may be mobile laterally but not in the long axis of the involved nerve. Separation of nerve fibers may occasionally be associated with temporary functional impairment or sensory disturbance. For practical purposes the neurilemoma is a benign tumor.

Encapsulated neurilemoma involved a major nerve trunk in 31 patients, and the nerve was injured in 5 instances. In 18 cases, a sensory nerve was identified but not always spared. The sympathetic chain was the site of the tumor in 4 cases, and removal resulted in regional sympathectomy in 3 of these. In 35 cases, the tumor was without obvious nerve involvement; 8 of these tumors occurred in the gastrointestinal tract. Superficial lesions were found 27 times and were simply excised. No catastrophic complications occurred in cases of nerve injury. Some degree of transient motor deficit often occurred even after careful enucleation, but no permanent functional impairment of an extremity was observed.

When neurilemoma involves a major nerve trunk, recognition of the tumor by the surgeon avoids needless destruction of the nerve in nearly all instances. Enucleation of neurilemomas results in no significant or permanent neurologic deficit and is not followed by recurrence. Tumors in the gastrointestinal tract and superficial lesions in minor sensory nerves are managed successfully by local excision.

▶ [The authors state, "This tumor continues to be misdiagnosed, mistreated and misspelled." The encapsulated form may be readily enucleated; "if a tumor involving a nerve trunk does not lend itself to enucleation, it is unlikely that it is a neurilemoma." Barfred and Zachariae (Scand. J. Plast. Reconstr. Surg. 9:245, 1975) make the same point in describing palmar median nerve neurofibromas that involved nerve fibrils and had to be removed by nerve resection. Grafts from both sural nerves were used in repair of 10-cm gaps. One patient is doing well with good recovery 8 years later and the other patient, after 2 years. In each case the motor nerve to the opponens was isolated so motor and sensory trunks could be grafted separately. — Ed.] ◀

Vascular Disease

HEMORRHAGES

► Brismar and Brismar (Acta Radiol. [Diagn.] (Stockh.) 17:180, 1976) emphasize the technique and findings of orbital phlebography in 6 cases of spontaneous carotid-cavernous fistulas. Carotid angiograms also were done; 1 fistula was fed only by 1 internal carotid artery. One was fed only by the accessory meningeal branch of the maxillary artery and 4 were fed by both external and internal carotids. Thrombosis was thought to be present in the cavernous sinus and its draining veins. "Spontaneous" closure and thrombosis may have been related to the angiography.

Debrun et al. (Nouv. Presse Med. 5:1294, 1976) consider the ideal treatment for carotid-cavernous fistulas and aneurysms to be catheterization with an inflatable balloon. In 3 of 6 cases of traumatic fistula they were able to preserve the internal carotid flow while obstructing the fistula. The balloon may be detachable, but sometimes this cannot be used and an ordinary Fogarty catheter is used, with sacrifice of the carotid flow. – Ed.

Cerebral Arterial Spasm: Part VIII. Treatment of Delayed Cerebral Arterial Spasm in Human Beings. George S. Allen[5] (Johns Hopkins Univ.) reports the treatment of 3 patients having neurologic deficits from delayed cerebral arterial spasm after the rupture of posterior communicating artery aneurysms, using continuous, simultaneous intravenous injections of phenylephrine and nitroprusside. Treatment was given after successful clipping of the aneurysms, and the results were assessed by cerebral angiography, done before and after treatment.

Angiograms obtained after treatment with nitroprusside and phenylephrine showed definite enlargement of the main arteries that had been in spasm, both visually and by measurement under magnification. Each patient had a worsening deficit before treatment. In 2 patients the deterioration was halted and recovery began shortly after the start of treatment. One patient with a large mass of infarcted brain did not improve clinically. The extracranial carotids also dilated after treatment. One patient continued to improve for 2 days after treatment was stopped, and her condition

(5) Surg. Neurol. 6:71–80, August, 1976.

then began to fluctuate again. Clinical improvement was slow in contrast with the dilation of cerebral arteries, which was clearly evident 4–5 hours after the start of treatment.

Patients suspected of having spasm should undergo angiography and be treated at the earliest sign of neurologic deficit. It is possible that the improvement observed in the present patients was not related to the treatment. The treatment is experimental and potentially can be extremely hazardous; its beneficial effect has not been fully proved. Spasm should not be treated until the aneurysm has been operated on, because dilating the cerebral vessels in the presence of a normal blood pressure could cause the aneurysm to rupture.

▶ [Mizukami et al. (Acta Neurochir. (Wien) 34:247, 1976) studied 6 cases of ruptured aneurysm, concluding on histologic bases that the original luminal narrowing is due to contraction of the medial smooth muscle. Prolonged narrowing is associated with intimal and medial thickening and thrombus. After more than 2 weeks, the lumen is dilated on angiography. This is accompanied by frank necrosis of smooth muscle cells.

Cameron and Haas (ibid., p. 261) tried the effect of a single intra-arterial injection of phenoxybenzamine after successful clipping of an aneurysm. The results were no better than with inert placebo. Propranolol tablets (β-adrenergic blocker) were no better than placebo. — Ed.] ◀

Postoperative Hypertension in the Management of Patients with Intracranial Arterial Aneurysms. Edward J. Kosnik and William E. Hunt[6] (Ohio State Univ.) have found elevation of systemic arterial blood pressure to be effective in alleviating ischemic symptoms attributable to cerebral vasospasm in patients with intracranial arterial aneurysms. The arterial blood pressure level was raised in 7 patients who had a postoperative cerebral flow crisis, with good results in most cases.

Man, 18, presented with sudden onset of headache, dizziness and blurred vision, with a blood pressure level of 112/68 mm Hg. Angiography showed an aneurysm of the right posterior communicating artery. Lethargy and neck stiffness resolved overnight and the aneurysm was repaired at craniotomy. A right 3d nerve palsy was present postoperatively. Blood pressure level was 110/74 mm Hg. Coma and decorticate posturing on the left appeared 3 days postoperatively. The blood pressure level was raised to 150/90 mm Hg with norepinephrine and colloid replacement was given in the form of 2 units of blood and 1,000 ml plasmanate over the next 12 hours; the patient became more responsive within a few hours. He was

(6)   J. Neurosurg. 45:148–154, August, 1976.

awake and talking 48 hours after onset of cerebrovascular crisis. Norepinephrine was stopped after a few days and the blood pressure level was kept at 150/90 mm Hg by hypervolemia. The patient was released 12 days postoperatively with no deficit other than the 3d nerve palsy.

These patients receive norepinephrine to raise the blood pressure level 40–60 mm Hg systolic or to produce definite clinical improvement; 16 mg norepinephrine is mixed with 500 ml normal saline and is given intravenously through a central venous line. Plasmanate also is begun, followed by whole blood transfusion. After the deficit clears, blood pressure is kept elevated for a day or two and then allowed to return to preoperative levels. Some patients have had a recurring deficit necessitating hypertensive therapy for up to 15 days. If the deficit can be reversed promptly by arterial blood pressure elevation, infarction can be prevented in some cases. Six of the current 7 patients improved markedly with hypertensive therapy. Treatment must be started as soon as deterioration is observed.

More experimentation is needed on this approach and the hazards must be clarified. The most serious hazard seems to be the institution of treatment too late, after the cerebrovascular system is so damaged that increasing perfusion pressure only increases brain swelling.

Use of ε-Aminocaproic Acid (EACA) in the Preoperative Management of Ruptured Intracranial Aneurysms. Ram P. Sengupta, Sing C. So and Francisco J. Villarejo-Ortega[7] (Newcastle Genl. Hosp., Newcastle upon Tyne) examined the value of EACA in preventing recurrent hemorrhage in one of two concurrent series of patients hospitalized during 1971–73 with ruptured intracranial aneurysm and subarachnoid hemorrhage confirmed by lumbar puncture. Of 142 cases reviewed, 76 were managed by bed rest and sedation and 66 also were treated with EACA, starting within 3 days after initial bleeding. The dose was 24 gm daily in 8 divided doses, usually given orally but occasionally intravenously. This dosage provides an effective blood level of EACA of 13 mg/100 ml, sufficient to inhibit fibrinolysis. Sex and age distributions were comparable in both groups.

There was no recurrent hemorrhage preoperatively in the

(7) J. Neurosurg. 44:479–484, April, 1976.

EACA-treated group but 17 control patients had rebleeding, most of them within 2 weeks after the initial ictus. Intracranial surgery was done on 88% of the EACA-treated patients and 60% of controls. Fifteen of the 31 unoperated controls rebled and 8 continued to deteriorate from the initial hemorrhage. Two control patients who rebled improved enough to be operated on. Two EACA-treated patients had thrombotic phenomena; 1 had middle cerebral artery thrombosis on the side opposite the aneurysm confirmed at autopsy and 1 had deep vein thrombosis in the calf and died of massive pulmonary embolism.

The role of EACA seems promising; it effectively prevents rebleeding during the postictal period, when aneurysm surgery is most hazardous. The pharmacologic aspects of this agent must be more clearly defined. The optimal effect of EACA occurs within the first 2 weeks after hemorrhage. It is not in itself a cure for ruptured intracranial aneurysm.

► [When subarachnoid hemorrhage is accompanied by vitreous hemorrhage, blindness may result. Sight may later be restored by vitrectomy, as in the case reported by Carruthers and Blach (Br. Med. J. 2:404, Aug. 4, 1976). — Ed.] ◄

Intracranial Aneurysms: Analysis of Results of Microneurosurgery. C. B. T. Adams, A. B. Loach and S. A. O'Laoire[8] (Radcliffe Infirm., Oxford, England) analyzed data on the first 100 patients with intracranial aneurysm treated by microneurosurgical methods during 1972–74. All patients but 1 were followed to 6 months after operation. The 56 women and 44 men had a mean age of 46 years. All but 3 patients presented with acute subarachnoid hemorrhage. The operation of choice was craniotomy and application of an aneurysmal clip or reinforcement of the aneurysmal wall with cotton wool and cyanoacrylate glue if clipping was not feasible. A check angiogram was done 2–3 days after operation in 81% of cases.

Sixty-four patients were working full-time at 6 months, whereas 12 had some residual deficit but had returned to some kind of work and 9 had poor results. Fifteen patients had died, 9 of postoperative cerebral vasospasm. Similar results were obtained in the hypotensive and hypothermic surgical groups. Eleven of 20 patients with untreated sys-

---

(8) Br. Med. J. 2:607–609, Sept. 11, 1976.

temic hypertension at operation had poor results or died, whereas treated patients had good or fair results. Mortality was less with operation in the 2d rather than in the 1st week after bleeding, but poor results were more frequent; no deaths occurred when the interval between hemorrhage and operation was more than 2 weeks. Most patients had either local or generalized vasospasm after operation. Generalized cerebral vasospasm correlated with a poor outcome from operation. Postoperative vasospasm was unrelated to the type of anesthetic used. Sodium nitroprusside did not seem to protect against the development of vasospasm in the doses used.

Surgical results depend especially on the interval between hemorrhage and operation. Modern surgical techniques have halved the total mortality but morbidity is unchanged. Results can be improved by delaying operation for 7 days and by treating hypertension before operation. Cerebral vasospasm is a major problem but affects the outcome of operation little unless it is generalized. Further improvement in the surgical results will depend on better blood pressure control, careful timing of operation, prevention of rebleeding and control of vasospasm.

► [Loach and de Azevedo Filho (Acta Neurochir. (Wien) 35:97, 1976) report good or fair results in 76% of 133 patients with aneurysms treated at Radcliffe Infirmary, Oxford, England. Mortality was 12%, and 12% of patients had poor results. Improvement may occur by delaying operation to the 2d week after bleeding and by better management of hypertensive patients before operation and of those who develop vasospasm postoperatively. Operation in the 1st week carried a 19% mortality and in the 2d week, 6%. No mortality occurred in the 24% who were operated on after 2 weeks. Results were worse with grade III and best with grade I patients; patients in grades IV and V were not operated on. These authors did not believe nitroprusside protected against subsequent vasospasm.

Pallidocaudate arteriovenous malformations (in the angle between the midline and the anterior perforated space) can be successfully attacked under deep hypotension, according to Pertuiset, et al. (Rev. Neurol. (Paris) 132:799, 1976). Sodium nitroprusside was used to lower the blood pressure for angiography (in addition to routine angiography, angiotomography and pneumoencephalography were done) to permit better delineation of the exact origin of the vascular pedicles. Then the surgical procedure was done via a coronal parasagittal flap, transcortical exposure of the ventricle and operation through the foramen of Monro to remove the malformation in the caudate head (even though the vascular supply was from the perforating arteries and hence away from the operative entry). Both patients are alive and without aggravation of their preoperative hemiplegia.

Among the items scarcely if ever mentioned to patients with aneurysms, who contemplate operation and its risks, is epilepsy. Cabral et al. (J. Neurol. Neurosurg. Psychiatry 39:1052, 1976) found the overall incidence of epilepsy to be 22% in a series of 152 patients with aneurysms. The incidence was 27.5% for 116 treated with an intracranial approach, whereas it was 5% for those treated with carotid ligation. The incidence was highest in those with severe brain damage in the territory of the middle cerebral artery (the most epileptogenic area). The authors are currently investigating the propriety of giving anticonvulsants routinely after operation for aneurysm.

Sarwar et al. (Radiology 120:603, 1976) tabulate findings of 16 cases of aneurysm in which the aneurysms "grew" or enlarged over a period of a few weeks to 8 years. Usually enlargement was correlated with clinical deterioration. The bleeding aneurysms are generally irregular and lobulated. — Ed.] ◄

Intracranial Surgery for Cerebral Artery Aneurysms: Five Years' Experience. David M. Kaufman and Kamran Tabaddor[9] (Montefiore Hosp. and Med. Center, New York) reviewed 133 operations done for intracranial aneurysm in 131 patients during 1971–76. Almost all the patients were admitted from the nearby community; some were extremely ill and many were too ill to be transferred. Operation was done by many different attending and resident neurosurgeons. Internal cerebral and posterior communicating artery aneurysms were treated in 57 cases, middle cerebral aneurysms in 32 and anterior cerebral and anterior communicating aneurysms in 39. Six patients were in poor condition at operation and all 6 died shortly thereafter.

Anterior cerebral-anterior communicating aneurysm surgery had a relatively high morbidity. The neurologic status of 12 patients deteriorated substantially before operation. The sensorium of 6 patients improved from stupor to lethargy between hospitalization and operation. Patients with aneurysms in the anterior circulation who were in good condition preoperatively had surgical morbidity of 28% and a mortality of 19%. Mortality was increased markedly with a depressed sensorium preoperatively, an age of 50 years or more and an interval of less than 15 days between rupture and operation.

These results reflect the serious illness encountered in this community-based medical center and the surgical outcome in consecutive and unselected cases. The results,

(9) J.A.M.A. 236:1707–1710, Oct. 11, 1976.

which do not compare favorably with those from foreign referral centers, are partially explained by disproportionate numbers of patients in poor-risk groups. The possible advantages of regionalization are apparent nevertheless. Further comparative studies should be done on an interinstitutional basis.

► [Choudhury (J. Neurosurg. 45:484, 1976) reviews the cases of anterior communicating aneurysms from the Aberdeen Royal Infirmary. In 28 of 37 cases (1971–73), proximal occlusion of the dominant anterior cerebral artery was done, with a 2- to 4.5-year follow-up. The mortality was 3.5% (1 patient), due to hemorrhage from improper clip application. Operation preferably was done 7–10 days after hemorrhage, only in patients in grades 1–3. Angiography in grades 4 and 5 "was of academic interest only," for such patients deteriorated and died (and were not included in the statistics). In the data presented, the problem of vasospasm in the presence of an aneurysm is not considered. Early operation is done in low-risk patients with repeated hemorrhages; urgent intervention is needed for cases with sizable intracranial hematoma or hydrocephalus. No late hemorrhages have occurred in this series. What happened to the 9 patients treated by direct clipping (because they did not have dominant anterior cerebral arteries) is not reported.

Gillingham (Rev. Inst. Nacl. Neurol. (Mex. 10:16, 1976) prefers complete investment of aneurysmal sacs of the middle cerebral artery with fine-mesh cotton gauze to avoid manipulation of the major trunk and neck of the sac, although its body may be clipped to allow dissection of the fundus. He believes operation should be within 10 days, with the aneurysm approached through splitting of the arachnoid of the sylvian fissure without exposure of the trunk and striate vessels. In the last 25 consecutive patients (1965–74) in grades 1–3 of Botterell's five grades, there have been only 2 deaths, both late, and only 4 patients are disabled and dependent, of which 3 were in grade 3 before operation. – Ed.] ◄

Surgical Treatment for Aneurysms of the Upper Basilar Artery.

Charles B. Wilson and Hoi Sang U[1] (Univ. of California, San Francisco) reviewed the results of treatment in 15 patients seen with aneurysms of the upper basilar artery during 1970– 75. All cases but 1 were diagnosed by vertebral angiography during study for subarachnoid hemorrhage. The approach was toward occluding the base of the aneurysm with a clip. When clipping was not feasible or when the applied clip did not approximate the parent artery, the entire lesion was encased either with muslin or with muslin and an adhesive.

Ten patients had postoperative angiography and 5 who had reinforcement alone have been followed for 8 months to

───────

(1) J. Neurosurg. 44:537–543, May, 1976.

5 years without having angiography. The 7 men and 8 women were aged 36 – 60 years. All but one of the aneurysms had bled. Two patients had major deficits caused by giant, partly thrombosed aneurysms. Operation was done using the operating microscope, induced hypotension and moderate hypothermia. Skull fixation was used and the approach was more anterior than that described by Drake (1969).

All of the first 6 patients had complications, whereas the last 9 did not. Two patients required evacuation of postoperative hematomas; 1 had residual but improving hemiparesis. Four patients had hemiparesis postoperatively; all had arterial spasm. Two patients had postoperative hydrocephalus requiring shunting and 1 also had shunt infection. One patient, in whom a perforating artery had been included in the clip, had choreiform movements postoperatively, ascribable to vasospasm with infarction. All patients had a postoperative oculomotor palsy. Eight of the 13 patients followed for up to 5 years were neurologically intact and 12 were intellectually intact. Four were impaired but ambulatory, with mild-to-moderate hemiparesis.

Developments in neuroanesthesia and microsurgical techniques have led to the successful surgical treatment of basilar bifurcation arterial aneurysms. Except in patients with aneurysms presenting with mass effects, operation has not been recommended for those in a condition lower than grade II.

The authors emphasize the benefits of experience in operating on these difficult-to-treat aneurysms.

Microsurgical Pterional Approach to Aneurysms of the Basilar Bifurcation. A subtemporal approach to basilar artery aneurysms is not entirely satisfactory. M. G. Yaşargil, J. Antic, R. Laciga, K. K. Jain, R. M. Hodosh and R. D. Smith[2] (Univ. of Zurich) felt that an anterior approach to basilar bifurcation aneurysms might be more suitable. Since 1971, 29 patients have had surgery for such aneurysms by this method. In all but 1 patient, the aneurysm could be readily clipped, with good visualization of adjacent small perforating vessels and of both posterior cerebral arteries.

TECHNIQUE. — A lateral frontotemporal-sphenoidal or "pterion-

(2) Surg. Neurol. 6:83 – 91, August, 1976.

al" craniotomy is performed through a curvilinear scalp incision extending from the zygoma to the frontal area. Four bur holes outline a diamond-shaped bone flap with its base between the zygomatic process of the frontal bone and the pterion. The arachnoid is opened at the proximal sylvian fissure and dissection is carried out proximally to the carotid bifurcation. Where the carotid is closely adjacent to the optic nerve, dissection should be done lateral to the carotid artery, between it and the oculomotor nerve. The interpeduncular cistern is opened by perforating its anterior wall, and dissection is carried caudally until the prepontine cistern is opened and both superior cerebellar arteries are clearly identified. Where the aneurysmal neck is broad-based and will not easily accept a clip, it is reduced by bipolar coagulation. Papaverine is applied to all major vessels. The dura is not closed tightly. Subgaleal drainage is routinely used. Moderate hypotension is produced with intravenous nitroprusside until the aneurysm is clipped. Patients receive 50 gm mannitol 30 minutes before surgery.

All but 1 of the 29 aneurysms could be clipped. Three patients died; in 1, a large thrombosed aneurysm could not be clipped. Several patients required shunting for communicating hydrocephalus.

There is minimal, if any, retraction of the temporal lobe with this approach. The oculomotor and trochlear nerves need not be dissected. Multiple aneurysms can be treated at one operation. The operation is technically difficult. It is unclear whether this operation offers definite advantages in terms of patient mortality and morbidity over previous approaches but the results obtained to date are encouraging.

Stereotactic Clipping of Arterial Aneurysms and Arteriovenous Malformations. The stereotactic method of aneurysm and malformation surgery avoids manipulation of blood vessels and retraction of the brain. Edward I. Kandel and Vyacheslav V. Peresedov[3] (Moscow) have performed 10 stereotactic clipping operations on 8 patients since 1973. The device used is shown in Figure 20; the stainless steel tube comes in diameters of 2.9 and 3.6 mm. The removable steel clips permit the clipping of vessels 1 – 7 mm in diameter. Preoperative angiography is performed and the blood pressure is reduced with Arfonad before clipping. The clipping procedure requires $1\frac{1}{2} – 2$ hours.

Four clipping operations were done in 3 patients with ar-

(3) J. Neurosurg. 46:12 – 23, January, 1977.

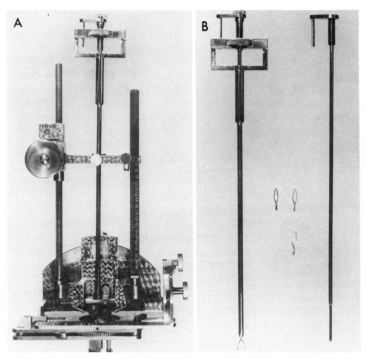

Fig. 20. — **A,** stereotactic clipping device in assembly with stereotactic apparatus. **B,** the clipping device is shown unassembled *(right)* and with open clip on the tip and first pivot *(left)*. Three clips of different sizes also are shown *(center)*. (Courtesy of Kandel, E. I., and Peresedov, V. V.: J. Neurosurg. 46:12–23, January, 1977.)

terial aneurysms. The narrow necks of most supraclinoid aneurysms of the internal carotid artery make them especially suitable for stereotaxic clipping. Six clippings of hemispheric arteriovenous aneurysms were performed in 5 patients; 4 aneurysms were of large or giant size. Four widespread aneurysms were supplied by several arteries and 2 by arteries from both sides. Only 1 relatively small aneurysm was supplied by a branch of the middle cerebral artery. Study of cerebral blood flow appears to be the objective criterion for evaluating clipping surgery in arteriovenous aneurysms. Efforts were concentrated on clipping feeding vessels for the palliative treatment of large and giant aneurysms. There was no mortality in this series and only 1 patient had hemiparesis that lasted several days. The patients generally endured the procedure easily and could walk 2–3 days postoperatively.

This new approach may be rational and advisable in carefully selected cases of arterial aneurysm in which a direct attack is too dangerous or technically impossible, in giant and deep-seated arteriovenous malformations as a palliative procedure for reducing aneurysm volume and in selected cases of arteriovenous aneurysms fed by a single artery, as a means of radical treatment. Brain trauma secondary to stereotactic clipping is less than during classic open surgery. It is assumed that future developments will make stereotactic clipping useful in vascular neurosurgery.

▶ [Cryosurgery can be used as an alternative to electrocoagulation in stereotactic operations on the brain, as a technique for destroying malignant gliomas and sometimes for benign processes. It should be regarded as a relatively minor operation when used for hypophysectomy according to Walder (Clin. Neurol. Neurosurg. 78:225, 1975). He reports on cryocoagulation used 39 times in 31 patients with arteriovenous lesions of the brain (up to a maximum of 25 times in a single operative session). Follow-up angiography is not used until after at least 3 weeks, because experimental studies show thrombosis may not occur for several weeks after the cold therapy. The malformation was totally eliminated in 16 of 31 cases, many of which were in areas of functional importance or unduly deeply located, or where lesions were thought not to be operable by orthodox surgery. In 5 of these, the malformation was totally eliminated in 2 and partially in 3. Thirty patients had an uneventful postoperative course; 1 died from pulmonary embolus. Recurrent hemorrhage occurred in 3 and caused death in 1 of these. The author believes cryotherapy has a place in treatment of arteriovenous malformations. – Ed.] ◀

Embolization of Cerebral Angiomas by Catheterization of Cortical Arteries is discussed by B. Vlahovitch and J. M. Fuentes[4] (Montpellier, France). The most striking progress in embolization of intracranial angiomas has been made by superselective catheterization of feeding arteries, especially for malformations of the external carotid region. The flow-guided balloon technique of Serbinenko is a promising approach to the internal carotid system.

Superselective angiography of the collateral branches of the internal carotid artery cannot always be achieved without risk, except by the peroperative catheterization of small cortical collaterals. Peroperative arteriography is necessary during embolization of a cerebrovascular malformation.

(4) Neuroradiology 11:243–248, 1976.

Generally, a flexible Teflon trocar is used for carotid arteriography. Brachial injection can be used for peroperative vertebral arteriography. Selective catheterization of submillimetric cortical arteries can be done using a flexible probe. The cerebral circulation is slow during deep anesthesia and seriography must be done with twice the usual number of exposures. In some cases, the principal feeding branch of an angioma can be catheterized with a 1-mm Teflon trocar, allowing a selective angiogram to be made; this seems better than to perform embolization only through the carotid artery in the neck.

Three patients having embolization by peroperative catheterization of the cortical arteries showed great improvement and in 1 case, the postoperative angiogram showed a significant reduction in size of the angioma. Luessenhop's technique seldom leads to complete exclusion of a cerebral angioma. There is no danger in using emboli smaller than 1 mm with peroperative selective catheterization. More knowledge is needed of the hemodynamics of the circulatory anastomotic plexus of angiomas, and progress must be made in the materials used for embolization. Peroperative catheterization of the cortical arteries provides interesting possibilities for embolizing some angiomas that are otherwise inaccessible using Luessenhop's technique or other superselective angiographic methods.

▶ [Pantopaque-soaked Gelfoam pledgets were used by Kasdon et al. (J. Neurosurg. 44:753, 1976) to eliminate a traumatic arteriovenous fistula of the scalp. The 3×3×20-mm strips were introduced into the ipsilateral external carotid artery via syringe and three-way stopcock redrilled to accept these pledgets.

A peculiar end result of attempted embolization of a traumatic carotid cavernous fistula is reported by McCormick et al. (ibid., p. 513). After intracranial clipping of the ophthalmic and internal carotid arteries, muscle emboli were put into the left carotid artery, followed by ligation of common, external and internal carotid arteries. Ipsilateral hemiplegia later developed, with death on the 4th postoperative day. Autopsy revealed occlusion of the right internal and middle cerebral arteries by a muscle embolus. It is believed to have gone into the fistulous left cavernous sinus, thence, via a patent foramen ovale (unrecognized during life), into the right carotid system. — Ed.] ◀

Arteriovenous Malformations of Vein of Galen: Microsurgical Treatment. M. G. Yaşargil, J. Antic, R. Laciga, K. K. Jain and S. C. Boone[5] (Univ. of Zurich) report the

(5) Surg. Neurol. 6:195–200, September, 1976.

use of a microsurgical technique in 9 patients with arteriovenous malformations of the vein of Galen. Four patients
had subarachnoid hemorrhage preoperatively. Most commonly, the arterial supply to the malformation was from the
anterior pericallosal arteries, the posterior cerebral and superior cerebellar arteries and the posterior thalamic perfo-
rators arising from the posterior cerebral artery. The supply
was often bilateral. Venous drainage was always through
the vein of Galen. After a transcortical approach proved unsatisfactory in 3 patients, an interhemispheric approach
along the falx cerebri was adopted. Three patients died, 2
after acquiring intraventricular hematomas after shunting
for hydrocephalus.

TECHNIQUE. — General anesthesia with controlled respiration is
used. A free bone flap is removed with the patient's neck slightly
flexed, exposing the superior sagittal sinus, torcular and right
transverse sinus. Under the operating microscope with a television
camera attached, the dura is opened in a stellate manner, sacrific-
ing as few bridging veins as possible. Cotton paddies are used as
wedges to separate the malformation from the surrounding brain.
The ambient cistern is opened laterally on the right, avoiding ventricular puncture. The caudal end of the splenium of the corpus callosum must sometimes be split. The feeders are coagulated and
divided, with a constant check on the completeness of occlusion
being maintained by observation of the vein of Galen for a blue
color. Where necessary, feeders from the posterior cerebral artery
are divided at the base of the malformation. Microclips are frequently used. The aneurysmal dilation of the vein of Galen is not
resected but in 1 patient it was necessary to occlude it. The blood
pressure, if it was lowered, is restored, and the dura is reapproxi-
mated but not closed tightly. A drain is placed in the subgaleal
space before closing the scalp.

Microsurgical techniques are a great aid to the successful
surgical management of such difficult lesions as arteriovenous malformations of the vein of Galen.

**Pure Meningeal Arteriovenous Fistulas with Corti-
cal Venous Drainage.** P. Castaigne, J. Bories, P. Brunet,
J. J. Merland and V. Meininger[6] (Hôp. de la Salpêtrière,
Paris) suggest a new classification of three groups of cortical
meningeal fistulas (Fig 21). The first are fistulas that drain
directly or through the intermediary of a meningeal vein
into a venous sinus. The second group, extremely rare fistu-

(6) Rev. Neurol. (Paris) 132:169–181, March, 1976.

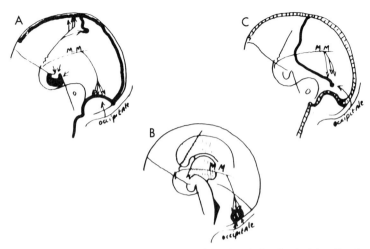

Fig 21. – Three types of cortical meningeal fistulas. **A,** fistulas draining directly or by the intermediary of a meningeal vein into a venous sinus. **B,** fistulas drained by a large dural venous sac that behaves like a true tumor. **C,** fistulas drained by a cerebral cortical vein. (Courtesy of Castaigne, P., et al.: Rev. Neurol. (Paris) 132: 169–181, March, 1976.)

las, are drained by a voluminous dural sac that behaves like a true tumor and most often are located in the posterior fossa. The third group are pure meningeal fistulas drained by a cerebral cortical vein and seem to represent a particular entity. Four cases of the latter fistulas are presented.

CASE 1. – Man, 53, without previous history, suddenly in 1975 experienced three generalized seizures, the second of which was followed by difficulty in reading and remembering for several days. The neurologic examination was normal. The EEG showed a bilateral temporofrontal irritable focus. Selective radiographic exploration of the branches of the external carotid revealed a dural arteriovenous fistula located behind and close to the wall of the lateral sinus. It was fed by the medial meningeal and the occipital arteries and was drained by a large cortical vein that connected the upper longitudinal and the cavernous sinuses. After treatment by embolization, the clinical signs disappeared. (Embolization of the occipital area that anastomosed the vertebral area required puncture directly beyond the origin of the vertebral area.)

In each of these 4 cases, the fistula was located on the dura mater and was fed by meningeal branches of the external carotid, but drainage was exclusively by a dilated cerebral vein that emptied into a venous sinus. Clinically, the fistulas were revealed by signs of involvement of the central nervous system. These cases were compared to 12 cases found in the literature that had a similar radiologic appearance. In these 12 cases, neurologic signs were the revealing symptoms.

Some meningeal fistulas have an indisputable traumatic cause. This was not so with these 4 cases, but in 1 of them it was a secondary factor from operation for intratemporal hematoma. An acquired origin seems probable.

Treatment of the fistulas rests on suppression of the shunt, accomplished surgically in 1 case and radiologically, through embolization, in the other 3 cases.

Cerebral Hematomas. Román Arana-Iñiguez, Eduardo Wilson, Ernesto Bastarrica and Mario Medici[7] (Montevideo, Uruguay) report a prospective study of 100 patients with primary cerebral hemorrhage, done to evaluate previously established guidelines for surgical treatment. Contraindications to surgery have included critical illness from the outset, a marked tendency to improve and deep hemorrhage. Surgery was usually done after clinical stabilization, on about the 5th day, unless sudden deterioration occurred in the first few days after presentation.

The diagnosis was confirmed at autopsy in 21 cases and at surgery in 33. The series included 82 gangliobasal hemorrhages, 11 lobar hemorrhages, 6 lobar and basal lesions and 1 unlocalized lesion. Over half the patients were male; deep hemorrhages were more frequent in female patients. The average patient age was 58.5. A past history of hypertension was obtained in 85% of 88 patients and of stroke in 16.8% of 91. Early papilledema was found in 7 patients, seizures in 7 and a well-developed pyramidal syndrome in 91. The EEG lateralized 50 lesions but was not helpful in determining the exact site of lesions. Angiography provided adequate information in 71 patients. All 6 air studies provided a precise topographic localization of the lesion.

The clinical picture stabilized at some point in all but 3 patients, and 49 patients were stable from the outset or after a period of less than an hour. All 19 patients who initially were severely ill died. Twenty-three patients improved

(7) Surg. Neurol. 6:45–52, July, 1976.

gradually to discharge, whereas 30 had a secondary exacerbation of their condition. Thirty-eight patients were operated on 16 hours to 45 days after the onset; 28 were treated when stable and 10 under emergency conditions. Five patients had postoperative complications and 2 of them died. Twelve surgical patients died, including 9 who were not initially severely ill and who were stable at surgery. Fifty-one patients died. Five of the 28 survivors who were followed over the long term were free of sequelae and 9 had only slight defects. Thirty-four deaths were neurologic in nature; 19 of these patients were initially in serious condition.

Cerebral hemorrhages tend to be resorbed and to be cured spontaneously. Surgery is indicated as a lifesaving measure, to reduce sequelae and to prevent secondary exacerbation. Surgery will not benefit patients who are critically ill from the outset; those with a small hematoma, especially if it is deep; or those who tend to improve with medical management, regardless of the location and size of the hematoma. Operation is done by cortical excision and exploration of the cavity and walls. Drainage is not used.

▶ [The authors believe that gangliobasal hematomas should not be operated on and that, in general, the condition of the patient should be stabilized before operation is considered. Some of the "guesswork" about the size of the hematoma and its entry into the ventricles can be resolved with the use of the computerized tomography (CT) scanner. Such an acute situation is not one suitable for transporting the patient to the CT scanner for a shared instrument some distance away, a feeling apparently not shared by those nonmedical people who control acquisition of these expensive machines. – Ed.] ◀

Cerebellar Hemorrhage: Reliability of Clinical Evaluation. About 10% of intracerebral hemorrhages occur in the cerebellum, and untreated patients have a high mortality. Gary A. Rosenberg and David M. Kaufman[8] (New York) sought to determine whether a clinical diagnosis of cerebellar hemorrhage justifies immediate surgical intervention without confirmation by radiologic contrast studies. Review was made of the data on 33 patients treated during 1970–75. All patients were aged 35 years or over and none had known illness that might produce a cerebellar mass.

Thirteen patients had cerebellar hemorrhage confirmed by angiography, surgery or autopsy. An avascular cerebellar mass was demonstrated angiographically in 9 cases, with confirmatory ventriculographic findings in 5 of them. In 3 patients with normal angiographic findings, ventriculography showed a cerebellar mass. Eleven patients in this group had operation. Four comatose patients died and only 2 of 7 lethargic patients lived longer than 2 weeks after operation. An infarction was found in 3 cases. In 10 patients, cerebellar hemorrhage was unsuspected initially but was subsequently demonstrated. Surgical procedures were done in 7 of these cases. Both comatose patients died, whereas 4 of 5 lethargic patients lived more than 2 weeks postoperatively. All these patients had cerebellar hemorrhage confirmed pathologically. Ten patients were strongly suspected of having cerebellar hemorrhage but had other conditions. Nausea, vomiting and corneal reflex depression were less frequent than in the other groups. Four patients in this group had a final diagnosis of brain stem infarction; all patients in this group recovered.

Diagnostic procedures are necessary to establish or exclude the diagnosis of cerebellar hemorrhage; ventriculography has been the most definitive diagnostic procedure. Both ventriculography and vertebral angiography are time-consuming, but judicious choice of one confirmatory study and good logistic planning should minimize delays in necessary surgery and avoid unnecessary posterior fossa explorations.

► [Messert et al. (Stroke 7:305, 1976) note the difficulty in diagnosis of cerebellar hemorrhage, which does not always produce unilateral headache, peripheral facial palsy, appendicular ataxia, defective corneal reflex and paresis of conjugate gaze. They value spontaneous unilateral eye closure as an additional striking manifestation and believe it is due to reflex avoidance of diplopia; obviously it cannot appear on the side of the facial paralysis. They present 2 case histories in which this sign was helpful.

According to Vincent (Minn. Med. 59:453, 1976), 10% of all intraparenchymal intracranial hemorrhages are cerebellar in origin. Hypertension was considered the major etiologic factor in 62% and anticoagulation in 14%. The most frequently observed signs were appendicular ataxia, ipsilateral gaze palsy, peripheral facial palsy, constricted reactive pupils and periodic respirations. Outcome of operation is most often dictated by the state of consciousness before operation. Computerized axial tomography and vertebral angiography are the best diagnostic procedures. Evacuation of hematoma may permit recovery, which otherwise infrequently occurs spontaneously. — Ed.] ◄

Subependymal Brain Stem Hematomas: Report of Two Cases is presented by I. Papo, U. Pasquini and U.

Salvolini[9] (Univ. of Ancona). Brain stem hematomas successfully operated on, most of them located in the pontine tegmentum, have been reported. Ventriculography indicated an expanding lesion in most cases; vertebral angiography failed to demonstrate any vascular malformation.

CASE 1. — Woman, 35, with severe headache, vomiting, blurred vision and an unsteady gait, exhibited bilateral papilledema and nystagmus, complete astasia-abasia and slight right-sided dysdiadochokinesia. Ventriculography showed an expanding lesion in the 4th ventricle. Craniectomy revealed slight bilateral tonsillar herniation and a hemorrhagic cyst in the right posterior pontine tegmentum. The cyst was entered and emptied, and its medial wall, which was formed by the ventricular ependyma, was removed. On follow-up, the patient had only an unsteady gait.

CASE 2. — Man, 23, with right-sided abducens paralysis lasting 1 month, had tomographic evidence of a lesion in the tegmental brain stem. Craniectomy showed no tonsillar herniation; the outlet of the 4th ventricle was free. On retraction of the cerebellar tonsils laterally, the rhomboid fossa showed yellowish discoloration and a subtle arteriolar network; its superolateral portion was blue and bulged into the lumen of the 4th ventricle. The ependymal layer was teased away and a clot removed. The cavity was 1-cm deep in the right pontine tegmentum. The abducens paralysis was unchanged after operation but a mild left-sided hemiparesis resolved.

Computerized axial tomography is valuable diagnostically. The brain stem hematomas that are amenable to surgery are likely to be caused by cryptic arteriovenous malformations in the outer brain stem tegmentum. Generally, a hemorrhagic collection from the peripheral pontine tegmentum tends to spread toward the lumen of the 4th ventricle, being limited only by the ependymal layer, which may be disrupted and therefore lead to subarachnoid hemorrhage. The subependymal hematoma has the appearance of an intraventricular expanding lesion. Operation is necessary if intracranial hypertension is present but seems less necessary when only cranial nerve deficits are present.

Recognizing Spontaneous Spinal Epidural Hematoma. Spinal epidural hemorrhage is an unusual cause of acute paraplegia in the elderly. Although devastating, it can be successfully treated in most instances if recognized early. Clark Watts (Univ. of Missouri) and Lito Porto[1]

(9) Neuroradiology 11:279–282, 1976.
(1) Geriatrics 31:97–99, September, 1976.

(Univ. of Texas Southwestern Med. School) report on a case and review 13 previously reported cases.

Woman, 73, was admitted with acute paraplegia about an hour after midline lower thoracic back pain developed while she was sitting. Hypesthesia to pinprick was present bilaterally to below the T10 dermatome and acute urinary retention was also present. X-rays showed moderate osteoporosis and spondylosis of the thoracolumbar spine and a myelogram showed a complete block at L2. A laminectomy from T11 to L2 showed an acute epidural hematoma, which was removed. No source of bleeding was found. The patient improved gradually and had only minimal weakness in the lower extremities 2 months postoperatively and no bladder or sphincter abnormality.

The usual features of previously reported cases included sudden spinal pain, paraplegia, a sensory level and urinary retention. Pain was usually at the level of the hematoma and generally was quite severe. It may become radicular in nature. Paraplegia usually developed within 6 hours of the onset of pain. Precipitating factors were not very remarkable. Laboratory findings are usually unremarkable except in patients on anticoagulant therapy. Manometric studies should not be done at myelography for fear that neurologic deficit be increased thereby. Eight of 12 patients, including the present patient, improved after surgery and 5 recovered completely. Of the 4 who did not improve, 3 died. Both patients not having surgery failed to improve and died. There were no surgical fatalities.

Spontaneous spinal epidural hematoma in the elderly may present with minimal or no trauma and is a potentially devastating condition. The diagnosis is made by myelography and the treatment is laminectomy.

Anterior Angiomas of the Spinal Cord and Their Treatment. In addition to pure anterior angiomas, A. Rey, M. Djindjian, R. Djindjian and R. Houdart[2] (Hôp. Lariboisière, Paris) include mixed angiomas that have a double anterior and posterior feeding. They represent slightly more than half of the angiomas and pose a difficult therapeutic problem. Their basic difference is that the entire intramedullary portion is fed by the anterior spinal axis.

The symptomatology of anterior angiomas is schematically different from that of posterior ones in age of occurrence of

(2) Rev. Neurol. (Paris) 133:13–21, January, 1977.

initial manifestations, in the acute clinical aspect of these manifestations and in their evolution. As a rule, the first disorders are observed in young patients, i.e., children, adolescents or young adults. Usually they are acute, e.g., paraplegia or paraparesis of quick onset, meningeal hemorrhage, alone or associated with medulloradicular syndrome. After the initial involvement, sometimes permanent paraplegia persists, giving a picture of hematomyelia or more often myelomalacia, but usually there is improvement and sometimes even complete regression. Ultimate development is marked by recurrences, each manifested at the same level as the preceding recurrence and leaving a worsened neurologic state.

Treatment of anterior angiomas is not simple. For a long time it was thought that they could be removed only at the expense of irreversible medullary lesions. Embolization has become a new effective therapeutic possibility in forms with a single anterior pedicle. It should be emphasized that we are not dealing with embolization of the artery in the proximal part, but with distal embolization of the artery at the very level of the malformation. This means that embolization is contraindicated in nondilated arterial forms, and it can be done only if the artery has sufficiently increased in size to obviate risk of its obstruction by a small embolus before malformation. Also to avoid such risks, partial and progressive embolizations are done. These are followed by clinical improvement and cure in some cases, but the risk of a new episode of paraplegia is not excluded, either spontaneously or with anticoagulants.

Fifteen patients were studied, with follow-up for 1 month to 2½ years. Radical removal of the angioma was possible in 12 cases with angiographic control in 7 cases. There was no benefit when the patient was operated on in the completely paraplegic stage (4 cases). However, in cases of incomplete paraplegia, there was no worsening and even some improvement.

The surgical approach for anterior angiomas depends on size of the angioma and the situation on the inside of the spinal cord. The angiographic findings permit classification of four types of intramedullary angiomas.

▶ [Ausman et al., from the University of Minnesota, reported to a Dallas seminar (J.A.M.A. 236:1335, 1976) on the use of tiny bits of Ivalon sponge to embolize a large arteriovenous malformation of the spinal cord. This synthetic sponge may be dried while compressed — and regains its original size and shape when it reaches its target via an embolization technique. — Ed.] ◄

Occlusions

Carotid Endarterectomy is discussed by Jesse E. Thompson and C. M. Talkington[3] (Baylor Univ. Med. Center). A completed frank stroke is a serious and incapacitating disorder. A carotid lesion is significant if there is a reduction in the diameter of the internal carotid artery of 40–50% or more as measured on the arteriogram. Arteriography remains the definitive diagnostic measure. The principal indication for carotid endarterectomy is transient cerebral ischemia. Patients with recent mild, stable strokes and those with old strokes who manifest new symptoms may also be candidates. Emergency endarterectomy is not often indicated. Significant bilateral lesions should be treated in separate stages. Indications for surgery also depend on a critical evaluation of operative risk. A shunt is used routinely, and regional or systemic heparinization is used during endarterectomy. Excessively high blood pressure, present postoperatively, must be treated aggressively. Use of a temporary inlying bypass shunt remains the most reliable means of cerebral support.

Anatomical restoration of blood flow may be achieved in over 98% of patients with partially occluded arteries, and the long-term patency rates approach 95%. Operative mortality in 1,140 endarterectomies done on 903 patients in an 18-year period was 2.3%; the rate in 338 operations for frank stroke was 5.9%. Of 126 survivors with frank stroke, followed for up to 13 years, 30.2% were normal and 58.7% were improved. Mortality in patients with transient ischemia should approach 1%. No more than 40% of total carotid occlusions are successfully treated, depending on the interval from onset to operation. Chronic total occlusion in the absence of symptoms is not an indication for operation. In acute total occlusion, operability depends mainly on the clinical picture of the stroke. No deaths occurred in 123 opera-

(3) Ann. Surg. 184:1–15, July, 1976.

tions on patients with unilateral carotid stenosis and contralateral occlusion, and there was only one operation-related deficit.

In some patients, an asymptomatic carotid bruit is probably not an innocent lesion if left untreated, and endarterectomy may be cautiously considered if arteriography demonstrates a hazardous lesion, provided multiple risk factors are not present and an experienced team is available. The surgical treatment of fibromuscular dysplasia of the internal carotid in symptomatic patients depends on the location of the lesion and any associated pathology. The relationship of carotid coils and kinks to symptoms of cerebrovascular insufficiency remains controversial.

▶ [The problem of what to do with unilateral extracranial carotid artery occlusion is also dealt with by Waltimo et al. (Stroke 7:480, 1976), but from the standpoint of prognosis without operation. In their series of 121 men and 34 women, only 15% were over age 59, and this age factor is presumed by the authors to explain the relatively high 5-year survival of 78% probability. Prognosis and functional recovery were better in nonsmokers, but hypertension was not of prognostic value. The state of the opposite carotid artery was not mentioned in this article.

Fibromuscular dysplasia has been associated with symptoms of impaired cerebral flow. In the case of Upson and Raza (N.Y. State J. Med. 76: 972, 1976), arteriotomy confirmed the thickenings inside while the external appearance was normal. Graduated internal dilatation with an arterial Fogarty catheter gave relief of symptoms and caused disappearance of the bruit. Postoperative angiography 8 months later showed minimal residual disease on the side operated on; so the opposite side was similarly treated successfully. These authors prefer the Fogarty catheter to the metal coronary artery dilators used by Thompson and Talkington.

Piepgras and Sundt (Ann. Surg. 184:637, 1976) have used silicone elastomer shunts in about a third of their 515 carotid endarterectomies. Despite intraoperative heparin anticoagulation, thrombus is found within the lumen of the shunt after removal. The authors have therefore impregnated the shunts by immersing them in heparin solution. In 244 operations with these treated shunts, there have been no problems caused by thrombotic occlusion, nor has thrombus been found in the lumen, despite prolonged use of the shunt (average, 40 minutes). It is of passing interest that unlike Thompson, Sundt believes shunts should not be used routinely, but only if indicated.

When both internal carotid arteries need operation the choice of which to do first is sometimes difficult. Clauss et al. (Arch. Surg. 111:1304, 1976) suggest they be done one after the other at the same operative sitting. They present good results in 12 patients. Myocardial disease may be a greater hazard than the primary carotid disease in such patients. In 8 patients, West et al. (Br. Med. J. 1:818, 1976) found pain in the head, face and neck along with Horner's syndrome. Angiography in some patients showed narrowing of the carotid artery compatible with dissection of the wall. Three patients had complete occlusion. The pain was widespread, burning or throbbing. Diagnosis of dissection was proved by operation in 1 patient with subsequent ligation. In another, the artery was found to be narrowed, but was not opened. Symptoms regressed within several months in most patients. — Ed.] ◄

Emergency Carotid Artery Surgery in Neurologically Unstable Patients. It is agreed that angiography and carotid artery surgery should be avoided in patients with acute, severe stroke but there is no consensus on the proper approach to patients with unstable, mild to moderate neurologic deficits. Jerry Goldstone and Wesley S. Moore[4] (Univ. of California, San Francisco) have adopted a more aggressive approach to such patients and report the results obtained in 11 patients seen in the past 1½ years. None of the patients had severe, devastating neurologic deficits or depressed consciousness. The indications for emergency angiography included crescendo transient ischemic attacks in 4 patients and stroke in evolution in 8.

Emergency angiography permitted identification of the responsible lesions in these patients and emergency carotid thromboendarterectomy produced prompt, complete recovery in all cases but 1. The patient who did not do well had a total carotid occlusion, did not have an operation and died of a cerebral infarction. Surgical management included general anesthesia with maintenance of normal arterial P_{co2} and blood pressure in the hospital. An internal shunt was used only when the internal carotid back pressure was below 25 mm Hg and in patients who have had a previous cerebral infarction on the side of operation. A shunt was used in 2 of the 4 patients with crescendo transient ischemic attacks, because of low back pressure, and in all 7 patients with stroke in evolution, because of concern for the presence of cerebral infarction. Intraoperative angiograms made at the end of surgery confirmed a satisfactory technical result in each case.

The primary goal of treatment in these patients is to prevent cerebral infarction or worsening of infarction. Patients with evolving stroke or with waxing or waning deficits should be immediately anticoagulated. An aggressive diagnostic approach is called for when the patient's neurologic status is rapidly changing or is atypical and not readily ex-

(4)   Arch. Surg. 111:1284 – 1291, November, 1976.

plained. Angiography and surgery are not advocated for patients with severe fixed neurologic deficits, especially when associated with depressed consciousness. Surgery is also not advocated to reestablish flow in a totally occluded internal carotid artery.

► [Unusual color photographs of the interior of the cervical carotid artery in cadavers have been published by Olinger (Surg. Neurol. 7:7, 1977). "Mountainous plaque," "rocklike formation," "stalagmite lesion" and "ridged plaque" are among the descriptions applied to the lesions of both common and internal carotid arteries. These and pictures of ulcerated and thrombosed lesions show the fallacy of determining operation only by the diameter of the stenosing lesion seen at angiography. The author apparently has not made the radical suggestion that the endoscope be modified for use in attacking the plaques in living patients. — Ed.] ◄

Reopening Some Occluded Carotid Arteries: Report of Four Cases. William A. Shucart and Eddy Garrido[5] (Tufts Univ.) recently operated on 4 patients in whom intermittent ischemic symptoms were referable to a cerebral hemisphere and in whom angiography showed complete occlusion of the ipsilateral internal carotid artery in the neck, with collateral filling of the ipsilateral intracranial carotid into the cavernous portion. Endarterectomy was performed successfully in each case, 1 – 5 weeks after demonstration of the complete occlusion. Angiography showed excellent retrograde filling of the cavernous part of the carotid artery on the occluded side in these patients. In each case the thrombus was easily removed from the cervical internal carotid artery and excellent backflow was reestablished. Angiography showed excellent patency of the entire internal carotid artery several weeks postoperatively in all cases. In no patient was a fixed neurologic deficit improved, but no further ischemic episodes occurred and patients in whom deficits appeared to be intermittently worsening did not deteriorate further.

An attempt can reasonably be made to reopen a symptomatic occluded cervical carotid artery if there is significant retrograde filling of the intracranial portion well down into the cavernous portion. The goal is to increase brain perfusion where the symptoms suggest an intermittent perfusion problem such as transient ischemic attacks, amaurosis fugax or stepwise worsening of a neurologic deficit. None of

(5)   J. Neurosurg. 45:442 – 446, October, 1976.

the present patients has had further symptoms from the operated hemisphere during follow-up for 6–24 months. If successful, this procedure is superior to the presently available alternatives and is much easier.

▶ [Selection of patients for angiography and hence for operation is difficult, especially in view of the report by Fields and Lemak (J.A.M.A. 235: 2734, 1976) concerning internal carotid artery occlusion. There was a 4% incidence of grave complication or death after angiography in those patients with carotid artery occlusion as compared to 2.1% in the general study population of The Joint Study of Extracranial Arterial Occlusion. The increase is ascribed to performance of angiography in the acute stage of occlusion, presumably contraindicated also by the dangers of operating on acute stroke patients. Surgery undertaken within a week of a cerebral infarction was associated with a 67% mortality.

Patients with carotid artery occlusion and no apparent neurologic deficit had a 43% mortality with nonsurgical treatment (mainly from stroke or myocardial infarction). About 12% of all those with unilateral occlusion have little or no deficit and are still doing well on follow-up. Review of cases with one carotid artery occluded and the other stenotic indicates much better results from medical management (63% alive after a 66-month follow-up compared to 34% after direct attack on the stenotic lesion or the occlusion). However, analysis also shows that the operative procedures were often faulty (lack of protection during operation or operation too soon after onset of symptoms) and the variation between institutions was extreme (1 complication and no deaths in 19 surgically treated patients in one center, compared to another center with 37 patients, 13 grave complications and 10 deaths). The authors believe that the new microsurgical bypass procedures will probably be of benefit to those with unilateral occlusions and ipsilateral transient ischemic episodes and to those with bilateral occlusions, minimal focal deficits and mental changes ascribed to decreased perfusion.

When postoperative carotid stenosis occurs (5 months to 13 years after endarterectomy), reconstructive techniques used by Stoney and String (Surgery 80:705, 1976) include endarterectomy for atherosclerosis and for intimal fibrosis, patch angioplasty and resection with anastomosis. Twenty-four of the 29 patients in their series came from the authors' series of 1,654 carotid endarterectomies. One patient developed transient aphasia; 1 died of stroke. The others have been free of neurologic symptoms except for 1 patient who had symptoms from a second recurrence 8 years after the first. In the discussion, it was pointed out that the incidence of recurrence is far less if vein graft patch is used routinely.

Humphries et al. (ibid., p. 695) have followed for up to 12 years 168 patients with asymptomatic carotid stenosis. Two developed typical neurologic symptoms, 26 had transient ischemic attacks and successfully had endarterectomies, 3 had strokes when they ignored transient attacks, 1 had stroke without warning and 136 remained asymptomatic. The authors believe asymptomatic carotid stenosis should be left alone unless an ischemic attack occurs. Opinions among the discussors of the article differed, with at least 1 favoring prophylactic operation on asymptomatic stenosis (no deaths and no infarctions); in symptomatic patients, in the last 200 operations, W. S. Moore reported neurologic morbidity of under 3% and operative mortality of 0.5%. — Ed.] ◄

Surgical Management of Vertebral-Basilar Insufficiency.

J. M. Cormier and C. Laurian[6] (Paris) reviewed the management of vertebral-basilar insufficiency in 114 men and 28 women, most of them aged 40–60 years. Arteriosclerosis was the major cause. Eighty-six patients did not have prominent neurologic disorders but did have signs related to reduced cerebral blood flow. Occlusion of the innominate artery was treated in 34 instances, occlusion of the right subclavian artery in 25, occlusion of the left subclavian artery in 68 and stenosis of the vertebral artery in 119. The surgical treatment depended in part on whether or not the lesions included the ostium. Ipsilateral common carotid lesions were treated in 24 instances and contralateral carotid lesions in 15 instances.

The operative mortality was 1.5%, and three deaths occurred later due to extension of arteriosclerosis. Local complications included 5 lymphoceles, 3 hematomas and 12 Horner's syndromes. Five laryngeal nerve paralyses and 9 phrenic nerve paralyses also occurred. One hemiparalysis was caused by a contralateral thrombosis, and 1 lateral hemianopsia occurred. General complications were due to coronary disease. The 79 asymptomatic patients did not worsen after surgery. Four of 93 symptomatic patients had neurologic exacerbations after surgery; 3 recovered completely.

By adapting the surgical approach to the extent of the lesions and to the patient's general condition, the operative mortality has been reduced to 1.5%, while the outcome has been improved. Even asymptomatic patients can be treated if conditions are favorable and life expectancy is reasonable. Use of the cervical approach appears justified in order to adapt the extent of surgery to the patient's condition.

► [Berguer et al. (Arch. Surg. 111:976, 1976) also use saphenous vein grafts for occlusive vertebral artery disease, but as bypasses, rather than for reimplantation of the vertebral or subclavian artery. They depend on angiography rather than arteriotomy to determine the extent of stenotic lesion. Each of the 4 patients in this report had a patent graft shown by angiography 1 week after operation, and follow-up will be by the Dopler ultrasound technique. Symptomatic improvement has been present for

(6) Int. Surg. 61:203–212, April, 1976.

the duration of follow-up (3 months thus far). Two patients had post-operative swelling due to lymphocele on the left, and in 1 patient transient Horner's syndrome also appeared.

Reversal of vertebral flow with neurologic symptoms was first termed "subclavian steal" by C. Miller Fisher in 1961. Ipsilateral vertebral artery ligation may be done in an extremely poor-risk patient, but Hafner (ibid., p. 1074) prefers to try to preserve the cerebral circulation. Common carotid artery to subclavian artery bypass with saphenous vein graft was most often done. Three patients had transcervical subclavian endarterectomy for lesions at or close to the orifice of the vertebral artery. There were 16 instances of transthoracic operation for Dacron prosthetic replacement from the aorta to the subclavian artery. Of 40 patients, 38 are alive and asymptomatic over periods averaging 60 months (15 months to 12 years). Extrathoracic procedures are preferred for elderly and poor-risk patients. – Ed.] ◄

Intracranial Neurosurgical Treatment of Occlusive Cerebrovascular Disease.

Jose L. Salazar, Abdul R. C. Amine and Oscar Sugar[7] (Univ. of Illinois) review data in 13 cases of anastomosis of the extracranial superficial temporal artery to the intracranial middle cerebral artery for transient ischemia. In another case, anastomosis was made between the occipital branch of the external carotid artery and the middle cerebral artery. Of 2 representative patients, 1 had stenosis of the right middle cerebral artery and occlusion of the left middle cerebral artery and the other had occlusion of the right internal carotid artery. Both patients have been followed for 8 and 10 months, respectively, after operation and both have been asymptomatic and subjectively improved.

Patent anastomoses were seen in 8 of 14 instances (in 7 of the 13 patients operated on) by angiography and ^{99m}Tc cerebral blood flow study. Six patients are free of transient ischemic attacks and are subjectively improved and have no neurologic deficit. One patient had mild dysphasia postoperatively from which he recovered. Occlusion of the anastomosis was demonstrated by angiography in 5 patients; 1 of these had a stroke in evolution; embolectomy of the middle cerebral artery was incomplete because of cerebral edema. Another patient was unchanged 7 months after an occluded anastomosis was seen. One patient essentially is asymptomatic, 1 died of myocardial infarction and 1 is alive with poor memory. One patient died 3 weeks postoperatively of

(7) Stroke 7:348–353, July–Aug., 1976.

myocardial infarction without having follow-up angiography.

Information on the long-term results of cerebral revascularization is inadequate but the short-term findings indicate enough promise to warrant a cautious extension of the procedure, and perhaps even an extension to vertebrobasilar insufficiency when this appears to steal blood from the carotid system.

▶ [A fine article by Sundt et al. (Mayo Clin. Proc. 51:677, 1976) describes experiences with 58 bypass operations on 56 patients. Patency of the shunt has improved from 25% (before November, 1973) to 95% since July, 1974 (58 patients), ascribed to improvement in microsuture techniques. Indications are transient ischemic attacks (TIAs), amaurosis fugax, "slow stroke" (progressive neurologic deficit over days or weeks, mimicking neoplasia), progressing stroke (hours to days), giant aneurysm and middle cerebral stenosis — all in the presence of occlusion of the internal carotid artery or severe stenosis in the siphon. Fibromuscular disease and moyamoya are probable indications in the presence of TIA or amaurosis fugax. Asymptomatic carotid occlusions or those associated with major infarctions are unlikely indications for operation.

Results in 100 cases are described by Chater and Popp (Surg. Neurol. 6:115, 1976). In an average postoperative follow-up of 20 months, 92% of the patients with TIA or reversible ischemic neurologic deficits were asymptomatic or had significant reduction in attacks. Doppler ultrasound studies showed good flow in 95 patients. Only 1 of 70 angiograms showed nonfunctioning anastomosis. Three patients died within the first 30 days after operation; none of the last 80 have died. The incidence of strokes in the ipsilateral hemisphere has been only 1%. In 20 patients with TIAs who were followed more than 36 months, only 1 had a stroke, and that was in the contralateral hemisphere.

Perhaps the most common occlusive disease for which the bypass is done is middle cerebral artery occlusion. Kaste and Waltimo (Stroke 7: 482, 1976) have described the long-term prognosis of 78 patients with occlusion of this artery or its major branches. The 46 men and 32 women were as young as under age 20 years and as old as aged 69; 69 were under age 60; 51 were under age 50 and the mean age was 44. Many elderly patients do not get to the author's department, and not all stroke patients have angiography. Acute-stage mortality was only 5%. Those who died were all men. Functional recovery was excellent; 72% who survived became independent in activities of daily living; 43% regained working capacity. (Strangely, more of these had left-sided occlusions!) Branch occlusion was more compatible with recovery than complete occlusion. Subsequent deaths were twice as often due to stroke than to cardiovascular disease. Unfortunately, it was not specified if the subsequent stroke was in the same artery, for, if so, that would tend to favor operation as a preventative measure.

Two cases of basilar and of middle cerebral artery thrombosis in boys aged 6½ and 5 years, respectively, are reported by Lillquist and Ingstrup

(Acta Paediatr. Scand. 65:119, 1976). The pathogenesis is unknown. Improvement occurred in both and is considered to be spontaneous. —Ed.] ◄

External Carotid-Vertebral Artery Anastomosis for Vertebrobasilar Insufficiency. Guy Corkill, Barry N. French, Con Michas, Cully A. Cobb, III, and Thomas J. Mims[8] (Univ. of California, Davis) report data on 2 patients in whom occlusive disease of the vertebral artery, responsible for vertebrobasilar ischemia, lent itself to direct surgical revascularization by anastomosis of the extracranial external carotid artery to the vertebral artery. The patients had previous brain stem infarction and current symptoms of vascular insufficiency in the basilar circulation and evidence of vertebral artery occlusive disease. Angiography showed ostial stenosis of the dominant right vertebral artery and retrograde flow down the left vertebral artery to the level of C2 in the first patient and to the level of a severely stenosed origin in the second. The carotid circulation was patent in both patients. Blood flow in the posterior circulation was augmented by extracranial anastomosis of the external carotid to the vertebral artery in the foramen transversarium at the C1 – C2 level by a lateral approach in the first patient and at the C4 – C5 level by an anterior approach in the second. Both patients had an improved neurologic status postoperatively.

Endarterectomy of the ostial stenosis in either of these patients would have involved clamping the only functioning vertebral artery in the presence of symptomatic incompetence of the collateral circulation. Such a procedure would be extremely risky and, in addition, ostial reconstruction requires a thoracotomy. The extracranial approach of external carotid-vertebral artery anastomosis is more likely to augment blood flow significantly in the posterior circulation because of the larger caliber of the vessels involved. End-to-side anastomosis involves less dissection of the recipient vertebral artery than does the end-to-end procedure, and the limited dissection required will enhance postoperative patency rates. The occipital artery is left intact if possible for future intracranial anastomosis if

(8) Surg. Neurol. 7:109–115, March, 1977.

required. The extracranial anastomosis in the neck avoids a thoracotomy in some cases and an intracranial procedure in others.

▶ [Khodadad (Surg. Neurol. 5:255, 1976) describes anastomosis between the end of the occipital artery and the caudal loop of the posterior inferior cerebellar artery in a man, aged 58, who had total occlusions of both vertebral arteries, 95% stenosis of the right internal carotid artery and total occlusion of the left one. Right carotid endarterectomy was done 2 months after a stroke produced right hemiplegia and aphasia from which he had made fairly good recovery. A month later, the occipital anastomosis was done. Two weeks later, angiography showed the occipital and posterior inferior cerebellar arteries, but did not show retrograde flow via the latter artery into the vertebral or basilar arteries. — Ed.] ◀

Selection of Patients for Extra-Intracranial Arterial Bypass Surgery Based on rCBF Measurements. The extracranial intracranial arterial bypass (EIAB) procedure is a new treatment for ischemic cerebrovascular disease; it is technically feasible and seems valuable in preventing stroke. Peter Schmiedek, Otmar Gratzl, Robert Spetzler, Harald Steinhoff, Robert Enzenbach, Walter Brendel and Frank Marguth[9] performed 167 regional cerebral blood flow (rCBF) studies before and after operation on 110 patients during 5 years to obtain objective data for determining which patients may benefit from EIAB. The rCBF was measured over 16 regions of one hemisphere by the ^{133}Xe intracarotid injection method. The 75 men and 35 women studied had an average age of 50. Diagnoses ranged from transient cerebral ischemic attacks to completed strokes.

Fifty-three of the 110 patients were selected for EIAB; of these, 47 had rCBF studies before and 40 after operation; 15 patients had two postoperative measurements made. Two of 22 patients having postoperative external carotid artery studies showed no evidence of bypass function. During hypercapnia, blood flow increased significantly in the area supplied by the anastomosis but was relatively constant in the extracerebral compartment. All eighteen postoperative internal carotid injection studies showed improved cerebral hemodynamics, and in 11 patients blood flow was improved over an extended area. Among 15 patients having further studies after an average of 11 months, 3 showed secondary occlusion of the bypass when the earlier postoperative study had shown bypass function. Six patients had further im-

(9) J. Neurosurg. 44:303–312, March, 1976.

provement in CBF, whereas in 6, the two postoperative studies gave identical results.

Measurement of rCBF allows an intelligent decision on the advisability of surgical intervention in patients with ischemic cerebrovascular disease. Patients with focal or relatively focal reductions of CBF seem to benefit from EIAB; those presenting with a generalized reduction of CBF, who show no clinical improvement and have a high rate of occlusion of the bypass, do not seem to benefit from EIAB.

▶ [An article by Gratzl et al. (J. Neurosurg. 44:313, 1976) describes clinical experience with extracranial intracranial anastomosis in 65 cases. All had preoperative angiograms, 47 had regional blood flow studies (some with test of autoregulation by increasing the blood pressure). Dextran-40 was given intraoperatively and postoperatively. Since regional blood flow studies have been relied on, morbidity and mortality with operation have not been encountered, in contrast to the numerous problems previously. This type of surgery is contraindicated in acute cerebral ischemia and when the region cerebral blood flow study reveals general reduction of cerebral blood flow as opposed to a localized ischemic focus. — Ed.] ◀

Experimental Carotid-Basilar Bypass. Michael Feely[1] (Cleveland Clinic) describes a procedure for anastomosing the carotid artery to the vertebrobasilar circulation in the dog.

Ten acute and 10 chronic studies were done on large mongrel dogs having carotid-basilar bypass. The carotid artery was dissected free over a 2-cm segment and, with the use of an operating microscope, a 2-cm opening was drilled in the occipital bone just above the foramen magnum to expose the basilar artery. A 10-cm length of saphenous artery was excised and a 5-mm segment of the basilar artery was occluded with clips; an arteriotomy was made and one end of the saphenous artery was joined to this and the other end was joined to the common carotid artery. The carotid artery distal to the anastomosis was ligated to facilitate later arteriography.

Successful anastomoses were done in 7 of 10 dogs; 4 lived for 3 months without any neurologic deficit. Carotid angiography showed a patent graft in 2 dogs 3 months postoperatively. One dog had carotid angiography 9 months after operation and had an occluded graft. Flow measurements, recorded in the graft at operation, showed flow rates of 5–9 ml/minute.

(1) Br. J. Surg. 63:186–188, March, 1976.

Meticulous surgical technique is needed to suture these vessels, with the use of long microsurgical instruments of the bayonet type. The larger basilar artery present in man would make anastomosis easier but the basilar artery is much less accessible in man than in the dog. The dog tolerates occlusion of a 1-cm segment of the basilar artery for 2–3 hours without subsequent deficit but there is no evidence that man would respond similarly. Probably another method of anastomosis, either partial arterial occlusion or insertion of a temporary shunt during surgery, would have to be used. In the future, this type of surgery may be used for treatment of patients with occlusive cerebrovascular disease.

Embolic Occlusion of the Superior and Inferior Divisions of the Middle Cerebral Artery with Angiographic-Clinical Correlation. Despite anatomical variations in the branching pattern of the middle cerebral artery (MCA), a superior division supplying 3 or 4 individual branches is present in 90% of anatomical specimens. L. Reed Altemus, Glenn H. Roberson, C. Miller Fisher and Michael Pessin[2] (Harvard Med. School) reviewed 84 angiographic examples of occlusion of the MCA or its branches and analyzed in detail 14 of these that satisfied angiographic criteria for division occlusion. Division occlusion by an embolus was defined either by showing a filling defect within the lumen or by demonstrating abrupt total occlusion of the division with simultaneous retrograde filling of all its major branches by collaterals.

Intraluminal filling defects were seen in 4 of 14 patients, whereas 10 showed total occlusion with reconstitution by retrograde flow. Collateral filling of superior division branches was furnished by branches of the ipsilateral anterior cerebral artery, whereas inferior division branches were reconstituted by multiple branches of the ipsilateral posterior cerebral artery or pericallosal artery, or both. Six of 7 patients with superior division occlusion showed severe hemiplegia and motor aphasia. All 4 with inferior division occlusion exhibited sensory receptive aphasia without motor weakness; 3 of the latter patients had a hemianopia.

Appreciation of the anatomy of divisions of the MCA helps

(2) Am. J. Roentgenol. 126:576–581, March, 1976.

in understanding the angiographic distribution of embolic fragments and in interpreting the clinical picture in what appears to be partial or incomplete divisional syndromes. Magnification and subtraction techniques should be used to visualize intraluminal emboli, and consideration should be given to visualizing the various routes of collateral circulation, especially if none is visible on unilateral carotid injection. This is particularly true of inferior division occlusion, where collaterals may be demonstrated only by opacification of the posterior cerebral artery. The cervical carotid, which may serve as a source of emboli, should be carefully studied.

► In an article in English in a German journal (Zentralbl. Neurochir. 37:1, 1976), Zülch explains his sometimes misquoted views on spinovascular insufficiency. He has developed a theory analogous to that of cerebrovascular insufficiency, with emphasis on watershed areas between the major supplying vessels that come in at C6 – C7 and at T8 – T10 (most often from the left). Other precarious zones may be below the high cervical supply coming from the vertebral anterior spinal branches or at T12 – L1, the terminus of a commonly seen vessel coming in at about L2. He emphasizes that he applies these concepts in the 10% of patients who lack the "maximum" vascular supply to these areas and agrees that the other 90% have a sufficient arterial supply that occlusion of one of the major radicular arteries will not produce a catastrophic myelopathy. – Ed. ◄

Pain

Geniculate Neuralgia: Diagnosis and Surgical Management are discussed by Jack L. Pulec[3] (Los Angeles). Geniculate neuralgia is a rare cause of pain in the ear. Typically it is characterized by severe paroxysmal neuralgic pain centered directly in the ear. The pain may be gradual in onset and of a dull, persistent nature, with occasional sharp stabs occurring. Section of the nervus intermedius and excision of the geniculate ganglion, done by a middle fossa approach without producing facial paralysis, vertigo or hearing loss, has been described in 15 patients. Patients suspected of having geniculate neuralgia should have a complete neuro-otologic examination, including audiography, electronystagmography, polytome roentgenography of the fallopian canal and petrous apex, and pantopaque myelography of the internal auditory canal and posterior fossa. Vertebral angiography should be done when indicated.

Woman, 42, had had severe left ear pain for 2 years that required codeine and morphine. Phenytoin and carbamazepine gave no relief. Exacerbations of severe lancinating pain had occurred, lasting up to 2 weeks at a time. Neuro-otologic examination showed no abnormality. Roentgenograms of the temporal bone and myelographic study of the posterior fossa showed no abnormality and hearing was normal for pure tones and speech. The left nervus intermedius was excised in the internal auditory canal through a middle cranial fossa approach. Pain remained at about the same intensity, and 50% of the lateral part of the posterior root of the 5th cranial nerve was sectioned through the retrolabyrinthine approach. Ear pain persisted and the geniculate ganglion was subsequently excised through the middle cranial fossa approach. Pain was then absent, and the patient has been free of pain for 2 years. Hearing and facial function were unaltered after the surgery.

Inclusion of the anterior 20% of the diameter of the motor portion of the facial nerve with geniculate ganglion excision causes no facial weakness and results in a more complete

(3) Laryngoscope 86:955–964, July, 1976.

excision of ganglion cells. The maximum amount of facial nerve trunk that can be removed without producing facial paralysis has not been determined. Tearing is absent on the involved side postoperatively but, in the absence of corneal anesthesia, this causes no problem.

Half the present patients had recurring inflammation of the skin of the external auditory canal and this may represent some as yet unidentified agent that might be responsible for development of the neuralgia.

▶ [I do not believe that neurosurgeons, as a group, should be doing this operation, but they certainly should know what is available for pain in the ear.

Section of the nerve of Jacobson for pain in the ear due to oropharyngeal cancer is advocated by Gehanno et al. (Ann. Otolaryngol. Chir. Cervicofac. 92:573, 1976). — Ed.] ◀

High Cervical Commissural Myelotomy in the Treatment of Pain was performed by I. Papo and A. Luongo[4] (Regional Genl. Hosp., Ancona, Italy) on 10 patients with unilateral or bilateral upper chest, arm and shoulder pain, or diffuse pain in the sacral region and in both lower extremities, who otherwise would have required bilateral cordotomy. Commissurotomy was performed at the C1 – C3 level by a combination of deep electrocoagulation and sharp splitting of the posterior columns. The OWL cordotomy set with an exposed coagulating tip 2.5 mm long and 0.4 mm in diameter was used. A standard laminectomy was done under general anesthesia, the pia was coagulated and cut in the midline and 6 – 7 coagulations are performed at a depth of 6 mm at different levels, with electric parameters of 30 ma, 20 – 25 v and 30 seconds. The posterior columns are then split between the C2 and C4 segments with a microsurgical hook up to a depth of about 5 mm. The risk of injuring the anterior spinal artery is avoided by this technique.

All patients had complete relief of pain after the operation, but in 5 patients the relief lasted only 2 – 4 weeks, and 6 patients had severe relapses of pain within 2 months. The only noncancer patient died of cardiocirculatory failure 8 weeks after surgery, having remained nearly pain free until death. A patient with bronchial carcinoma died at 5 weeks without pain. Two other patients were fairly well relieved until they died 3 months after surgery, but 1 had had unilat-

(4)   J. Neurol. Neurosurg. Psychiatry 39:705 – 710, July, 1976.

eral spinothalamic cordotomy at the same operation. Respiratory and bladder troubles were never observed. Nearly all patients had temporary ataxia for 3–4 weeks and 2 noted paresthesias in the lower limbs. The right posterior column was injured in 1 patient, with distressing dysesthesia resulting. Three patients had a well-defined band of mild hypalgesia from the C2 to the T10 dermatomes. Changes in pain sensation disappeared in about 3 weeks.

This experience is rather disappointing. Cervical myelotomy has extremely limited indications, but might be considered in some patients with unilateral or bilateral arm, shoulder and upper chest pain, especially when respiratory function is impaired and the life expectancy is short. The mechanism of action of myelotomy is unclear; many ascending systems seem to be involved. Experience with dorsal myelotomy by the method of Šourek is limited.

▶ [One wonders about the verification of the depth of the pain commissures in the cervical cord in these patients.

Commissurotomy has been tried more often in the lumbosacral cord. A case in point is that of Whitten (V. Med. Mon. 103:280, 1976). A woman, aged 32, developed allesthesia after laminotomies, disk removals, neurolysis, rhizotomy and cordotomy for severe lumbar radicular pain. She developed pain in the anesthetic left leg after stimulation (pin, pressure, squeezing) of the right leg. Relief of the cross-reference of pain by commissurotomy has persisted, but the effects of cordotomy have worn off and she now has pain again in the left leg despite the myelotomy.

Autopsies of patients with cordotomy for intractable pain are relatively rare. Moffie (Clin. Neurol. Neurosurg. 78:261, 1975) describes the findings in the spinal cords of 4 patients with percutaneous cordotomy for relief of pain from cancer. In all 4, relief of pain was accomplished. In 2, there were well-placed lesions in the anterior quadrants of the spinal cord as planned. In the other 2, the lesions were found in the posterior quadrants, but the relief of pain was just as good. It appears to be of no importance where the lesion is placed as long as sufficient fibers are interrupted. Such accessory pathways for pain, as well as the homolateral uncrossed pathways, might well explain why recurrence of pain is so common after cordotomy if sufficient time is allowed to elapse. – Ed.] ◀

Peripheral Nerve Stimulation in Treatment of Intractable Pain. James N. Campbell and Donlin M. Long[5] (Johns Hopkins Hosp., Baltimore) reviewed the results of implantation of peripheral nerve stimulators (PNS) in 15 women and 8 men (mean age, 45 years) treated in 1974–75. All had persistent disabling pain despite all traditional

(5) J. Neurosurg. 45:692–699, December, 1976.

medical and surgical therapy. None had major psychopathology. If transcutaneous electric stimulation was unsuccessful, a trial of percutaneous nerve stimulation was carried out, often with an electrode left in place for 24–48 hours. Patients who obtained excellent pain relief on two separate trials were considered candidates for permanent PNS implantation. Electrodes were implanted on peripheral nerves at the loci at which percutaneous stimulation had provided pain relief. There were 1 ulnar nerve, 15 sciatic nerve, 5 brachial plexus and 2 median nerve implants in the series. A radiofrequency receiver was placed in a subcutaneous pocket at a convenient site, and an external transmitter was connected to an antenna several days postoperatively. Patients modified the stimulus intensity to maximize pain relief. Questionnaires were obtained an average of 12 months after surgery.

Four patients had excellent results, whereas 5 had partial successes and 14 were considered treatment failures. Eleven of the failures occurred in patients with low back pain syndrome with sciatica or pain from metastatic disease. Two of the excellent results were in patients with peripheral nerve trauma that had not responded to multiple operations. One infection occurred, and there was one noninfectious tissue reaction. Use of the stimulator by patients who responded changed little from the time immediately after implantation to the time of follow-up. Nearly all patients used the device more than 12 hours a day. No patient had muscle cramps from stimulation. Hyperesthesias in 2 patients disappeared with stimulation. Stimulation did not interfere with walking, sexual functioning, driving, sensation or muscle strength

The best predictor for success in using the PNS implant to treat intractable pain is the patient's diagnosis. Patients with peripheral nerve injuries are the most promising group for this procedure, but it is not indicated for the treatment of low back pain syndrome or pain from metastatic disease. The incidence of complications appears to be relatively low.

Cryoanalgesia: New Approach to Pain Relief. Experimental work has shown that a 2d-degree type of nerve injury follows freezing and that normal function will return if inflammation and scarring are minimal. The use of such agents as alcohol and phenol on peripheral nerves is disappointing, since incomplete nerve destruction often causes a painful neuritis. J. W. Lloyd, J. D. W. Barnard and C. J. Glynn[6] (Abingdon, England) thought that the blocking of peripheral nerves by application of a cryoprobe might be superior to these techniques.

PROCEDURE. – The Spembly-Lloyd nerve blocking unit, incorporating a cryosurgical system coupled to a nerve stimulator to position the probe accurately, is utilized. The refrigerant used is nitrous oxide, and at an operating pressure of 600 psi a minimal temperature of -60 C can be achieved within the iceball generated at the probe tip. Local anesthetic is injected at a previous visit to assess its effects. The cryoprobe is applied either through a track made through the tissues or after nerve exposure, and two freeze-thaw cycles are carried out, each freeze timed for 2 minutes from the establishment of a steady low temperature of about -60 C.

Sixty-four patients were treated by cryoanalgesia. The median duration of pain relief was 11 days, with a range of up to 224 days. All but 1 patient had failed to respond to previous treatment. Twelve patients with intercostal pain had pain relief for a median of 14 days. Seventeen with low back pain, treated by closed application, had pain relief for a median of 10 days; 5 obtained no relief. All 6 patients with facial neuralgia obtained relief, lasting a median of 21 days. Nine cancer patients were treated by closed application, and 8 were relieved for a median time of 14 days. Fifteen patients with pain of unknown cause were treated with cryotherapy, applied to the affected nerve or directly into painful foci. Four patients obtained no relief. The median duration of pain relief in this group was 10 days.

Cryoanalgesia produces an effective reversible nerve block, with a median duration of 11 days. This has particular significance in the postoperative period. No patient has manifested neuralgia subsequent to treatment. Cryoprobe application to a peripheral nerve blocks all transmission, and this may be important in situations where motor function must be preserved. Cryoanalgesia is a simple technique that appears to have a place in the management of acute pain. Its role in the relief of chronic pain is being further evaluated.

(6)   Lancet 2:932 – 934, Oct. 30, 1976.

Miscellaneous

Testing Cerebrospinal Fluid Shunt Capacity and Adequacy by the Lumbar Route in Adults. When improvement does not occur after cerebrospinal fluid shunting or there is deterioration after initial improvement, it is often impossible to distinguish clinically between disease and a malfunctioning shunt. Pumping of the shunt to assess patency is misleading in nearly 40% of cases. Leakage to the epidural space is an important source of error in testing shunts by the lumbar route and there is doubt as to the validity of the infusion test in noncommunicating hydrocephalus. Bjørn Magnaes[7] (Univ. of Oslo) describes a lumbar shunt testing procedure that includes control of leakage to the epidural space and the measurement of four variables. The patients studied had ventriculoatrial shunting with a Pudenz medium-pressure system. Infusion cisternography was performed in patients with communicating hydrocephalus and ventriculography in those with noncommunicating hydrocephalus. Cerebrospinal fluid opening pressures were measured with the patients sitting and in the lateral position.

Eighteen of the 51 adult patients with communicating hydrocephalus studied had a well-functioning or malfunctioning shunt determined with high probability based on clinical conditions. Eighty-two valid tests without leakage to the epidural space were performed in these 18 patients. Observation times ranged from 6 months to 2½ years. Leakage to the epidural space was detected during 5 tests. Five patients later had symptoms that indicated a failing shunt, and tests then showed preshunt values. One patient exhibited primary shunt failure. Fourteen adults with noncommunicating hydrocephalus were studied. Ventricular cerebrospinal fluid opening pressures were reduced after shunting. A high lumbar pressure during the lumbar infu-

(7) Surg. Neurol. 6:327–333, December, 1976.

sion test could lead to an incorrect conclusion of shunt capacity. All patients with benign internal obstruction of the cerebrospinal fluid space and several with neoplastic obstruction had nearly equal pressure levels for all variables. Cisternography showed activity in the supratentorial subarachnoid space in all these patients.

The lumbar infusion test gives information on shunt capacity, whereas the opening pressures in the lateral and sitting positions reflect shunt adequacy. A reduction in shunt capacity precedes a rise in opening pressures when shunts become inadequate. Cisternography is unreliable in determining shunt adequacy in the middle ranges of shunt capacity. In noncommunicating hydrocephalus, the lumbar infusion test results in a correct conclusion as to shunt capacity provided the subarachnoid space is patent and the test is terminated before the ventricular system is empty.

▶ [A round table on chronic nonneoplastic hydrocephalus in adults was held in Lausanne in June, 1975, and the papers given there appeared in volume 22 of *Neuro-chirurgie* (pp. 103–216) in 1976. The first section deals with clinical features, including hydrocephalus after meningeal hemorrhage, operation and aqueductal stenosis. Memory difficulties and Parinaud's syndrome in relation to decompensating hydrocephalus are discussed, followed by a rare instance of histologic study of the brain in normal-pressure hydrocephalus. There was diffuse pia-arachnoidal fibrosis associated with multiple ependymal lesions and periaqueductal gliosis.

The second part, on complimentary examinations, includes data on scintigraphy of the choroid plexuses, isotopic cisternography, myeloscintigraphy and isotopic ventriculography. Tomographic study of the brain and ventricles is shown to be useful for follow-up as well as initial diagnosis. Cortical biopsy can be done at the time of shunting and may show increased extracellular space in the cortical neuropile.

Physiopathology and treatment are covered in the third part of this issue. Basic mechanisms of chronic hydrocephalus are described, including increased fluid absorption and decreased fluid pulse pressure but no consistent change in cerebral blood flow, although best results seem to occur if preoperative flow is low. The cerebrospinal fluid absorption test seems a good indicator of successful operation. Recordings of intraventricular pressure indicate hyperpressure waves, but these have no obvious prognostic meaning.

Most participants in the meeting use cardiac shunts, but other techniques include lumboperitoneal shunts, ventriculocisternostomy and aqueductal catheterization; choice of valve type especially dealt with low-pressure or other types of valves. Infections were rarely encountered, but subdural hematoma occurred in 5–10% of cases. Most authors contended the shunt should be discontinued during treatment of the hematoma.

Milhorat et al. (J. Neurosurg. 44:735, 1976) used a ventricular perfusion technique to determine the rate of cerebrospinal fluid formation in a child, aged 5 years, who had had bilateral choroid plexectomy at 5 weeks for communicating hydrocephalus. At 5 months, he had a ventriculoperitoneal shunt that later failed to function. Prior to successful shunt revision, study showed a normal rate of fluid formation, 0.35 ml/minute. It is concluded that significant amounts of cerebrospinal fluid are formed at extrachoroidal sites. This may be so, but there is no proof that the other two choroid plexuses are not forming more than their usual share.

A new tool for the study of cerebrospinal fluid is cholera toxin! Epstein et al. (Science 196:1012, 1977) find that this toxin injected into the ventricles of dogs increases cerebrospinal fluid production (e.g., 17 $\pm$ 6 to 73 $\pm$ 7 μml/minute), presumably by stimulating adenylate cyclase that in turn increases cyclic adenosine monophosphate. If one could use an inhibitor of adenylate cyclase, one might be able to decrease cerebrospinal fluid formation in hydrocephalus, but the effects of such chemicals on other parts of the body are unknown. Cholera toxin, it is found, also promotes electrolyte transport in the gut and kidney and increases endolymph production in the ear. – Ed.] ◄

Microsurgical Treatment of Hemifacial Spasm. Hemifacial spasm is an uncommon condition of embarrassing, fatiguing facial twitching, usually cryptogenic but occasionally associated with subtentorial lesions. Jannetta reported excellent results from separating the facial nerve from a large branch of the anterior inferior cerebellar artery in the cerebellopontine angle with use of the operating microscope. H. L. Hankinson and Charles B. Wilson[8] (Univ. of California, San Francisco) have treated 5 patients by Jannetta's microsurgical method since 1970. The 5 women were aged 44 – 66 years and had had symptoms for 3 – 15 years. They have been followed for 3 months to 5 years. The operation was done under general anesthesia with the patient semiprone. A 3-cm craniectomy was made through a vertical incision medial to the mastoid process, and the responsible artery was teased away from the facial nerve before a Teflon sponge was interposed to hold the artery away from the junction of the facial nerve and brain stem.

The first patient had had an unsuccessful operation a year earlier. Reoperation was followed by immediate disappearance of hemifacial spasm. All 5 patients have had normal facial nerve function and a complete absence of spasm for the duration of follow-up. With one exception, preoperative 8th nerve function has been retained. In all cases the postoperative course was uncomplicated.

(8) West. J. Med. 124:191 – 193, March, 1976.

The basic pathologic lesion in hemifacial spasm appears to lie either at the nuclear level or distally. Microdissection of arterial structures from the facial nerve in the posterior fossa is a safe and effective means of dealing with cryptogenic hemifacial spasm and is the method of choice in treating this entity. The patient must accept a risk of hearing loss from operatively induced vascular impairment of the inner ear, but this risk has been reduced with increasing experience.

Effect of T-Myelotomy on Spasticity. Bischoff described interruption of the reflex paths between the anterior and posterior horns, by means of a lateral longitudinal incision of the cord from the L1 to S2 roots, to relieve severe spasticity in the lower extremities. Residual neurologic function was not always preserved, and the approach was changed to a dorsal midline myelotomy with lateral extension to protect any preserved bladder and motor function. Joseph F. Cusick, Sanford J. Larson and Anthony Sances, Jr.[9] (Med. College of Wisconsin) have used this T-myelotomy in 12 patients since 1973, with the additions of evoked potential recordings and microsurgical technique.

A laminectomy was done from T10 through L1 and a bipolar platinum disk electrode was placed over the dorsal cord surface at the superior limits of the laminectomy. A ring electrode and cutaneous electrode were used to stimulate the digital nerve, and a bipolar electrode was used to record from nerve roots near the conus medullaris. In 2 patients the myelotomy was carried through the conus medullaris unilaterally to relieve painful bladder spasms. A midline incision 2-3 mm deep was extended down to the gray matter with a fine microsuction tip, and a knife was used for the lateral cuts (Fig 22).

Nine patients were paraplegic from spinal cord trauma and 3 had severe flexor spasms from multiple sclerosis. All tolerated the procedure well. Spasticity was completely relieved in all but 2 patients, but 1 patient had a delayed return of spasticity; this was 1 of 2 in whom the S1 root was poorly identified. Pain associated with flexor spasms was totally relieved and painful bladder spasms were completely relieved in both affected patients. Reflex emptying of the

(9) Surg. Neurol. 6:289–292, November, 1976.

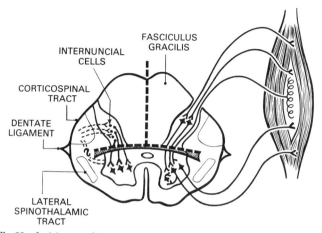

Fig 22. – Incisions used in myelotomy. Lateral incisions not only interrupt reflex arcs between anterior and posterior horns but also result in section of major connections between corticospinal tract internuncials and anterior horn cells. (Courtesy of Cusick, J. F., et al.: Surg. Neurol. 6:289–292, November, 1976.)

bladder was not significantly impaired by the operation. Three of 4 patients who could maintain erections had short-term deterioration of this function postoperatively. Evoked potential recording was useful in identifying the L5–S1 cord segments.

The T-myelotomy is a good means of producing sustained relief of lower limb spasticity, but it appears to be limited to patients who do not have voluntary muscle activity. It is well suited for patients whose spastic muscles are paralyzed or so paretic that paralysis from treatment is tolerable. Recording of evoked potentials during the procedure is useful for monitoring posterior column function and has facilitated a more accurate delineation of the limits of the myelotomy.

▶ [According to Anderson and Raines (Neurology 26:858, 1976), phenytoin (Dilantin) and chlorpromazine (Thorazine) may be useful in suppressing muscle rigidity in some disorders of upper motor neuron lesions. Experiments in cats appear to show that chlorpromazine suppresses fusimotor drive, whereas phenytoin suppresses muscle spindle feedback, presumably by suppressing the peripheral receptors. – Ed.] ◀

Myelotomy for Control of Mass Spasms in Paraplegia. Shokei Yamada, Phanor L. Perot, Jr., Thomas B. Ducker and Isabel Lockard[1] advocate a procedure utilizing inter-

(1) J. Neurosurg. 45:683–691, December, 1976.

mittent dorsal midline incisions for controlling spasms in paraplegia. The procedure interrupts the lumbosacral reflex arcs and also spares certain useful motor connections destroyed in other procedures. A knife with a double-edged blade 0.5 mm wide and not more than 0.35 mm thick is used for the operation.

TECHNIQUE — Under general anesthesia and with the patient prone, a laminectomy is performed at T10–12, and the dura is opened in the midline. The arachnoid is reflected from the operative site under microscopic observation, and venous tributaries are coagulated. The pia and the midline posterior surface of the midportion of the L1 segment are cut to a depth of 2–3 mm for a distance of 3 mm. The myelotomy knife is inserted for 4.0 mm cephalically as far as the central canal and the blade turned to the 3 o'clock position. The gray matter is then cut at the lower end of the incision, and the knife is turned another 90 degrees at the upper end of the incision and then moved caudad 3 mm and withdrawn. The procedure is repeated five or six times at intervals throughout the L1-S1 cord segments; the upper limit of each incision is 5 mm below the lower limit of the preceding one. In the L3, L4 and L5 segments, the knife is inserted to a depth of 4.5 rather than 4.0 mm. The dorsal roots are stimulated before and after sectioning the gray matter of each cord segment.

Fourteen paraplegic or tetraplegic patients aged 23–55 years, seen during 1969–74 with spasms of the lower limbs, with or without decubiti, had this operation. All patients were free from severe spasms postoperatively, although 1 required a second operation to extend the myelotomy. Deep tendon reflexes were abolished or made hypoactive in all patients, but postural reflexes were retained. No patient was bedridden after surgery, and 5 were able to walk. Decubiti healed spontaneously in 3 of 7 patients. With one exception, sensation was not altered by the operation. Several patients have been trained for bladder self-control since surgery. Erections were not impaired by the operation.

Mass spasms were well controlled in all patients by this myelotomy. Cord measurements must be strictly observed during the operation.

Chronic Cerebellar Stimulation in Cerebral Palsy. It was hypothesized that chronic stimulation of the cerebellar cortex, especially that of the paleocerebellum, in patients could augment the inhibitory function of cerebellum in certain syndromes, such as spasticity, that appear to result from disinhibition of motor or behavioral activity. I. S. Cooper, Manuel Riklan, Ismail Amin, Joseph M. Waltz and Thomas Cullinan[2] (St. Barnabas Hosp., Bronx, N. Y.) reviewed the results obtained in the first 50 patients treated by chronic cerebellar stimulation for moderately incapacitating cerebral palsy, followed for 6–36 months.

An electrode plate of silicone-coated mesh is applied at suboccipital craniectomy to the anterior or posterior cerebellar lobe or to both lobes. More recently, bilateral anterior lobe placements have been used. The most common frequency of stimulation has been 200 cycles per second, given at 1- to 8-minute intervals through the 24-hour period.

The mean patient age was 23.1; most patients had previously been operated on and 4 had had brain surgery without significant benefit. No patient could walk normally but 11 could ambulate. All patients but 8 had normal EEGs.

Spasticity was considerably reduced in the limbs, trunk and neck after a mean of 37 days of cerebellar stimulation. Follow-up of 28 patients at 5 months indicated a progressive

Fig 23.—**A,** patient preoperatively is unable to lower arms and sit unsupported in upright position. **B,** patient 3 months postoperatively. Note improved posture and relaxation of both arms. **C,** patient 32 months after initial surgery riding tricycle, an activity impossible before operation. (Courtesy of Cooper, I. S., et al.: Neurology (Minneap.) 26:744–753, August, 1976.)

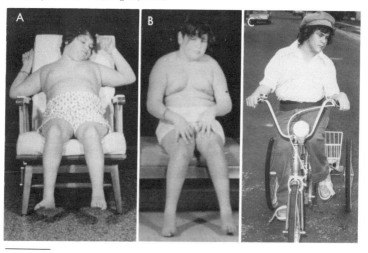

decline in spasticity, and a cumulative effect was evident. Athetosis in the arms and legs was reduced and the gait improved progressively. Tendon reflex hyperactivity improved only slightly for the group as a whole. The proportion of totally dependent patients fell from 20 to 7% at 5 months.

Definite improvement in speech production was apparent in about half the patients evaluated. Major effects on mental functioning were observed. The changes in 1 patient are shown in Figure 23. The 1 postoperative death was due to brain hemorrhage. No other surgical mortality has occurred in 140 patients with cerebral palsy operated on to date. No abnormal cerebellar function has been seen in patients followed for up to 3 years, but some minor difficulties have arisen from individual reactions to stimulation or from technical complications.

Preliminary data indicate that chronic cerebellar stimulation is a promising method for the attenuation of long-standing symptoms in patients with moderate to severe cerebral palsy. The cumulative effects of cerebellar stimulation may be due to the re-gating of the sensory communication systems modulated by cerebellar inhibition or to the accumulation or depletion of certain neurotransmitter substances consequent on the long-term neural stimulation.

Significance of Purkinje's Cell Density in Seizure Suppression by Chronic Cerebellar Stimulation. Cooper et al. recently proposed that chronic stimulation of the paleocerebellum and neocerebellum in man relieves cerebral seizures and muscular hypertonia. In epileptics who have been maintained on anticonvulsant agents for long periods, seizure suppression by cerebellar stimulation may depend on the degree of cerebellar degeneration. Rodwan K. Rajjoub, James H. Wood and John M. Van Buren[3] (Natl. Inst. of Health) compared the results of such stimulation with Purkinje's cell densities determined from cerebellar cortical biopsy specimens obtained during electrode installation.

Cerebellar autopsy specimens were taken from 4 patients with focal and grand mal epilepsy, and biopsy specimens were taken from 3 epileptic patients during cerebellar electrode installation. The patients had stimulation with 3–12

(3) Neurology (Minneap.) 26:645–650, July, 1976.

ma capacitively coupled monophasic pulses with exponential decay and 1-msec duration, at a rate of 10 pulses per second, alternating between two electrode arrays every 8 minutes. Control autopsy specimens were taken from 5 epileptic patients (mean age, 47 years) within 14 hours after cardiac arrest.

The mean Purkinje's cell density of cerebellar autopsy specimens from control patients was 3.56 cells/mm/16-μ section, compared with 1.35 cells in epileptic patients, a significant difference. Densities among the specimens from epileptic patients were significantly lower than those from controls; however, densities among specimens obtained from epileptic patients during electrode installation were not significantly different from those obtained from autopsy specimens of deceased epileptic patients. Isomorphic gliosis of the cerebellar cortices was found in 2 biopsy specimens obtained during electrode installation, but there was surprisingly little additional change. No rod cell transformation of the microglia was seen. Two patients had marked reductions in seizures with cerebellar stimulation and 1 had a moderate reduction. The patient who had marked loss of Purkinje's cell density before stimulation appeared to have better seizure control than the patients exhibiting only a mild reduction in Purkinje's cell density.

Another cerebellar-mediated mechanism, perhaps the postulated cerebellorubroreticular system or one involving nonspecific thalamic nuclei, may play the dominant role in cerebellar stimulation-induced seizure suppression. Depressed cerebrospinal fluid γ-aminobutyric acid concentrations have been found during cerebellar stimulation in epileptics, suggesting that Purkinje's cell discharge may be depressed during stimulation. Cerebellar biopsy is useful at electrode installation and rebiopsy is indicated if revision of the stimulation apparatus necessitates a later posterior fossa exploration.

Sensory Jacksonian Seizures. Progression of a somatic sensory seizure, as experienced by the aware patient, can often be reported in fine detail. Richard A. Lende and A. John Popp[4] (Albany Med. College) mapped and analyzed sensory jacksonian seizures in 27 male and 15 female pa-

(4) J. Neurosurg. 44:706–711, June, 1976.

tients seen in a 20-year period. The patients studied had 54 seizure patterns; several had more than 1 seizure pattern, and 1 patient had 4 different sensory marches. In the typical seizure, an abnormal sensation appears without apparent stimulus at a localized cutaneous site, marches on the sensory surface of the affected part and progresses to other members. Some motor activity may occur but there is no impairment of awareness and the march disappears without apparent reason.

The perceived origins of the sensory marches are transcribed onto a schema for the somatic sensory cortex in Figure 24. Ten seizures originated in the head area, 24 in the upper extremity and 20 in the lower extremity. Only 2 pa-

Fig 24. — Proposed sites of the cortical origins of sensory jacksonian seizures. (Courtesy of Lende, R. A., and Popp, A. J.: J. Neurosurg. 44:706–711, June, 1976.)

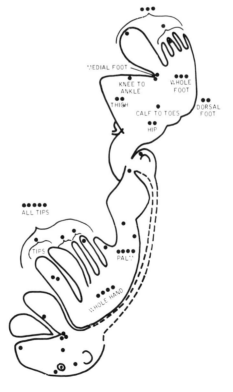

tients had an onset in the thumb alone and only 1 had an onset in the great toe. Four attacks originated in the hip or thigh, or both. Once a somatic site of onset was established, it tended to persist despite change in the pathologic lesion. Progression of attacks was not rectilinear, radiate or disorganized. The front of the discharge appeared to follow a path of predilection toward the anatomic limit of a functionally coherent unit, such as a digit, hand or arm. Only 50% of the attacks originating in the hand eventually progressed to the face. Progression was occasionally bidirectional, but the general tendency was seizure spread toward the base of a member. In some cases a cutaneous area appeared to be "skipped" by the march. A motor component was present in 20 patients, and 16 of these had close anatomical and temporal correlation between the motor and sensory components of the attack. In only 4 instances did motor activity precede the sensory perception. Most of the 24 histologic diagnoses that were made were vascular abnormalities or tumors.

A cortical construct summarizing these sensory marches conformed more closely to Woolsey's evoked potential map of the chimpanzee cortex than to the cortical sensory sequences described for man. Complete diagnostic studies are indicated in patients presenting with sensory jacksonian seizures, because of the frequency of related focal pathology.

▶ [The functional representation on the medial aspect of the frontal lobes in man is described and pictured by Van Buren and Fedio (J. Neurosurg. 44:275, 1976). Sensory and motor responses to stimulation of the medial aspect of the frontal lobe were complex postural synergies of the trunk and proximal contralateral extremities (occasionally bilateral). Sensory responses from the cingulate gyrus were referred over the body and extremities with a questionable contralateral preponderance. Many facets of speech impairment from stimulation of the supplementary motor area are similar to those of the lateral aspect of the frontal lobe. It seems likely that the basis of speech inhibition from stimulation of the frontal lobe is interference with striatal function. — Ed.] ◀

Value of Brain Biopsy in Neurodegenerative Disease in Childhood. Studies of the value of brain biopsy in childhood have been extremely limited. E. Boltshauser and J. Wilson[5] (Hosp. for Sick Children, London) reviewed experience with brain biopsy in a children's hospital during 1968–74. Forty-five children, 22 boys and 23 girls with suspected progressive neurologic syndromes, had biopsy. The

(5) Arch. Dis. Child. 51:264–268, April, 1976.

mean age was 3 years 9 months and the age range was 4 months to 15 years. Biopsy was done with general anesthesia; a trephine disk 2.4 cm in diameter was removed from the area anterior to the right coronal suture, and a block of about 1 cc of brain was obtained, including cortex and white matter. All biopsy specimens were taken from the right frontal lobe and 1 patient also had a left frontal biopsy. Diathermy was not used and anticonvulsants and antibiotics usually were not given after biopsy.

Nineteen patients had nonspecifically abnormal histologic findings, 6 had specific abnormalities and 20 had histologically normal findings. One child with normal findings may have had a variant of phenylketonuria. Ten of those with nonspecific findings had convincing evidence of an evolving neurologic syndrome; a specific diagnosis later was made in 3 of them. Specific abnormalities included spongy degeneration in 3 cases and metachromatic leukodystrophy, Alexander's leukodystrophy and macrogyria in 1 case each. Only in the case of metachromatic leukodystrophy was neurochemical analysis diagnostically helpful. Three children, 1 with a history of epilepsy, had grand mal seizures postoperatively; 1 had mild left-sided hemiparesis and 1 had a subgaleal cerebrospinal fluid collection. Cortical atrophy was not correlated with the histologic findings in this series; half the children with evidence of cortical atrophy had normal biopsy findings. Two of 7 children with cerebrospinal fluid protein levels above 30 mg/100 ml had normal biopsy findings and 3 had nonspecifically abnormal findings.

The number of conditions in which brain biopsy is the diagnostic procedure of choice is extremely small; these conditions may be suspected on clinical grounds. The neurodegenerative disorders of childhood that are currently identifiable in life only by brain biopsy include spongy degeneration, Alexander's leukodystrophy, myoclonus epilepsy (Lafora's body type) and infantile neuraxonal dystrophy.

Identification of Motor and Sensory Funiculi in Cut Nerves and Their Selective Reunion. The results of repairing a divided mixed nerve are usually less satisfactory than those of repairing pure sensory or motor nerves because of an inability to identify the various funiculi and the inevitable and nonfunctioning union of sensory fibers to motor fibers. Identification by electric stimulation of individual funiculi is suitable only in conscious patients and is a difficult clinical procedure. H. Gruber, G. Freilinger, J. Holle and H. Mandl[6] (Univ. of Vienna) describe a new approach based on a histochemical technique for acetylcholinesterase activity, which differentially strains motor and sensory funiculi and is applicable to recently cut nerves.

Both stumps of the severed nerve are freed for about 2 cm and marked by colored subepineural threads. A 2- to 3-mm disk is cut from each stump and fixed in 6% formaldehyde buffered by 0.1 M Na-cacodylate at pH 7.2 for not more than 1 hour. Sections are placed in the Karnovsky-Roots medium for cholinesterase activity with 10^{-4} M iso-octamethyl pyrophosphoramide (OMPA) added to inhibit nonspecific cholinesterase and are incubated for 20–24 hours. About half the myelinated fibers in motor funiculi are stained, whereas nearly all the myelinated fibers in sensory funiculi are unstained. In both types of funiculus there is some irregular staining of unmyelinated fibers. Repair is usually carried out 2–3 days after the primary operation. Funiculi are identified from the microphotographs oriented by the colored threads. The motor funiculi are sutured individually, whereas the sensory funiculi, especially the smaller ones, are sutured together in groups.

This histochemical procedure is limited to acute nerve injuries because of the rapid onset of nerve fiber degeneration. The intricacy of the procedure and the long time required are fully justified by the enhanced security of suturing functionally adequate funiculi. Cases so far have been confined to injuries of the median and ulnar nerves in the distal forearm, but the method can be used for any mixed peripheral nerve. Only in the more distal parts of a nerve or only a few centimeters before a motor branch leaves a nerve trunk, however, are the motor and sensory funiculi separated sufficiently.

▶ [Ihm and Samii (Acta Neurochir. (Wien) 34:185, 1976) show that, at least in rabbits, long homografts do worse than short homografts. Autologous grafts do much better. There is no benefit from using a long autologous graft as compared to a short one. Homografts that are tissue compatible with the experimental animal (beagle) do better than grafts which are not tissue typed (Singh: ibid., p. 195). – Ed.] ◀

▶ ↓ A comparison of end-to-end sutures and cable grafts is given by Haftek in the following article. – Ed. ◀

(6) Br. J. Plast. Surg. 29:70–73, January, 1976.

Autogenous Cable Nerve Grafting instead of End-to-End Anastomosis in Secondary Nerve Suture. Tension on the suture line in repairs of divided peripheral nerves has an extremely bad effect on nerve fiber regeneration. End-to-end suture in secondary procedures is very rarely possible when a gap of 2 cm or more is present. Autogenous nerve grafting gives results nearly as good as end-to-end suture in the repair of large gaps of peripheral nerves. In 1967, J. Haftek[7] (Military Med. School. Lódź, Poland) began using autogenous cable nerve grafts in some cases with small gaps and recently has used short grafts more often in cases where end-to-end anastomosis would previously have been performed.

During 1967 – 74, 53 short cable nerve grafts were done in cases with gaps less than 3.5 cm in length. Grafts were glued to the nerve stumps with autogenous plasma clot or sutured under the operating microscope with the use of fine silk (8 – 0 to 10 – 0) on atraumatic needles. During the same period, 74 end-to-end nerve sutures were performed by the same surgeon. Patients have been followed for 1 – 7 years. Short cable grafts have good results in 75% of cases, fair results in 19% and poor results in 6%. End-to-end anastomosis gave good results in 34.5% of cases, fair results in 25.5%, poor results in 27% and bad results in 13%.

The results of nerve grafting are much better than those of end-to-end anastomosis. The procedure is not extremely difficult technically and is sometimes easier than end-to-end suture, especially with a long gap present. Use of the operating microscope is extremely important. Autogenous plasma clot gluing is of great value in joining nerve ends and grafts. The good results of nerve grafting are related to a lack of tension in the suture line, with resultant good revascularization of the repaired nerve trunk. Autogenous cable nerve grafting is the method of choice for the secondary repair of peripheral nerves. Adequate resection of nerve ends and extremely careful coaptation of grafts to individual nerve bundles are the critical steps in cable nerve transplantation. More experience with the technique is needed before final conclusions can be drawn.

► [Only 30 of 332 patients with peripheral nerve injuries studied by Do-

(7) Acta Neurochir. (Wien) 34:217 – 221, 1976.

lene (Acta Neurochir. (Wien) 34:235, 1976) involved the radial nerve. Most were secondary to humeral fracture. Operation showed 16 cases of fibrosis, treated by funiculolysis. Good reinnervation occurred, and only 1 patient (2.5-year interval between injury and operation) failed to show improvement even 2 years postoperatively. Grafts up to 20 cm long were taken from the sural nerve for repair of defects in 14 patients. Positive electromyographic findings usually preceded actual muscular contraction, which usually appeared in 2–5 months for grafts of 10 cm or less, 6–8 months for grafts of 11–15 mm, 8 months for a graft of 16 cm and 13 months for a graft of 20 cm. Function of the extensor of the thumb was always the last to appear.

Taylor and Ham of Australia (Plast. Reconstr. Surg. 57:413, 1976) used a 24-cm length of superficial radial nerve with its attached blood vessels for grafting into a median nerve injury of the opposite arm (which also had an inoperable radial nerve injury). The vascular anastomoses were successful in restoring blood flow to the recipient arm (damaged at the time of nerve injury), and the graft was sutured with interfunicular sutures; the anterior and central funiculi were chosen because the radial graft was only 3 mm wide, compared to 7 mm for the median nerve stump proximally. Sonography and angiography later proved the success of the vascular surgery; nerve regrowth has given some protective sensation in the hand. – Ed.] ◄

Psychosurgery: National Commission Issues Surprisingly Favorable Report. Barbara J. Culliton[8] reports that about 400 psychiatric patients in the United States have had psychosurgery each year for the past 5–10 years and that many favorable patient impressions have been recorded in studies conducted during the past year for the National Commission for the Protection of Human Subjects of Biomedical and Behavioral Research, a commission formed partly in response to fears that psychosurgery would be used to tame the violent, including leaders of unpopular causes. The Commission has released a report approving psychosurgery in carefully defined circumstances; its issuance of recommendations encouraging support of research in psychosurgery is surprising. The Commission was impressed by the findings of Teuber et al. in 34 cingulotomy patients and by those of Mirsky and Orzack in 27 psychosurgery patients. Many patients in these studies were cured of long-standing, refractory illness and derived considerable benefit from psychosurgery, especially those treated for depression or depression and pain.

The effect of psychosurgery may be due more to chemical than to purely physical changes in the brain. The patients

(8) Science 194:299–301, Oct. 15, 1976.

who do best may end up with a rather selective loss of cognitive functioning. It also is possible that successful psychosurgery is nothing more than a placebo effect. Generally, psychosurgery in the United States has been regarded as part of medical practice rather than as an experimental procedure and has not been subjected to as much rigorous research as is needed if questions concerning its value are to be answered. The Commission believes that psychosurgery can be good for mental health, but there is also a sense of uncertainty and continuing potential for abuse; it recommends that psychosurgery be done only where an institutional review board is available. The incidence of psychosurgery is not expected to increase dramatically but it may increase a little because of the Commission's report. The report also may stimulate research to determine whether psychosurgery works and, if it does, why.

▶ [Open prefrontal leukotomy is *not* the procedure of choice for operation in severe psychiatric illness, according to Smith et al. (Med. J. Aust. May 15, 1976, p. 731). Benefits were obvious, but operative mortality was 6.9%, operative complications 18.6% and long-term sequelae 9.3%. Stereotactic or electrode implantation techniques are much less dangerous and are to be preferred. — Ed.] ◀

Subject Index

Index to Authors